GP Psychotropic Handbook
third edition

GP Psychotropic Handbook
third edition

Stephen Bazire

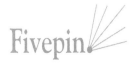

Published by Fivepin Limited.
91 Crane Street, Salisbury, Wilts, SP1 2PU

British Library Cataloguing in Publication Data
A catalogue record for this book is available from the British Library

Stephen Bazire, 2003
ISBN 0-9544839-1-X

Printed in the UK by The Bath Press, Bath

Contents

5. — Drug-induced psychiatric disorders 189

6. — Other useful information 204

Index 206

Foreword

Before using this book . . .

This book is designed to act as a psychiatric drug information source, directory of sources and 'Aide Memoire' for the general practice team involved with the care of patients with mental health problems and learning disabilities.

Its aim is to complement the *British National Formulary* and does not seek to replicate information in standard texts, eg. with the 'Treatment options' chapter you should refer to standard national texts for information on doses, cautions etc. The book aims to provide a handy reference source and the sections are subsequently arranged in a problem-orientated manner and with a minimum level of knowledge assumed. Information given can be followed up in the appropriate sources as time allows. References, where quoted, are usually of a good recent review article. Lists are as comprehensive as possible but could never claim to be fully complete. The listing of a drug use in this book does not in any way imply that it is licensed or safe for this use and all information is presented in good faith.

Throughout I have tried to be as objective as possible. It must be up to the reader to make up his or her mind on a topic but I hope the statements will have pointed you in the right direction and the time saved in looking papers up will allow more thought.

Acknowledgements

Writing a book such as this is a tremendous challenge. Help and encouragement, constructive criticism and advice is, thus, always very welcome, and in this respect, I would like to thank the many members of the UK Psychiatric Pharmacy Group for their enthusiasm, encouragement and support, including of course members of the current committee. I must also thank many members of Norfolk Mental Health Care NHS Trust, plus the local PCTs (including the marvellous pharmaceutical advisors) for providing a stimulating and caring environment within which to work. Thanks also as ever to my pharmacy staff at Hellesdon and Colegate for the help and humour, Vicky & Lou for the index, my GP Dr Thurlow for keeping me ticking over, John Tams and Dido for the company, Paul Woods, and finally Jill, Rosemary and Christopher for putting up with me, although I occasionally have to put up with you lot as well.

Finally, many thanks to my old chum Dr Chris Barclay, who helped with the original idea for the book and paid the price by ending up doing his own books, thus losing his remaining free time.

Stephen Bazire *BPharm, MRPharmS, DipPsychPharm, MCPP*

Pharmacy Services Director, Norfolk Mental Health Care NHS Trust,
Hellesdon Hospital, Norwich NR6 5BE, England
e-mail: sbazire@ukppg.org.uk
Website for service users www.nmhct.nhs.uk/pharmacy

1.
Drug treatment options in psychiatric illness

This chapter details drugs which are licensed for the conditions listed and other drugs sometimes used by specialists, but which are not licensed for this purpose. Advice should be sought for fuller details of non-Product Licence uses. Drugs are classified as follows:

BNF listed — are drugs listed in the *British National Formulary* as indicated for that condition. See the appropriate section in the *BNF* for a review of a drug's role in therapy and its prescribing details. Information provided here is in addition to that in the *BNF* and may prove useful.

Combinations — are those which have been used to benefit patients. They carry the risks of additive side-effects and interactions.

Unlicensed/further information — drugs listed here are those which are sometimes used (particularly, but certainly not only, by hospital specialists) and which have some clinical efficacy but where no specific Product Licence exists within the UK. The distinction is often slightly blurred, eg. use of antipsychotics for aggression may be considered to be treating some undiagnosable or suspected psychotic aspect of a patient's behaviour. Information in this category is provided to help the GP understand why other prescribers (usually hospital specialists) may have prescribed what they have, although even this book won't help all the time. It is, of course, the responsibility of prescriber to ensure all precautions are taken when prescribing drugs for unlicensed purposes.

1.1   Aggression — see also self-injurious behaviour (SIB) (*1.28*), borderline personality disorder (*1.10*) and APE (*1.24*)

Uncontrolled or episodic aggression can be a problem in the management of patients, particularly in those with a learning disability, dementia (see *1.11*), PTSD (*1.23*), PMS, trauma and other conditions. Drug therapy may be helpful where suppression of aggression is considered important on safety grounds.

BNF listed

Lithium (Camcolit®, Priadel® etc)

Several trials have shown lithium to have a significant effect on reducing aggression in people with learning disabilities such as conduct disorder, eg. reducing both aggression and the frequency of episodes. In practice, other factors often make the effect difficult to detect. However,

a two-month trial (at plasma levels of 0.6–0.8mmol/l) may be justified, particularly in people with learning disabilities uncontrolled by environmental factors.
Prescribing points:
- ❖ See main entry for lithium under bipolar disorder (see *1.9*).
- ❖ Care is needed with lithium plasma level monitoring in this client group, as toxicity is often difficult to recognise (suggest plasma level tests at least every three months, and particularly in hot weather).

Unlicensed/further information

Antipsychotics

Antipsychotics/neuroleptics   are   not licensed specifically for aggression but are frequently used (some might say over-used) for the control of aggression. Evidence for their efficacy is suggestive rather than conclusive, possibly based on their sedative effects and that they risk inducing tardive dyskinesia. With a growing evidence-base, **risperidone** is becoming a drug of choice for aggression from a variety of causes, especially in lower doses initially. In the elderly, zuclopenthixol has been shown to be effective in the treatment of aggression and one careful study of behavioural disturbances in learning disability patients showed zuclopenthixol (2–20mg/d) to be significantly superior to haloperidol (0.5–5mg/d) at notably modest doses.

SSRIs

Low central serotonin activity may occur in aggression and so use of some SSRI anti-depressants has some rationale, eg. there have been some studies with citalopram (in aggressive and impulsive adolescents) and fluoxetine, and cases with sertraline showing reduced aggression. This may be useful in the future when more studies have confirmed the effect.

Others

Benzodiazepines (the incidence of para-doxical aggression is probably as low as 1%), beta-blockers, carbamazepine, gaba-pentin, valproate (17 studies show a promising effect) and vitamin supplements (the prison trial in violent offenders) have also been used.

1.2 Agoraphobia — see also anxiety (*1.5*) and panic disorder (*1.22*)

Agoraphobia (an anxiety disorder), is an overwhelming and disabling anxiety provoked by being alone or in public places. Panic attacks may accompany the phobia, and depression may be present in up to a half of patients. A serotonin deficiency has been shown.

Role of drugs

Drug treatment may be effective in many patients. Psychotherapy is considered an essential component of the treatment package. A meta-analysis of 54 published studies has shown that symptoms are improved by tricyclics and high potency benzodiazepines, although there may be a short-term deterioration (minimised by starting at lower doses). There is a weak but significant placebo response to drugs. SSRIs may exacerbate the symptoms initially.

BNF listed

Citalopram (Cipramil®)

Citalopram is licensed in the UK for the symptoms of panic disorder, with or without agoraphobia (see *1.22*).

Prescribing points:

❖ Start at 10mg/d for a week, before moving up to 20–30mg/d (maximum 60mg/d) to minimise any initial anxiety.
❖ May take 3 months to reach optimal effect.

Escitalopram (Cipralex®)

Escitalopram is licensed in the UK for the symptoms of panic disorder, with or without agoraphobia (see *1.22*).

Prescribing points:

❖ Start at 5mg/d for a week, before moving up to 10mg/d (maximum 20mg/d) to minimise any initial anxiety.
❖ May take 3 months to reach optimal effect.

Paroxetine (Seroxat®)

Paroxetine is licensed in the UK for the symptoms of panic disorder, with or without agoraphobia (see *1.22*).

Prescribing points:

❖ Start at 10mg/d for a week, before gradually moving up to the optimum dose of 40mg/d (maximum 50mg/d) to minimise any initial anxiety.

❖ May take 3 months to reach optimal effect.

Unlicensed/further information

Benzodiazepines

Diazepam and clonazepam have been used and shown to help, particularly with anxiety symptoms.

Others

MAOIs and tricyclics have been used, but suffer from high drop-outs from adverse effects, particularly initially.

1.3 Alcohol dependence and alcohol abuse — see also alcohol withdrawal syndrome (*1.4*)

Symptoms

The main diagnostic symptoms of alcohol dependence include primacy of drinking over other activities, increased tolerance to alcohol, symptoms of repeated withdrawal, stereotyped patterns of drinking, compulsion to drink and drinking to relieve withdrawal symptoms.

Risk factors

Some risk factors for alcohol abuse or being an alcohol dependent drinker include:
1. Occupations, eg. brewers, company representatives, alcohol retailers, doctors and pharmacists.
2. Genetic component (up to 30–40% influence).
3. Marital and social problems, eg. stress.
4. Personality, eg. anxious.
5. Psychopaths and criminals, eg. taking alcohol before criminal events.
6. Psychiatric illness, eg. depression, anxiety, phobia etc.
7. Use for hypnotic or analgesic purposes.
8. Adverse childhood or adolescent experiences.
9. Parental misuse of alcohol.
10.Sweet taste preference.

Alcohol contents of some drinks

One unit of alcohol = 1/2 pint standard beer or cider, pint stronger beer, one *pub* measure of sherry, table wine, spirits etc. A 75cl bottle of wine is 8 to 12 units, Sherry is 12–14units/bottle and whisky or spirits about 30–32u/bottle. Most canned

or bottled beers are two or less units per can, except the stronger ones such as Tennents Super, Carlsberg Special Brew, Holsten Export, Kronenberg 1664, Tennents Extra etc, which are 3–4 units per can. The body metabolises one unit of alcohol per hour; peak levels occurring one hour after the drink is consumed. One unit gives a man a blood level of about 15mg alcohol/100ml and a woman 20mg/100ml. Absorption is rapid with low volume drinks, eg. spirits and slower with higher volumes, eg. beer.

Alcohol metabolism

A maximum of 4–5 units of alcohol per day plus two drink-free days per week should be possible without developing a drink problem, or less than 25 units/week for a man or 20 units/week for a woman. Greater than 35 units per week is generally considered harmful.

Role of drugs

Drugs may play a part in the overall plan, such as the treatment of associated psychiatric morbidity (eg. such as withdrawal DTs, dementia, Korsakov's psychosis, Wernicke's encephalopathy), affective disorders, suicide and hallucinations. Disulfiram can have a role to play in experienced hands and in selected patients. Acamprosate and naltrexone are superior to placebo and may have some role. Vitamin deficiency must be corrected rapidly.

BNF listed

Acamprosate (Campral EC®)

Acamprosate is licensed for abstinence maintenance therapy for up to one year in motivated alcohol dependent patients. It takes about seven days to reach therapeutic levels and so should be started soon after detoxification. Continued alcohol consumption negates the therapeutic effect but it can still be effective with occasional relapses. Acamprosate may reduce intake via reduced reward, a possible anticraving effect. Many good trials have shown a significant if modest (10–15% reduction in relapse over the first year) therapeutic effect. It is certainly not a miracle 'cure' for repeatedly failed detoxification patients and should be combined with continued counselling.

Prescribing points:

❖ Start within 7 days of detoxification.
❖ An excellent independent self-help treatment support programme (Campral EC Plus) is supported by the manufacturers.
❖ It is most effective when combined with psychosocial and behavioural therapies.

Disulfiram (Antabuse®)

Disulfiram irreversibly inhibits the ALDH (Hepatic Aldehyde-NAD reductase) enzyme, leading to accumulation of toxic acetaldehyde from incomplete alcohol metabolism. Disulfiram's main use is as adversive conditioning and maintenance therapy in alcoholics. The *BNF* tends to underestimate doses needed so it is usually best started with a loading dose of 400mg/d with 365mg/d the average dose used. Depots or implants have no significant pharmacological action and any deterrent effect is probably psychological rather than pharmacological.

Prescribing points:

❖ For maintenance, it can also be given as a twice a week dose (ie. daily dose × 7 divided by 2) as the enzyme block is irreversible and the clinical effect lasts about 7–10-days.

❖ Antabuse® tablets are dispersable and can be given as a liquid in a supervised setting (eg. with relatives, neighbours, clinics etc).

B Vitamins

Vitamin deficiency may occur due to inadequate diet, impaired absorption, increased metabolic demand and impaired utilisation. The deficiency needs correcting as it can lead to Wernicke-Korsakoff syndrome, where 25% of sufferers make a complete and 50% a partial recovery. This deficiency is usually treated in hospitals with Pabrinex®, oral thiamine or Vitamins B and C strong. Thiamine (Vitamin B1) is considered primary and priority treatment to reverse the mental confusion secondary to thiamine deficiency (Wernicke's syndrome).

Prescribing point:

❖ See the CSM advice on allergic reactions in the *BNF* (section *9.6.2*).
❖ Oral thiamine is poorly absorbed (maximum around 10mg/d) and so injections are necessary over the first few days after withdrawal to ensure adequate vitamin replacement.

Combinations

Acamprosate+disulfiram

A combination of the two may improve outcomes, although the only study had a high number of drop-outs.

Unlicensed/further information

Naltrexone

Naltrexone is an established drug in the USA for this indication. It has a significant effect on reducing drinking by reduction in desire, and may have a good an outcome as acamprosate. The once-a-day dose helps, although it has higher side-effects.

Others

Numerous other drugs have been tried by specialists for alcohol dependence eg. buspirone, carbamazepine, SSRIs (a modest but detectable effect) and valproate.

1.4 Alcohol withdrawal syndrome — see also alcohol dependence (*1.3*)

Symptoms

Alcohol withdrawal syndrome (AWS) can present with psychological symptoms (eg. anxiety and restlessness), psychotic symptoms (eg. hallucinations), tremor, sweating, tachycardia, gastrointestinal symptoms, fits, illusions, clouding of consciousness and delirium tremens (DTs) or Wernicke-Korsakoff syndrome (including short-term memory loss). These last for about 48 hours after the last drink. Withdrawal fits may first occur within 24 hours. AWS may be self-limiting or progress to delirium tremens. In DT, fits may occur (either primary or secondary to hypoglycaemia, hypomagnesaemia or hyponatraemia) as may suicidal ideation, gross disorientation, delusions, violence, marked tremor etc. DT symptoms peak on the third or fourth day, physical complications are common, eg. pulmonary infection and hepatic encephalopathy, and it needs to be treated as a priority.

Role of drugs

AWS can be fatal and drug use to reduce seizures and correct vitamin deficiency is essential, usually at specialist centres but there has been some investigation and routine use of careful home or out-patient detoxifications. Short-term benzodiazepines are the most useful.

BNF listed

Benzodiazepines

Chlordiazepoxide and **diazepam** are established treatments for use by specialists in hospital. Chlordiazepoxide is very effective in preventing AWS fits, using up to 60–160mg/d over ten days, then reducing gradually and being wary of potential cumulative effects. Both are standard in the USA where clomethiazole is not available.

Prescribing points:

❖ Long-term therapy in alcoholics must obviously be avoided but short-term use is highly effective.

❖ Beware of an extended metabolism in liver damage (see *Chapter 3.6.2*) and of respiratory depression.

❖ Dosage should be individualised according to symptom severity, co-morbidity and any history of seizures.

Clomethiazole/chlormethiazole (Heminevrin®)

Regarded as safe and effective treatment of AWS at up to 16capsules/d, reducing over 6 or 7 days. It has a relatively low addictive potential but dependence (mainly psychological) can be seen in some patients on longer-term therapy, although with care this can be avoided.

Prescribing points:

❖ Obviously, clomethiazole is not a long-term treatment for alcohol dependence.

❖ Maximum duration of treatment is nine days.

Vitamin B supplementation

Initial treatment should include, preferably, IM multivitamin preparations as oral absorption can be highly variable. B vitamins act as co-enzymes for essential carbohydrate metabolism. Deficiency of nicotinamide, riboflavine (B_2) and pyridoxine (B_6) can cause neuropathies.

Prescribing points:

❖ Oral thiamine is poorly absorbed (usual maximum around 10mg/d) and so injections (Pabrinex®) are essential to ensure adequate vitamin replacement over the first 3 days after withdrawal.

Unlicensed/further information

Carbamazepine (Tegretol®)

This is considered by some specialists to be an effective and useful treatment for alcohol withdrawal symptoms. It is not licensed specifically for this in the UK (although it is of course licensed as an anticonvulsant) but is licensed in some European countries (eg. Ireland). It's advantages are that it is non–addictive and it's metabolism is little affected by liver dysfunction, although higher blood levels may occur with alcohol, enhancing side-effects. It is also sometimes used by specialists for out-patient detoxifications due to its safety and lack of abuse potential.

Others

Beta-blockers and clonidine (both may reduce withdrawal symptom severity), antipsychotics (may lower seizure threshold), gabapentin and valproate have been used.

1.5 Anxiety and agitation

Symptoms

There are numerous symptoms of generalised anxiety disorder but they can be classified into two main groups, psychological and physical:

Psychological symptoms include fearful anticipation, irritability, poor concentration, restlessness, sensitivity to noise, disturbed sleep (lies asleep worrying, wakes Intermittently, unpleasant dreams, but not usually early morning waking) and poor memory (due to poor concentration).

Physical symptoms are mainly due to overactivity of the sympathetic system or increased muscle tension, eg. gastrointestinal (dry mouth, difficulty swallowing, wind, loose motions etc), CNS (tinnitus, blurred vision, dizziness), respiratory (constricted chest, difficulty inhaling, over-breathing), cardiovascular (palpitations, heart pain, missed beats, neck throbbing), genitourinary (increased micturition, lack of libido, impotence), muscular tension (tension headache, tremor) and panic attacks (sudden episodes of extreme anxiety or apprehension).

Anxiety must be differentiated from depression (which is more severe, suicidal thoughts, depressive thinking), early schizophrenia (anxiety will be caused by delusions), dementia (test memory closely), drugs/alcohol abuse including withdrawal (eg. if severe on waking consider alcoholism) and physical illness (eg. thyrotoxicosis, hypoglycaemia).

Role of drugs

Anxiolytics used as a "first-aid" measure are quite rational but it is difficult to assess the longer term effectiveness of these drugs as anxiety tends to vary for reasons other than drug treatment. Decisions on the need for longer-term treatment must be made on an individual basis. The risk: benefit analysis will be influenced where the anxiety compromises the person's ability to function and the potential for dependence in that individual.

Reviews

General (Gale and Oakley-Browne, *BMJ* 2000, **321**, 1204–7, 26 refs; Hallström, *Hosp Med* 2000, **61**, 8–9; Bell and Wilson, *Prescriber* 2000, **11**, 46–48), practical advice on diagnosis and treatment (Birtwistle and Baldwin, *Prescriber* 2001, **12**, 89–101), anxiety in the elderly (Krasucki, *Prescriber* 1998, **9**, 21–31) and in primary care (Livingstone and Jarvie, *Prescriber* 2002, **13**, 17–28).

BNF listed

Benzodiazepines

Benzodiazepines may be extremely useful for chronic anxiety and should not be overlooked, especially if short-term (up to 4 weeks) or intermittent. Users have a greater risk of road traffic accidents (especially if combined with alcohol) and of increased hip fractures, especially in the elderly during the first month of treatment (even with the short-acting benzodiazepines).

Benzodiazepines are indicated for short-term or 'first aid' relief of severe anxiety. Other treatment methods should then be started, eg. relaxation, psychotherapy, treating any underlying depression etc. The *BNF* (see *4.1.2*) sets out cautious advice for the use of benzodiazepines, eg. for short-term use, not used in depression or personality disorder etc.

Alprazolam (Xanax®)
A black-listed benzodiazepine.

Chlordiazepoxide
This has a slow onset of action and many active metabolites.
Prescribing points:
❖ Consider carefully the risk:benefit ratio for long-term treatment.
❖ Care in the elderly due to an extended half-life.

Clobazam
See epilepsy (*1.15*).

Clorazepate dipotassium
Black-listed benzodiazepine.

Diazepam
Diazepam is the standard longer-acting benzodiazepine, with sedative, anxiolytic and muscle relaxant properties (amongst others). It has a long half-life and many active metabolites.
Prescribing points:
❖ Consider carefully the risk:benefit ratio for long-term treatment.
❖ Care in the elderly due to extended half-life.

Lorazepam
A potent shorter-acting benzodiazepine. Dependence seems to be a particular problem with this drug and it has received a bad press because of this, but remains useful for short-term management and in acute and severe anxiety.

Prescribing point:
❖ Consider carefully the risk:benefit ratio for long–term treatment.

Oxazepam
A shorter-acting benzodiazepine, the ultimate metabolite of diazepam and some other benzodiazepines but with no active metabolites itself.
Prescribing point:
❖ Consider carefully the risk:benefit ratio for long-term treatment.

Others

Beta-blockers
Propranolol, oxprenolol etc at 20–60mg/d may be useful for somatic anxiety symptoms such as tachycardia, sweating, tremor etc. and for short-term problems. They appear non-addictive but physical withdrawal symptoms on long-term treatment would be possible.
Prescribing points:
❖ Useful for physical symptoms.
❖ The *BNF* doses of 80–120mg/d may be too high in many patients and can lead to cardiac symptoms and so lower starting doses are recommended, eg. 20–60mg/d.
❖ Remember not to prescribe to anyone with asthma.

Buspirone (Buspar®)
A non-benzodiazepine anxiolytic with negligible sedative, hypnotic, anticonvulsant and muscle relaxant properties. Overall, a limited number of placebo-controlled trials have shown some efficacy. It has a slow onset of action but its effects are similar to benzodiazepines at four weeks. Longer-term treatment may not be as effective as with benzodiazepines but abrupt withdrawal has not been shown to produce withdrawal symptoms. Buspirone does not act on benzodiazepine receptors and has no effect on withdrawal in a benzodiazepine-dependent person. It has a low 'peak' effect and so the abuse potential is low.

Prescribing points:

❖ Generally considered to be of moderate potency but can be highly effective in some people.

❖ Needs four weeks at 10mg TDS before becoming fully effective, so don't give up too soon, or expect too much before then.

Hydroxyzine (Atarax®)

An antihistamine related to the phenothiazines, which at 75–100mg/d may be mildly useful in some cases.

Paroxetine (Seroxat®)

This is licensed in the UK for anxiety, at a dose of 20–50mg/d.

Prescribing points:

❖ Start at 10mg/d for the first few days or weeks to minimise initial exacerbation of anxiety, with 20mg/d the optimum dose.

❖ Careful with discontinuing (see 2.2.2).

Venlafaxine (Efexor XL®)

Now licensed for anxiety, a dose of 75mg/d seems the minimum and optimum, with 150mg/d possible in resistant cases. It has also be shown useful for co-morbid depression and anxiety.

Prescribing points:

❖ Start at 37.5mg/d for the first few days to minimise initial exacerbation of anxiety.

❖ Careful with discontinuing (see 2.2.2).

Unlicensed/further information

Antidepressants

Other **SSRIs** such as citalopram, sertraline and fluoxetine have been shown to be of some clinical effect in anxiety, provided they are started at a low dose to minimise initial anxiety. **Tricyclics** are generally considered useful for persistent or disabling anxiety not part of an adjustment/stress reaction. They may take several weeks to act but may be very potent. **Trazodone** is sedative but may have some use. **Mirtazapine** (15–45mg/d) has been shown to have a rapid effect in anxiety, especially given at night.

Antipsychotics

All have low proven efficacy and marked side-effects but the sedative antihistaminic effects of phenothiazines such as pericyazine (Neulactil®) may be useful, with a low dependence potential.

Useless

Caffeine

See section (*1.32*) for the potential problems of excess caffeine consumption, which may negate any other strategies tried. In anxiety there may also be an abnormal sensitivity to caffeine.

1.6 Attention deficit hyperactivity disorder (ADHD)

Symptoms

ADHD presents as extreme and persistent restlessness, sustained and prolonged motor activity and difficulty in maintaining attention. Such children are impulsive, reckless, prone to accidents, have learning difficulties (partly due to poor concentration), often with antisocial behaviour and a fluctuating mood. Onset is before 7 years of age. Symptoms usually fade out by puberty but learning disability and antisocial behaviour may persist into adult life (resulting sometimes in poor achievement levels), and adult ADHD may be misinterpreted as eg. an antisocial personality disorder.

Role of drugs

Pharmacotherapy with stimulants, whilst somewhat controversial, has been shown to be highly effective against core symptoms if used carefully and monitored regularly. Methylphenidate is clearly the first-line treatment, with a relatively immediate effect. Lack of response to one stimulant does not necessarily predict lack of response to another. Dietary restrictions, eg. dairy products, cereals, food additives etc. may help a small number of children. There is a natural reluctance to prescribe stimulants for children but this must be weighed against the disadvantage of poor performance at school, and the long-term damage that may cause the individual.

BNF listed

Dexamfetamine (Dexadrine®) CD

This has been used in doses of 5–40mg/d by hospital specialists, and is clearly superior to placebo.

Prescribing point:

❖ Hospital specialist advice needed.

Methylphenidate (Ritalin®, Equasym®, Concerta XL®)

Established as first-line treatment, doses of 10–60mg/d (in divided daily doses, usually TDS with the last dose no later than 4pm) can be rapidly effective. The main side-effects in ADHD are insomnia, appetite disturbance, stomach ache, headache and dizziness. The once-daily novel sustained-release preparations eg. Concerta XL® obviate the need for multiple daily doses (which may be forgotten at school).

Prescribing points:

❖ Predictors of response include younger age, demonstrable inattention, near normal IQ and low anxiety.
❖ Hospital specialist advice may be needed.
❖ Concerta XL® needs only to be taken once a day.

Unlicensed/further information

Atomoxetine (Strattera®)

Not available at the time of writing, atomoxetine is a non-stimulant noradrenaline reuptake inhibitor, and so is different to existing stimulants. It is due to be launched in late 2004 and may also be licensed for ADHD in adults. Open studies show comparative efficacy to methylphenidate. Decreased appetite and cardiovascular effects have been seen since it was launched in USA early in 2003.

Clonidine

Doses of 0.1–0.3mg/d may be useful in reducing core symptoms in resistant cases.

Tricyclic, SSRIs etc

Tricyclics, SSRIs, venlafaxine (especially for adult ADHD) and related drugs are considered by specialists as third-line treatments, in children non-responsive or intolerant of stimulants. They are less effective than stimulants on behaviour and similar to placebo on performance. They produce drowsiness, anorexia, sadness and irritability but have less insomnia side-effects. Tricyclics are more toxic in overdose and in routine use, particularly cardiac side-effects where deaths have been reported. Close monitoring is suggested. Bupropion is showing some promise in recent trials. Atypical antipsychotics such as risperidone may be particularly useful as adjuncts.

1.7 Autistic disorder

Symptoms

Autistic disorder, or autism, is a neurodevelopmental disorder. It is characterised by an excessive or morbid dislike of others or society, sometimes with a morbid self-centred attitude. Such children do not respond with normal human emotions towards other people. The main features include 'autistic aloneness', poor speech and language disorder development, an obsessive desire for sameness and bizarre behaviour or mannerisms. Up to 25% develop seizures in adolescence and 75% have an IQ in the retarded range. 60+% need long-term residential care. Onset is not later than 30 months of age. A gluten-free diet may be dramatically helpful, especially if implemented early, before full symptoms develop.

Role of drugs

Antipsychotics may be of limited use in more severe cases to help control some of the more distressing symptoms in conjunction with other strategies. Autistic individuals seem to be very sensitive to neuroleptics and so lower doses may be needed, a therapeutic window of effect having been proposed.

SSRIs and other antidepressants

Many SSRIs have been shown superior to placebo for core symptoms, ritualistic behaviour and anger. There has been some use to reduce withdrawal, hyperactivity and self-injurious behaviour. The mantra "start low and go slow" is the best advice.

Unlicensed/further information

Antipsychotics

Low-dose antipsychotics have been shown to reduce behavioural symptoms (eg. aggression and SIB) and improved learning, with excess sedation, irritability and dystonic reactions noted with some. Recent RCTs have shown **risperidone** 0.5–3mg/d to be well tolerated and effective for tantrums, aggression and SIB. Other atypical antipsychotics may also be useful, although with less published evidence.

Others

Methylphenidate, mirtazapine, levetiracetam, naltrexone and valproate have been used in difficult to manage cases.

Useless

Secretin

Despite much publicity, a complete lack of demonstrable effect has been shown in a series of randomised and open trials and it remains a waste of time and money.

1.8 Benzodiazepine dependence and withdrawal

Although short-term use at standard doses is usually without substantial risk of toxicity and dependence, higher dose and longer-term use is not without this risk. Lorazepam, diazepam and flunitrazepam may be more liable to abuse (probably due to the more rapid absorption and higher receptor potency) than chlordiazepoxide, nitrazepam and oxazepam. The main symptoms from **high-dose** benzodiazepine withdrawal are memory impairment, seizures, mood lability and muscular weakness. Many patients may have underlying psychiatric illness which is controlled by the benzodiazepine and withdrawal may uncover this. Withdrawal should not be attempted in elderly maintained symptom-free by low and steady doses, in epilepsy and where quality of life is significantly improved. A combination of drugs and cognitive behavioural therapy has been shown to be significantly better than either treatment separately, with no medication continued for at least 2 weeks.

BNF listed

Diazepam

Transfer from the current benzodiazepine to diazepam (if necessary) is a common and useful strategy, as diazepam is a longer-acting benzodiazepine and possibly easier to withdraw from.

Prescribing point:

❖ Reduce doses no more often than every 5–7-days. It is usually an advantage not to do the last few dose reductions too quickly.

❖ Doses can be reduced by breaking tablets (eg. down to 1/4 of a 2mg tablet), diluting the syrup or using oral syringes.

Usual users of prescribed benzodiazepines

1. **Older medically ill**:
Benzodiazepine usually prescribed by a non-psychiatrist. Seldom abused, dose not escalated, effective long-term. Care with subtle cognitive changes that can occur.
2. **Psychiatric patients with panic or agoraphobic disorders**:
Seldom abused, doses not escalated, necessary long-term.
3. **Psychiatric patients with recurrent dysphoria**:
Long-term indication for use less clear. Abuse of other drugs often occurs.
4. **Chronic sleep disordered patients**:
Drug may be active or be prevent a rebound syndrome.

Minimising the risk of dependence

Carefully select patients (eg. avoiding especially dependence prone).
Keep the doses low.
Stop where possible, eg. use shorter courses.
Use intermittent or variable doses.
Use tricyclics if depression is mixed with anxiety.

Withdrawal symptoms in the dependent patient

Primary: **Psychological/mild**
Tension (to avoid pre-treatment levels), restlessness, agitation, panic attacks.
Physical — dry mouth, sweating, tremor, sleep disturbance, lethargy, headache, nausea.
Mental — impaired memory and concentration, confusion.
Secondary: **Moderate** — perceptual changes (ie. hypersensitivity to light/sound), dysphoria, flu-like symptoms, anorexia, sore eyes, depersonalization, depression, abnormal sensations of movement.
Severe (rare)
Convulsions, psychoses (eg. visual hallucinations), delusions.

Patients where withdrawal should not be attempted

Elderly maintained symptom-free by low and unchanging doses.
Chronic physical disorders controlled by BDZs (eg. epilepsy).
Where quality of life is so improved by BDZs that long-term use, preferably with intermittent variable doses, is justified eg. chronic or severe anxiety or insomnia and an inadequate personality, people who relapse to alcohol and other more dangerous substances when BDZ-free.

Antidepressants (tricyclics, SSRIs etc)

The *BNF* recommends use of antidepressants for co-morbid depression.

Prescribing points:

❖ Antidepressants can be potent anxiolytics in their own right (see anxiety, *1.5*).
❖ Care is needed with a potentially lowered seizure threshold.

Unlicensed/further information

Many drugs can be used to help manage benzodiazepine withdrawal, either to minimise withdrawal seizures or to help any breakthrough anxiety (see anxiety *1.5*).

Buspirone (Buspar®)

Buspirone may relieve benzodiazepine withdrawal symptoms, as well as being an anxiolytic (but with a slow onset of action) in its own right. Introducing buspirone before a tapered BDZ discontinuation may be successful.

Carbamazepine (Tegretol®)

This has been used to reduce the chance of withdrawal seizures and can additionally minimise withdrawal symptoms (eg. emotional lability), especially if withdrawal is abrupt.

Valproate (Epilim® etc)

Valproate may reduce the intensity of symptoms in protracted withdrawal as well as acting as an anticonvulsant. Specialist advice would be needed.

1.9 Bipolar mood disorder (manic–depression) prophylaxis

— see also mania (*1.17*), depression (*1.12*) and rapid-cycling bipolar disorder (*1.26*)

See also depression (*1.11*), mania/hypomania (*1.17*) and acute psychiatric emergency (*1.24*) for the treatment of any particular relapse or episode. Bipolar mood disorder effects up to 5% population, is often unrecognised, misdiagnosed and inadequately treated. The mean age of onset is 30 years, and it still takes most people with bipolar an average of 3 professionals and over 6–10 years to get a proper diagnosis and start mood stabilisers. It has often been misdiagnosed as substance misuse, ADHD and personality disorders. Bipolar has the highest suicide rate amongst mental health disorders, the first attempt often being before diagnosis. Lithium is the only mood stabiliser shown to reduce suicide rates.

Role of drugs

Lithium, valproate and carbamazepine are acknowledged as being effective in the prophylaxis of bipolar disorder and a major problem within psychiatric services is the premature discontinuation of these agents resulting in sometimes catastrophic relapse. Optimum outcomes are usually achieved with appropriate and consistent prescribing of mood stabilisers combined with social and psychological support.

BNF listed

Carbamazepine (Tegretol®)

Long-term therapy in bipolar disorder is well established, either as an alternative to lithium, or occasionally in combination in treatment-resistant cases. It is reported to be better for early onset illness and with an alternating pattern of mood. Predictors of the best response include severe mania or depression, anxiety and dysphoria, rapid cycling and a negative family history, typically those symptoms shown by lithium non-responders. Its effectiveness is generally apparent soon after therapy starts. Trough plasma levels of ≥7mg/L are strongly associated with better outcomes. There is no evidence of a rebound syndrome.

Prescribing points:

❖ Retard® preparations may be useful to reduce side-effects due to reduced peak plasma levels.

❖ Once- or twice-a-day therapy is quite appropriate.

❖ Plasma level monitoring for higher doses (eg. above 600mg/d) is recommended.

Monitoring schedules for lithium regimens	Test and recommended frequency
Plasma lithium level	3 months
T3 T4 and TSH	6 months
If TSH raised	4–6 weeks

Lithium (Camcolit®, Priadel® etc)

Prophylactic use of lithium in bipolar disorder is well-established and with care lithium can be highly successful and safe. The usual reasons for starting lithium are two illnesses in two years or three in five years. The usual reasons for not starting are the danger of overdose, side-effects, potential poor compliance and uncertainty about the future course of the illness. Lithium has been shown to **reduce suicide**, excess mortality, relapse and severity, if used properly and carefully in correctly selected patients.

Compliance:

The efficacy of lithium in bipolar disorder is beyond doubt, but studies have indicated that its effectiveness can be significantly compromised by poor compliance (including short-term discontinuation and erratic consumption) and poor monitoring. The main reason for lithium failure is non-compliance/concordance, and the patient (and any partner) needs to be aware of the long-term commitment needed.

Discontinuation:

Relapse in bipolar illness following lithium discontinuation is well established. Treatment with lithium should be for at least two years (and more probably three years at the minimum) and that up to two years it may have at best no beneficial effect (premature stopping resulting in premature recurrence of mania). In addition, withdrawing stable patients may result in subsequent lithium refactoriness. **Rapid discontinuation** (over less than 4 weeks) is more **likely** to lead to relapse of depression or hypomania than gradual (over 4–12 weeks) reduction.

Prescribing points:

❖ Lithium is the only mood stabiliser shown to have an anti-suicide effect. It is an effective drug but potent and must be treated with respect and care.

❖ Lithium is a high-risk strategy for adjunctive treatment of depression. Don't add it in too quickly for resistant depression — try 3 antidepressants first, and only use if the person will take regularly for 2 years.

❖ Over 10% of all psychiatric negligence claims involve lithium monitoring (or rather the lack of it).

❖ Plasma level monitoring **every three months** is strongly recommended, more often if risk factors exist, eg. interacting drugs, hot weather etc.

❖ Plasma levels of 0.4–0.8mmol/l are generally considered safe and effective and there is no evidence that doses above 1.0mmol/l are needed except in rare cases.

❖ **Do not stop lithium abruptly**. If withdrawing lithium, slow **tapering over four to twelve weeks** is essential/recommended.

❖ Rapidly changing levels may also be detrimental — take all dose changes gently as well.

❖ Once daily lithium reduces side-effects, especially renal damage, and simplifies dosage requirements.

❖ If a woman finds out she's pregnant whilst taking lithium, don't panic (and refer to *Chapter 3.8*).

Olanzapine (Zyprexa®)

Olanzapine is licensed in the UK for moderate to severe manic episodes, and also now as a mood stabiliser. The starting dose is 15mg/d as monotherapy and 10mg/d in combination. A Cochrane review concludes that olanzapine is effective in mania, possibly more so than valproate but with more weight gain and somnolence.

Combinations

Lithium +/− carbamazepine +/− valproate

These have been used in combination by some specialists. An additive anti-thyroid effect may occur with lithium and carbamazepine, lowering T4 and free T4 levels, so check regularly.

Unlicensed/further information

Antipsychotics/neuroleptics

These may be useful in some patients, ie. prophylaxis of bipolar affective disorder, reducing hypomanic relapses and time in hospital. **Risperidone** may be useful in mania and bipolar, as may clozapine and quetiapine.

Lamotrigine (Lamictal®)

Lamotrigine may soon be licensed in UK for the long-term management of bipolar depression, at doses of 50–200mg/d.

Valproate salts (Depakote®, Epilim® etc)

Valproate semisodium is licensed for acute management of mania. In the only major one-year trial against lithium and placebo, valproate was superior as a mood stabiliser against placebo for all secondary measures but only just failed statistically on the primary measure of time to mood episode. It clearly has mood stabilising effects and is an established alternative to lithium and carbamazepine.

Prescribing points:

❖ Depakote® is more tolerable than sodium valproate at high dose and has a proper dosing schedule for mania, but no valproate preparation is licensed for mood stabilisation so at lower valproate doses, any valproate preparation can be used.

Others

Topiramate, tamoxifen, tiagabine, oxcarbazepine and calcium-channel blockers have been used in resistant cases.

1.10 Borderline personality disorder (BPD)

Symptoms

The main symptoms of borderline personality disorder (BPD) are of a deeply ingrained maladaptive pattern of behaviour, recognisable from adolescence and continuing through most of adult life. Such people show continued boredom, anger, unstable relationships, impulsive self-harmful behaviour (eg. gambling, stealing, binge-eating), variable moods, recurrent suicide threats or behaviour and uncertainty about their personal identity. BPD may account for up to 7.5% of psychiatric admissions, with a raised incidence of psychiatric morbidity and mortality. Bipolar mood disorder has been misdiagnosed as BPD, especially if combined with substance misuse.

Role of drugs

Drug use in some people with BPD is supported by the literature. The drugs will not alter established character traits or the effects of abuse, but they may produce modest benefits, with the occasional striking result. They may possibly be more effective if combined with psychotherapy. Drug therapy, however, is fraught with problems. Side-effects may be grossly exaggerated to avoid treatment and patients be actively anti-medication. Care in patients with suicidal tendencies is necessary.

Unlicensed/further information

Antipsychotics

In patients with borderline personality disorders, **small** doses of antipsychotics/neuroleptics may produce significant benefit and may allow psychotherapy to proceed more effectively. Low dose **risperidone** (mean 3.5mg/d) has been shown to be useful for aggression, overall functioning and other psychopathological symptoms, as have **olanzapine**, and Depixol® (20mg monthly). Generally, high–potency drugs in low dose are preferred by patients (due to a lack of the abhorred sedative effects).

Other drugs

Carbamazepine and lithium have been used for the aggressive components of BPD, with SSRIs and tricyclics also sometimes used. Benzodiazepines may be useful but can be abused or rarely cause disinhibition. SSRIs and valproate may reduce irritability, anger and aggression.

1.11 Dementia including Alzheimer's, Lewy Body disease etc

1.11.1 Senile dementia

Dementia is a progressive and irreversible reduction in the level of previously attained intellectual, memory and personality/emotional functioning. Clinical features include: disturbed behaviour (disorganised, inappropriate, distracted, restless, antisocial, rigid thinking, stereotyped behaviour, anger, neglect, incontinent), lack of insight, impaired thinking (slow, impoverished, delusions, incoherent, concrete, rigid), poverty of speech, low mood, poor cognitive function (forgetfulness, cannot learn, poor attention, disorientation in time and later place) and impaired memory.

1.11.2 Alzheimer's disease

This is a form of dementia characterised by senile plaques and neurofibrillary tangles, with reduced levels of acetylcholine and other transmitters in the brain. It usually shows as a steady deterioration. The main features of its insidious onset are forgetfulness, lack of spontaneity, disorientation, depressed mood, decline in self-care, poor sleep (waking disorientated and perplexed) and intellectual impairment (dysphasia, dyspraxia, language decline).

1.11.3 Lewy Body disease/dementia

This is a variant of Alzheimer's disease, more common in men and with an extreme sensitivity to antipsychotics (CSM warning in *Current Problems* 1994, **20**, 6), which may result in a sudden onset of Parkinsonian side-effects, confusion, deterioration and sudden death.

Role of drugs

There are numerous causes of dementia, some of which can be treated, eg. vitamin depletion (eg. B_{12}, folic acid, thiamine), infections (encephalitis, neurosyphilis) and drug toxicity. The anticholinesterases are now first-line treatment through correcting the cholinergic deficit that occurs in dementia, although other transmitter systems may also be faulty. Other drugs may help to control some of these symptoms, eg. depression, disinhibition etc. but their effect is of minimal importance. There are growing concerns that whilst the anticholinesterases help in the short-term, there are still major (and often unexpected) problems when these drugs begin to lose their effectiveness.

Reviews: general (Fairbairn, *Prescribers' J* 2000, **40**, 77–85; Hughes and Livingstone, *Prescriber* 2000, 85–95), anticholinesterases (Holden and Kelly, *Adv Psych Treat* 2002, **8**, 89–96), guidelines for the appropriate use of cholinesterase inhibitors (Van Den Berg *et al*, *Drugs & Aging* 2000, **16**, 123–38).

BNF listed

Acetylcholinesterase inhibitors (AChEs)

Donepezil (Aricept®)

Donepezil is licensed for the symptomatic treatment of mild or moderate Alzheimer's disease. Dosage is simple (5mg once a day, increasing to 10mg/d after a month if required). The few peripheral side-effects include diarrhoea and muscle cramps but no LFT or blood monitoring is required. Stabilisation or some improvement may be seen initially. There is no evidence yet that the course of the disease is slowed, so when the drug is discontinued, the deterioration may be rapid. It may also be effective in the later stages of disease.

Galantamine (Reminyl®)

As well as being an AChE, galantamine stimulates pre- and post-synaptic nicotinic receptors. The target dose is usually 12mg BD, and a Cochrane review concluded 16–32mg/d produces a consistent effect at 3–6 months.

Prescribing points:

❖ Start at 4mg BD (morning and evening) for 4 weeks, then 8mg BD for 4 weeks, then increase to 12mg BD if necessary after a further 4 weeks.

Rivastigmine (Exelon®)

Rivastigmine inhibits both the acetylcholine and butylcholine esterase enzymes. A Cochrane review concluded that 6–12mg/d was the target dose.

Prescribing points:

❖ Start at 1.5mg BD, increase to 3mg BD after 2 weeks if tolerated, then increase at 1.5mg BD increments to 6mg BD at not less than 2-weekly intervals.

Co-dergocrine (Hydergine®)

This vasodilator may slightly improve performance but a meta-analysis of the 46 studies showed an effect little superior to placebo in probable Alzheimer's disease.

Prescribing point:

❖ Do not expect an improvement.

Memantine (Ebixa®)

Memantine has a unique license for management of moderate to severe Alzheimer's Disease and a recent trial (n=252, *NEJM* 2003, **348**, 1333–41) also showed that it may reduce deterioration in moderate to severe Alzheimer's Disease by blocking the neurotoxic effects of glutamate. It may have some efficacy also for the symptoms of vascular dementia.

Prescribing points:

❖ Start at 5mg/d then increase by 5mg/d per week up to a maximum of 20mg/d.

Unlicensed/further information

Many drugs have been tried but few have succeeded to any extent. Most drug therapy is to help treat some of the symptoms of dementia rather than the dementia itself.

Antidepressants

At lower doses, antidepressants can be used to treat any understandable concurrent depression, although side-effects can be a problem, particularly the anticholinergic side-effects of the tricyclics in a person who already has a cholinergic deficit. SSRIs come into their own here, with studies showing **citalopram** (Cipramil®) to improve confusion, mood, restlessness and irritability in dementia. **Trazodone** (Molipaxin®) may help some people with persistent screaming.

Antipsychotics/neuroleptics

In their role as "major tranquillisers", these have been used for many years as symptomatic treatment of aggressive, agitated behaviour and as sedatives. They have been shown to reduce behavioural disorders but with the risk of side-effects. Lower doses of **risperidone** (0.25–1mg/d) seem effective for aggression and behavioural disturbances, without impairing cognitive performance. Starting at 0.25mg/d using the syrup helps improve tolerability. **Olanzapine** (2.5–10mg/d) and **quetiapine**

(50–150mg/d) may also be useful. Patients with **Lewy Body** dementia (*1.11.3*) may be **extremely sensitive** to antipsychotics and use may result in a sudden onset of Parkinsonian side-effects, profound confusion and deterioration and can lead to death.

Ginkgo biloba

There is now good evidence that gingko biloba is only slightly less effective than the anticholinesterases for Alzheimer's Disease.

Other drugs

Others tried include clomethiazole (Heminevrin®) as a hypnotic for confused or agitated patients, NSAIDs (with accumulating evidence that use for 2 years or more significantly reduces the chance of developing Alzheimer's), conjugated estrogens or diethylstilbestrol for aggression in elderly demented men and piracetam (Nootropil®) as an adjunct to an anticholinesterase.

1.12 Depression — see also bipolar mood disorder (*1.9*)

Depression is a common illness, affecting 3% of the population per year, 25% of whom do not see a GP and in many that do, the true diagnosis is not evident. Use of sub-therapeutic doses of antidepressants means that the number identified and then treated with full antidepressant doses is even lower, a tragedy for this eminently treatable condition.

Symptoms

Patients usually show a mixture of biological symptoms (insomnia or hypersomnia, poor sleep, diurnal variation in mood, low appetite, fatigue or loss of energy, constipation, loss of libido, weight loss or gain) and psychiatric symptoms (depressed mood, loss of interest or pleasure, poor memory, psychomotor agitation or retardation, recurrent thoughts of death or suicide, anxiety, feelings of worthlessness or guilt, including delusions etc). The normal reaction to death of a loved one is not usually considered as depression.

Causes

Precipitating factors can include drugs and drug abuse, physical illness and stress (bereavement, loss of job, birth of child, break-up of a relationship, work stress, poor social background, time of year etc).

Role of drugs

The overall cost of depression (eg. work, family, other illnesses) is very high.

Although most depressions will resolve with time, antidepressants have a major role in hastening this recovery and reducing suffering during the indeterminate time before recovery. Adequate doses (see later) of antidepressants are needed for clinical effect, and continuation for an appropriate period (see later) should prevent relapse. Antidepressants are effective in most people, are not addictive (see *1.32*) and do not lose efficacy with prolonged use (except perhaps in a few people).

Optimum use

The main problem with the use of tricyclic antidepressants in primary care seems to be that too low a dose is often used. There is **no** published evidence that 75mg/d of a tricyclic is effective as an antidepressant, although a few people seem to respond to lower doses and can relapse on withdrawal (probably because about 1 in 20 people lack the CYP2D6 enzyme that metabolises tricyclics, giving high blood levels with low doses). If the older tricyclics are used, it may be difficult to reach therapeutic doses due to intolerable side-effects.

Follow the "Six D's depression" for the medication management of depression:

1. Diagnosis: making, or being able to make, a diagnosis always helps.

2. Drug-related causes eliminated: eg. excessive caffeine intake, other drugs liable to cause depression (see *5.5* for a list), physical reasons (eg. low folate, hypothyroidism) etc.

3. Drug and Dose: The choice of drug is of less importance than ensuring it is used at therapeutic levels (eg. standard dose SSRI, 150mg/d tricyclic equivalent etc). Allow **four to six weeks at therapeutic dose** for optimum effect. If no response occurs within 4–6 weeks, there is little point in continuing so consider another antidepressant, eg. tricyclic, SSRI, venlafaxine, mirtazapine (the easiest to switch to or from), moclobemide, trazodone. (See section on switching antidepressants *2.2.2.*).

Bipolar depression — extra care is needed with drug and dose in a depressed phase of bipolar disorder (manic-depression, see *1.9*). Avoid sudden dose changes, start with drugs with the lowest risk of switching the person to mania or mixed states (eg. SSRIs, mirtazapine and bupropion but avoid tricyclics) and use mood stabilisers if not already in use. If a switch starts to occur, reduce the antidepressant dose immediately and allow the mood to settle for a month or so.

4. Duration — first episode: After an initial response, inadequate or no treatment for the next six months in controlled trials has resulted in relapse rates as high as **50%** (cf. 20% relapse with adequate treatment). Continuation doses should be the **same or close** to the therapeutic dose. Patients should be advised that continuation therapy substantially reduces relapse and that the drugs are not addictive (see *1.32*). Numerous recommendations for the duration of this treatment phase have been proposed, but the only study to look at this systematically concluded that for a first episode, **6 months** continuation from full recovery significantly reduces relapse, but that unless risk factors for depression remain, there is no real advantage continuing beyond six months. The depression should be carefully monitored when the drug is then tapered and withdrawn.

Duration — several episodes: 50–85% of people suffering an episode of major depression will go on to have a further recurrence, usually within two to three years. Thus maintenance therapy is indicated for many if relapse occurs. Risk factors include recurrent dysthymia (low grade depression), concurrent non-affective psychiatric illness, chronic medical disorder and a history of relapses. Increasing severity of subsequent episodes is predicted by serious suicide attempts, psychotic features or severe functional impairment. A prophylactic effect beyond three years has been shown for many antidepressants. With recurrent episodes less than two years apart, treatment for at least five years is warranted. As full doses are needed for maintenance it is usually easier to use SSRIs, as full antidepressant dosage of these drugs is usually more tolerable to the patient. In the elderly, therapy for up to two years after recovery may be needed.

The general consensus seems to be:

First episode: 6 months continuation after recovery significantly reduces relapse

Second episode: 2–3 years continuation after recovery

Third episode: consider 5 years or longer

Fourth or subsequent episode: continuous antidepressants unless there is a good reason to stop

5. Discontinuation: As and when discontinuing therapy is considered appropriate, slowly reduce doses over **a minimum of four weeks**. Discontinuation syndromes have been reported with most antidepressants (most with paroxetine, venlafaxine and tricyclics), including gastrointestinal and somatic distress, sleep disturbance, movement disorders and hypomania, which is not due to relapse nor accompanied by craving for the drug. These symptoms usually appear within 1–14 days of stopping treatment and then improve within a week or so without reintroduction of the drug. Recurrence of depression begins within 3–15 weeks and continues to worsen. Treatment of withdrawal symptoms includes reinstatement at low dose and then tapering, use of an anticholinergic for symptomatic relief or just letting the symptoms resolve (see *2.2.2 for a range of practical strategies).*

Choice of antidepressants

All the main drugs appear to have roughly similar efficacy and so choice will be based upon:

1. Features of depression, eg. agitation etc.
2. Suicide risk (avoid TCAs and MAOIs).
3. Concomitant drug therapy (see *Chapter 4).*
4. Concurrent illness.
5. Side-effect tolerability eg. weight, sexual etc.
6. Cost.
7. Special considerations, eg. cognitive impairment, driving etc.

Nearly all antidepressants can be given once a day.

Loss of antidepressant efficacy has been reported in 9–33% people and explanations may include non-compliance, loss of placebo response, inadequate prophylactic dose, pharmacological tolerance, change in severity and unrecognised rapid cycling. The most effective initial strategies are:

- to increase the dose
- switch to another drug.

Antidepressant drugs have been alleged to be associated with the emergence of suicidal tendencies. The risk of suicide appears to be the same with tricyclics as with the newer drugs, but the rates of death are higher with tricyclics.

BNF Listed

Selective Serotonin Reuptake Inhibitors (SSRIs)

The SSRIs are first choice drugs in depression in most patients due to their low overdose risk, safety in heart disease and low side-effects (eg. lack of anticholinergic, sedation and weight gain effects).

The SSRIs are more similar than different and are all effective antidepressants but the ADR profiles (eg. nausea, sexual dysfunction, discontinuation) and potential for interactions can be different. SSRI therapy discontinuation rates are lower than with the TCAs (10% overall, 25% due to side-effects).

With the SSRIs, there is an almost flat dose response curve and so there is little clinical benefit from increasing doses above the recommended starter and usually only results in increased side-effects. Usually only about 1 in 20 will benefit from a dose above the standard.

Citalopram (Cipramil®)

Well-established across the globe, citalopram is indicated for depression and preventing relapse/recurrence. A meta-analysis of 30 RCTs showed it to be effective and well-tolerated from 20–60mg/d, with a very low incidence of drug interactions. The green and yellow pack has proved a great success in the author's home city of Norwich.

Prescribing point:

- ❖ Antidepressant dose is 20mg/d, but an increase to 40mg/d may be useful in severe depression, but don't give it much longer than 4/52 at the higher dose.
- ❖ Starting at 10mg/d (ie. half a 20mg tablet) for the first few days improves tolerability and reduces drop-outs.

Escitalopram (Cipralex®)

Escitalopram is the pharmacologically active enantiomer of citalopram and at least twice as potent on a mg for mg basis. There have been suggestions that the inactive enantiomer might actually have a depressant effect.

Prescribing point:

- ❖ Antidepressant dose is 10mg/d, which may have slightly fewer side-effects than citalopram 20mg/d, although citalopram is relatively low on side-effects.
- ❖ Starting at 5mg/d (ie. half a 10mg tablet) for the first few days improves tolerability and reduces drop-outs.

Depression treatment algorithm

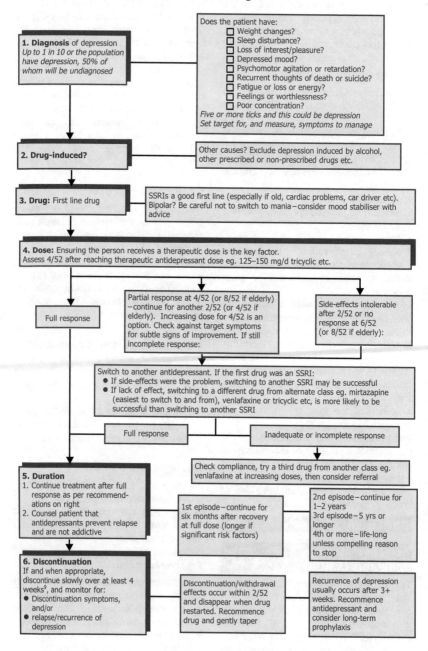

1. Diagnosis of depression
Up to 1 in 10 or the population have depression, 50% of whom will be undiagnosed

Does the patient have:
☐ Weight changes?
☐ Sleep disturbance?
☐ Loss of interest/pleasure?
☐ Depressed mood?
☐ Psychomotor agitation or retardation?
☐ Recurrent thoughts of death or suicide?
☐ Fatigue or loss or energy?
☐ Feelings or worthlessness?
☐ Poor concentration?
Five or more ticks and this could be depression
Set target for, and measure, symptoms to manage

2. Drug-induced?

Other causes? Exclude depression induced by alcohol, other prescribed or non-prescribed drugs etc.

3. Drug: First line drug

SSRIs a good first line (especially if old, cardiac problems, car driver etc). Bipolar? Be careful not to switch to mania – consider mood stabiliser with advice

4. Dose: Ensuring the person receives a therapeutic dose is the key factor.
Assess 4/52 after reaching therapeutic antidepressant dose eg. 125–150 mg/d tricyclic etc.

Full response

Partial response at 4/52 (or 8/52 if elderly) – continue for another 2/52 (or 4/52 if elderly). Increasing dose for 4/52 is an option. Check against target symptoms for subtle signs of improvement. If still incomplete response:

Side-effects intolerable after 2/52 or no response at 6/52 (or 8/52 if elderly):

Switch to another antidepressant. If the first drug was an SSRI:
● If side-effects were the problem, switching to another SSRI may be successful
● If lack of effect, switching to a different drug from alternate class eg. mirtazapine (easiest to switch to and from), venlafaxine or tricyclic etc, is more likely to be successful than switching to another SSRI

Full response

Inadequate or incomplete response

Check compliance, try a third drug from another class eg. venlafaxine at increasing doses, then consider referral

5. Duration
1. Continue treatment after full response as per recommend-ations on right
2. Counsel patient that antidepressants prevent relapse and are not addictive

1st episode – continue for six months after recovery at full dose (longer if significant risk factors)

2nd episode – continue for 1–2 years
3rd episode – 5 yrs or longer
4th or more – life-long unless compelling reason to stop

6. Discontinuation
If and when appropriate, discontinue slowly over at least 4 weeks[9], and monitor for:
● Discontinuation symptoms, and/or
● relapse/recurrence of depression

Discontinuation/withdrawal effects occur within 2/52 and disappear when drug restarted. Recommence drug and gently taper

Recurrence of depression usually occurs after 3+ weeks. Recommence antidepressant and consider long-term prophylaxis

Fluoxetine (Prozac® etc)

The best-established SSRI world-wide, fluoxetine was the first drug to make taking an antidepressant 'trendy'. Although 20mg/d is the standard dose, resistant depressions may respond to 40–60mg/d. A long half-life may prove a problem in the elderly, although missed doses become less important in continuation and prophylactic therapy and discontinuation effects are minimal. Little need for dose escalation is apparent from prescribing studies, indicating that the standard 20mg/d dose is appropriate.

Prescribing point:

❖ Adult antidepressant dose is 20mg/d. There is probably little point in going above 20mg/d as the response rate is little better.

The Serotonin Syndrome

This is a relatively rare condition caused by central serotonin hyperstimulation. It presents as changes in mental status, restlessness, myoclonus, hyperreflexia, shivering and tremor. Hypertension, convulsions and death have been reported.

Mainly reported with various combinations of tryptophan, MAOIs, (with or without lithium), SSRIs and TCAs (either together or in quick succession).

Treat symptomatically, eg. discontinue medication (usually resolves in 24 hours) and support, eg. cooling blankets etc. and refer any suspected cases to psychiatric specialists.

Fluvoxamine (Faverin®)

Fluvoxamine has been compared with, and shown to be as effective as, many standard tricyclics (eg. imipramine) but it may have a higher incidence of nausea and vomiting than other SSRIs. Once daily dosing at night produces less side-effects than OM or BD dosing.

Prescribing point:

❖ Antidepressant dose is probably 200mg/d, although no one is very sure.

Paroxetine (Seroxat®)

Paroxetine is licensed for depression, including that accompanied by anxiety and it has been shown to be effective compared to standard tricyclics, SSRIs and placebo. 20mg/d is the minimum dose, 50mg/d the usual maximum. On discontinuation or rapid dose reduction, withdrawal symptoms lasting three weeks or longer have been reported to occur within 48 hours (see switching antidepressants in *Chapter 2.2.2 point 13*).

Prescribing points:

❖ Standard antidepressant dose is 20–30mg/d, with little advantage in going beyond this.
❖ A gradual discontinuation is strongly recommended (see *Chapter 2.2.2*).
❖ The CSM has recommended it not to be used in the under 18's for depression (fluoxetine is the CSM-recommended alternative).
❖ Starting at 10mg/d (ie. half a 20mg tablet) for the first few days improves tolerability and reduces drop-outs.

Sertraline (Lustral®)

The pharmacological profile of sertraline is similar to fluoxetine, but with a shorter half-life and has a low incidence of drug interactions.

Prescribing point:

❖ Antidepressant dose is 50mg/d although prescribing studies indicate 100mg/d is as frequently used.
❖ Starting at 25mg/d (ie. half a 50mg tablet) for the first few days improves tolerability and reduces drop-outs.

Tricyclic antidepressants (TCAs)

Tricyclics are still one of the commonest causes of fatal and non-fatal drug poisoning in the world. The risk of suicide attempts appears to be the same with TCAs as newer drugs such as fluoxetine or trazodone, but the rates of death are higher with TCAs (especially dosulepin and amitriptyline). About 300 people a year die from tricyclic overdoses in the UK.

Amitriptyline

A widely used tricyclic with potent anticholinergic, sedative and weight gaining properties.

Prescribing points:

❖ Antidepressant dose in 95% adults is 125–150mg/d.

Clomipramine (Anafranil®)

A potent tricyclic which has also been used to treat depression with an obsessional component.

Prescribing points:

❖ Antidepressant dose in 95% adults is 125–150mg/d.

❖ Once daily dosage can be appropriate.

Dosulepin/dothiepin (Prothiaden®)

Established UK tricyclic. The author finds its continued popularity slightly surprising considering it's severe toxicity in overdose and standard side-effect profile. It has significant sedative effects and impairment of concentration and memory (eg. compared with lofepramine). A retrospective toxicity study showed dosulepin to be more toxic than other tricyclics, particularly due to its pro-convulsive and cardiac arrhythmic effects. It is frequently prescribed in the community at sub-therapeutic antidepressant doses (eg. 75mg/d) which must be a major cause of treatment failure.

Prescribing points:

❖ Antidepressant dose in 95% adults is 125–150mg/d.

❖ Dosulepin should not be used in someone actively or potentially suicidal.

Doxepin (Sinequan®)

A standard tricyclic with moderate sedation, which may have fewer anticholinergic and cardiac effects than older tricyclics.

Prescribing point:

❖ Antidepressant dose in 95% adults is 125–150mg/d.

Imipramine

An established standard tricyclic suitable for once daily administration. Stimulant side-effects may be trouble-some as may the anticholinergic effects, especially in the elderly.

Prescribing point:

❖ Antidepressant dose in 95% adults is 125–150mg/d.

Lofepramine (Gamanil®)

Established UK tricyclic. It may have relatively less side-effects than other tricyclics, eg. it has minimal sedative effects and impairment of concentration and memory compared with dosulepin. The data on safety in overdose is incontrovertible, with lofepramine itself seeming to block the cardiotoxic effects of the main metabolite desipramine.

Prescribing points:

❖ Antidepressant dose in 95% adults is 210–280mg/d.

❖ Relatively safe in overdose.

Maprotiline (Ludiomil®)

Maprotiline is essentially a tricyclic antidepressant and its cardiac effects are certainly similar to the older tricyclics. It has the greatest incidence of **seizures** in overdose (and even at standard doses) than all other antidepressants available in Europe, made worse by its unusually long half-life.

Prescribing points:

❖ Antidepressant dose in 95% adults is 125–150mg/d.

❖ Restrict to use in patients where the risks of seizures and overdose are absolutely minimal.

Nortriptyline (Allegron®)

A mildly sedative tricyclic with low cardiotoxic side-effects.

Prescribing points:

❖ Antidepressant dose in 95% adults is 125–150mg/d.

❖ Suitable for once daily administration.

Trimipramine (Surmontil®)

Trimipramine has notable sedative properties which can be useful for hypnotic and anxiolytic purposes. Once daily dosing is effective. It has been shown to be as 'cardiologically safe' as doxepin at low divided doses (eg. 50mg/d) although these will be sub-therapeutic doses for depression.

Prescribing point:

❖ Antidepressant dose in 95% adults is 125–150mg/d.

Switching antidepressants

For a table on swapping antidepressants and the gaps needed, see *2.2.2.*

Related antidepressants

Mianserin

Mianserin is a true tetracyclic with a good safety in overdose, low cardiotoxicity and useful marked sedative properties.

Prescribing points:

❖ Antidepressant dose is up to 90mg/d.
❖ Full blood counts at regular intervals are still recommended despite no good evidence of a problem.

Mirtazapine (Zispin®)

Mirtazapine is an antidepressant described as a NaSSA. It increases noradrenaline transmission directly and indirectly enhances serotonergic transmission, but as it also blocks $5HT_2$ and $5HT_3$ receptors has minimal serotonergic side-effects, eg. nausea, headache, sexual dysfunction etc. It has been shown to be as effective as other antidepressants in both moderate and particularly in severe depression, with improved sleep shown. The main side-effects seem to be somnolence and markedly increased appetite/weight gain in a small number of patients. Three studies have shown a robust slightly faster onset of action (for once a claim of a faster onset that can actually be proven).

Prescribing points:

❖ Starting at 30mg/d (rather than 15mg/d) may minimise the initial sedative effects.
❖ Easy to switch to and from should you need to.

Moclobemide (Manerix®)

Moclobemide inhibits only the MAO-A and not MAO-B enzyme in the brain. Both MAO-A and MAO-B metabolise tyramine but only MAO-A is active in the brain. An excess of tyramine in the body will displace moclobemide from MAO-A, allowing tyramine metabolism to occur, MOA-B remaining free. This results in a 'cheese-reaction' usually only at amounts above 100–150mg of tyramine (see interactions chapter), **highly** unlikely under normal conditions. It is effective in depression, comparable in efficacy to tricyclics but usually better tolerated.

Prescribing points:

❖ Antidepressant dose is at least 300mg/d, and possibly up to 600mg/d.
❖ A traditional MAOI card is **not** needed.

Reboxetine (Edronax®)

Reboxetine is a selective noradrenaline reuptake inhibitor and has no dopamine, histamine, adrenergic nor serotonin effects but a weak anticholinergic action. There is little published data but in short-term studies it appears as effective as imipramine and fluoxetine in major depression. A higher level of social functioning has been shown with reboxetine. Relapse prevention has been shown in a one year study *vs* placebo. There is no effect on reaction time. Due to a lack of placebo-controlled studies, it is not recommended in the elderly.

Trazodone (Molipaxin®)

An antidepressant with low cardiotoxicity and anticholinergic side-effects but a higher incidence of drowsiness and nausea.

Prescribing points:

❖ Antidepressant dose is probably 150mg/d.
❖ Best taken with food to reduce peak blood levels.
❖ More useful as a hypnotic.

Venlafaxine (Efexor®, Efexor-XL®)

Venlafaxine inhibits the reuptake of serotonin, noradrenaline (which becomes significant from about 150mg/d) and dopamine (from about 225mg/d). Although doses of 75mg/d are generally required for an antidepressant effect, titrating up to 150mg/d seems optimal and higher doses seem particularly useful in resistant depression. It can cause nausea, headache and dizziness, as well as dry mouth, somnolence and elevated bp. Discontinuation effects on rapid withdrawal have been reported.

Prescribing points:

* ❖ Doses of 75–150mg are the minimum needed for depression, but it has little advantage over an SSRI at this dose. From 150–225mg, it becomes more of an SNRI, above 225mg/d it becomes an SNDRI, so escalating doses may be worth it.
* ❖ Switching to and from SSRIs needs some care to minimise serotonin effects.
* ❖ Nausea is dose-related and usually transient. Use of the once-daily XL formulation minimises this.
* ❖ Discontinuation should be gradual over several weeks.
* ❖ Not now recommended for depression in under 18's (fluoxetine is the CSM-approved alternative).

MAOIs

Isocarboxazid (was Marplan®)

A hydrazine derivative which irreversibly blocks the MAO enzyme.

Prescribing point:

* ❖ Adult antidepressant dose is at least 30mg/d.

Phenelzine (Nardil®)

A hydrazine derivative which irreversibly blocks the MAO enzyme.

Prescribing point:

* ❖ Adult antidepressant dose is around 60mg/d.

Tranylcypromine (was Parnate®)

A non-hydrazine amphetamine-related drug with stimulant effects and a greater incidence of adverse drug interactions.

Prescribing point:

* ❖ Adult antidepressant dose is around 30mg/d.

Others

Flupentixol (Fluanxol®)

In low doses, either orally or sometimes as a depot, flupentixol can have some antidepressant properties. Its efficacy has, however, been queried as the speed of action is more in line with an anxiolytic effect and an equally good case can be put forward for other antipsychotics.

Prescribing points:

* ❖ Antidepressant dose is 1mg/d.
* ❖ Anxiolytic properties may be important.

Lithium (Camcolit®, Priadel® etc)

Use of lithium as monotherapy in the treatment and prophylaxis of unipolar depression has been well established and has been associated with low mortality. Use for less than 2 years in bipolar depression has been shown to have a negative effect.

Prescribing points:

* ❖ Lithium is a high risk strategy for adjunctive treatment of depression. Don't add it in too quickly for resistant depression—try 3 antidepressants first, and only use if the person will take regularly for 2 years.
* ❖ Over 10% of all psychiatric negligence claims involve lithium monitoring (or lack of it) — monitor plasma level monitoring **every three months**.
* ❖ Plasma levels of 0.4–0.8mmol/l are generally considered safe and effective and there is no evidence that doses above 1.0mmol/l are needed except in rare cases.
* ❖ Do not stop lithium abruptly. If withdrawing lithium, slow **tapering over twelve weeks** is essential/recommended. Rapidly changing levels may also be detrimental — take all dose changes gently as well.
* ❖ If a woman finds out she's pregnant whilst taking lithium don't panic — see *Chapter 3.8*. See main entry under Bipolar mood disorder (*1.9*).

Tryptophan (Optimax®)

A naturally occurring amino acid and precursor to serotonin, tryptophan is usually used in combination with tricyclic or other antidepressants. Due to a previous association with eosinophilia-myalgia syndrome (EMS), it is now only licensed in the UK for resistant depression, usually started by hospital specialists, in patients with severe depression continuously for more than two years, after adequate trials of standard drug treatments and as an adjunct to other treatments. Such restrictions seem very harsh compared to the risks involved and possible benefits. However, observe for the signs and symptoms of EMS (eg. muscle or joint pain, fever and rash). The doctor and patient must be registered with OPTICS (Optimax Information and Clinical Support), with progress reported at 3 and 6 months, then 6-monthly. Eosinophil levels should be measured at start of therapy, 2, 4, 6, and 12 months, then 6-monthly.

Prescribing points:

❖ Antidepressant dose is about 2–3g/d.
❖ Can be prescribed by GPs provided it is initiated or recommended by a hospital specialist (see *BNF* and the *SPC*).

Augmentation

A number of drugs with no intrinsic antidepressant activity may be highly effective as adjunctive therapies eg. **folic acid** (low folate has been associated with melancholic depression), **levothyroxine/thyroxine** (up to 0.1mg/d) and **liothyronine** 25–50mcg/d (subclinical hypothyroidism may predispose to depression), **modafinil** (recent papers) and **pindolol** (see adjuncts below).

Combinations/adjunct therapy

Antidepressants+antipsychotics

Low doses of risperidone added to an SSRI and olanzapine combined with fluoxetine have been shown to be useful for psychotic depression.

Benzodiazepines+SSRIs

A Cochrane review concludes that short-term benzodiazepines may lead to lower drop-outs from SSRIs by reducing initial anxiety and improving sleep.

Lithium+antidepressants

There have been reports of sertraline and fluoxetine improving resistant depression with lithium. In one study, where lithium or placebo was added to lofepramine or fluoxetine and where the TCA/SSRI had been ineffective by itself, 50% responded to lithium augmentation whereas only 25% responded to addition of placebo. Adequate lithium levels (0.4mmol/l or more) were necessary and often response indicates a previously undiagnosed bipolar mood disorder.

Lithium+tryptophan+tricyclic (eg. clomipramine) or an SSRI

This is variously known as the MRC Cocktail, 'Triple Therapy', Newcastle Cocktail and the London Cocktail:

Clomipramine (150+mg/d) or an SSRI
+ Tryptophan (2–4g/d)
+ Lithium (standard levels)

The combination appears effective in severe resistant depression but the combination should only be used with extreme care.

SSRI+pindolol

There is some evidence that the addition of pindolol to an SSRI (particularly paroxetine) increases the speed of onset of an SSRIs antidepressant action significantly. Usually, the pindolol can then be stopped gradually after about 6 weeks but may need to be continued for some time longer.

SSRIs+tricyclic

Several open studies have shown this to be a potentially useful combination in **resistant** depression but some SSRIs (fluoxetine, fluvoxamine and paroxetine) may **significantly raise tricyclic levels and toxic reactions have occurred**. Great care is needed with this combination.

Tricyclics+MAOIs

Although this combination is known to be effective in some resistant patients, the *BNF* rightly urges extreme caution as deaths have been reported and should only be initiated with care in an in-patient setting by skilled specialists with careful monitoring.

Venlafaxine+mirtazapine

Venlafaxine at high-dose may be potently effective for severe depression, but frequently produces side-effects such as sexual dysfunction and anxiety. Mirtazapine (15–30mg/d) blocks the serotonin receptors that cause these effects and may allow high dose venlafaxine to be tolerable without losing efficacy. There is very little safety data for this combination.

Unlicensed/further information

Bupropion (Zyban®)

Bupropion is licensed in USA for depression, but only for smoking cessation in UK. It appears as effective at doses of 100–300mg/d (optimum 250–300mg/d), with less sexual dysfunction and nausea, but a higher incidence of seizures at higher doses. It may cause less mood switching in bipolar disorder.

Carbamazepine (Tegretol®)

This is sometimes used by specialists as an adjunct/mood stabiliser, but the evidence for its efficacy as an antidepressant is poor.

Estradiol/estrogen

Lack of stimulation of estrogen receptors may cause depression and several trials have shown estradiol patches to produce a rapid, remarkable and sustained effect in **postnatal depression**.

Lamotrigine (Lamictal®)

Lamotrigine 50–200mg/d has been shown to be highly effective in bipolar depression and is licensed in USA for this, with a UK license expected for 2004.

Methylphenidate (Ritalin etc®)

A rapid onset of action may be useful in the short-term management of acute depression.

St. John's wort

Although not licensed in UK, St. John's wort is a widely used self-medication for depression. A meta-analysis of studies indicates that *Hypericum perforatum* extracts are significantly superior to placebo and as effective as standard antidepressants for **mild to moderate** depression, but data on moderate to severe depression is less convincing.

1.13 Dysthymia — see also depression (*1.12*)

Symptoms

Dysthymia is a low-grade chronic melancholic depression (often with anxiety) of insidious onset, chronic course (lasting at least two years) and high risk of relapse. The life-time prevalence rate may be around 3–6%, and higher in the elderly. It has been considered by some to be similar to depressive personality disorder or anxiety.

Role of drugs

It is clear that antidepressants are effective in dysthymia, with no proven significant differences between classes, and should form part of an overall treatment strategy including, eg. IPT and marital therapy. A greater sensitivity to side-effects has been noted in dysthymia, with tricyclics most likely to cause these. If one class of antidepressants does not work, switching to another may give a 40–60% chance of response. A low (10–20%) placebo response is seen.

Unlicensed/further information

Fluoxetine (Prozac®)

Fluoxetine 20mg/d may produce a significant improvement in dysthymic symptoms after eight weeks.

Mirtazapine (Zispin®)

Mirtazapine 15–45mg/d may be effective in 75% of patients with dysthymia.

Moclobemide (Manerix®)

Moclobemide (mean 675mg/d) has been shown to be significantly more effective for dysthymia than imipramine (mean 220mg/d) and placebo, with fewer side-effects.

Sertraline (Lustral®)

Two out-patient studies have shown sertraline (50–200mg/d) to be superior to placebo and as effective as imipramine (50–300mg/d), but better tolerated.

St John's wort

SJW seems effective in mild to moderate depression, including dysthymia.

Tricyclics

Amitriptyline has been studied over 6–12 weeks and found at doses of 150–300mg/d to be 2–3 times more effective than placebo.

Venlafaxine (Efexor®)

An open study showed venlafaxine (up to 225mg/d) effective in 10 of the 14 patients who completed a 9-week trial, although adverse effects were a problem in another trial.

1.14 Eating Disorders

1.14.1 Anorexia nervosa

Symptoms

The main diagnostic symptoms of anorexia nervosa are:

1. Amenorrhoea in females (absence of three consecutive menstrual cycles).
2. Refusal to maintain body weight over minimum normal for age and height (marked loss in body weight $>25\%$ may occur).
3. An intense/morbid fear of becoming obese.
4. Disturbance in body perception, eg. person feels fat even when emaciated.

Anorexia usually starts in the late teens, with distorted body image and relentless dieting. Anorexics may avoid carbohydrates, induce vomiting, abuse laxatives, take excess exercise, binge eat and suffer depression and social withdrawal.

Prevalence

It has been estimated that about 1% of secondary school girls have the full syndrome with 2–3% a partial syndrome. High rates occur in dancers, models and media-related people.

Role of drugs

Drugs are of little perceived value in anorexia and non-drug treatments are the first choice. Anorexia is not very responsive to drugs as such and none are licensed specifically for anorexia, although many have been tried.

Unlicensed/other information

Antipsychotics

Some improvement in body perceptions and improved insight has been reported with olanzapine.

Antidepressants

Antidepressants are used by specialists as a part of the maintenance therapy once stabilisation has occurred. Amitriptyline and clomipramine have been tried at relatively high doses, as have the SSRIs, especially citalopram and fluoxetine.

Nutritional feeding

Additional feeding may be needed in life-threatened cases although this will almost inevitably be in residential care or in conjunction with a hospital specialist.

Pre-menstrual treatments

Pre-menstrual exacerbations may occur and so treatment of these is a well-known technique.

1.14.2 Bulimia nervosa

Symptoms

The main diagnostic symptoms of bulimia nervosa are:

1. Recurrent binge eating (rapid and uncontrolled consumption of food in a discrete period of time).
2. An urge to overeat (including lack of control over eating during binges).
3. Regular self-induced vomiting/laxative abuse/strict dieting/fasting etc.
4. Persistent over-concern with body shape and weight.

There must be a minimum of two binge episodes per week for at least 3 months. Weight and menses can be normal.

There is a strong association between bulimia and major affective illness. There is often a very disturbed attitude to weight and shape.

Role of drugs

Drugs have a role as adjuncts in individualised programmes along with nutrition and psychotherapy. The greatest care is needed with side-effects, potential for overdose, notoriously low compliance rates and ensuring proper therapeutic trials (ie. adequate dose and duration). Antidepressants are superior to placebo (but with high drop-outs) but do not work as antidepressants. Adequate doses are needed, eg. at least 150mg/d equivalent of a tricyclic or higher dose SSRI for at least four weeks. Side-effects (especially anticholinergic) can be severe and result in non-compliance. Maintenance with drugs has a lower relapse rate if group psychotherapy is also included.

BNF listed

Fluoxetine (Prozac®)

60mg/d has been shown to have a significant effect on binge eating, purging, eating attitudes and food craving and attitude and behaviour. Fluoxetine seems not to work purely as an antidepressant as the improvement is independent of depression scores and uses higher doses, although any depression may also improve.

Prescribing points:

❖ It's long half-life may help with missed doses.
❖ Care will be needed building up to the therapeutic dose of 60mg/d.

Unlicensed/further information

Pre-menstrual treatments

Pre-menstrual exacerbations of bulimia can be a major feature of the condition and pyridoxine and progestogens in particular may help to minimise these.

SSRIs

Only fluoxetine is licensed, but other SSRIs, eg. fluvoxamine, have been used.

Tricyclics

Tricyclics such as amitriptyline, doxepin and imipramine have all been used but are of debatable potency, particularly compared to fluoxetine.

Others

Other drugs tried include ondansetron, sibutramine and topiramate.

1.15 Epilepsy

The annual incidence of epilepsy is 50–70 cases per 100 000 (excluding febrile seizures), with a lifetime prevalence of 2–5% of the population. Of those with epilepsy, 30–40% have seizures at an unacceptably high rate or have additional problems.

Role of drugs

Anticonvulsants are the first-line and single most important treatment for epilepsy, with a range of newer drugs adding to the options, although few have displaced the established agents. Generally, diagnosis and drug treatment should be guided by specialists.

Plasma level monitoring

For anticonvulsants this is *often overused* and should be restricted to:

1. Patients on **phenytoin.**
2. **Polypharmacy** (more than one drug) where dosage adjustment is necessary due to poor control or dose–related toxicity.
3. People with **learning disabilities**, where assessing toxicity is difficult.
4. Patients with **renal or hepatic** disease.
5. **Pregnant** women.
6. Where poor compliance/concordance is suspected.

BNF listed

Drugs licensed for monotherapy

Carbamazepine (Tegretol®)

A broad spectrum anticonvulsant widely used in the UK. It has been compared with valproate in complex partial and secondary generalised seizures in a large adult study, where they were of similar efficacy, but with carbamazepine better for complex partial seizures and with fewer long-term side-effects. The sustained release tablets can be used as a once a day dosage, along with careful monitoring if seizures continue (although lower trough concentrations mean some patients may need twice daily dosing).

Prescribing points:

❖ Twice daily dosage is appropriate, with even once a day seemingly effective.
❖ Use of the sustained release tablet may reduce side-effects and improve control, although overall doses may need to be adjusted slightly upwards.
❖ Don't withdraw suddenly.

Lamotrigine (Lamictal®)

An anticonvulsant licensed as mono-therapy and add-on therapy for a variety of seizures such as complex partial, secondary GTC and primary GTC seizures (may be very useful in the latter) and child-hood (2–12 yrs) epilepsy. About 30% of epileptics treated with lamotrigine have a 50% or more reduction in seizures. Mild CNS side-effects as per other anticonvul-sants have been reported, although these are of similar incidence to placebo. Lamo-trigine is the only anticonvulsant with an effect on the excitatory system and it may reduce neuronal death.

Prescribing points:

❖ Starter packs are available for con-current valproate and non-valproate initiation.
❖ The 2–5% risk of rash can be minimised by starting at 25mg/d for 2/52, then increasing gradually (see *BNF*/SPC).

Oxcarbazepine (Trileptal®)

This is related to carbamazepine, but may be better tolerated and useful in people not able to take carbamazepine, or where interactions are relevant.

Prescribing point:

❖ If switching, use 1mg carbamazepine to 1.5mg oxcarbazepine (or 1:1 for doses of carbamazepine > 800mg/d).
❖ Start at 150mg/d, increasing by 150mg/d on alternate days to 900–1200mg/d.

Phenytoin (Epanutin®)

A broad spectrum anticonvulsant still widely used in the UK. Phenytoin is not now routinely recommended for use in children as it can cause permanent learning difficulties.

Prescribing points:

❖ Plasma level monitoring is essential, especially as due to non-linear kinetics, sometimes even small dose increases can cause dramatic plasma level rises.
❖ Best to keep to the same preparation.

Valproate salts (sodium valproate, valproic acid) (Epilim®, Epilim Chrono®, Convulex® etc)

An invaluable drug for primary generalised epilepsy, absence seizures and GTC fits in children and myoclonic seizures. Mono-therapy in partial seizures is less well established. There is little correlation between blood levels and therapeutic effect and so **routine** blood level monitoring is of **limited use** except in suspected toxicity. Serious toxicity is rare

Seizures Classification

Type	International classification	Other names	Manifestation	Age of onset	Duration	Recovery
Generalised	Generalised Tonic-clonic (GTC)	Major motor	Sudden loss of consciousness, intense (tonic) muscle spasms, then intermittent seizures. Also flushing and incontinence	Any	1–5 mins	Varies, up to 1 hr
	Absence (typical or atypical)	Petit mal	Sudden cessation of activity. Eyes rolling. Unresponsive. Immediate recovery, no awareness	3–15 years limit	Secs	Immediate
	Myoclonic or partial seizures with motor symptoms	Minor motor Infantile spasms Myoclonic jerks	Sudden jerk of limbs. May be followed by GTC or atonic seizures	During 1st yr of life (3–9 mo)	Secs to mins	Varies
	Atonic	Akinetic attacks 'Drop attacks'	Sudden loss of consciousness	2+ years (3–7 most common)	Mins	Varies

Seizures Classification (Continued)

Type	International classification	Other names	Manifestation	Age of onset	Duration	Recovery
Focal	Simple partial (partial seizures with simple symptomatology)	Focal (localised) Simple motor sensory	Spasmodic convulsions. Hallucinations of flashing lights, numbness, parasthesia dysphagia and visual phenomena. No loss of consciousness	Any	Mins	Varies
Partial	Complex partial (partial seizures with complex symptomatology)	Temporal lobe Psychomotor	Unconscious behaviour (chewing, lip smacking, walking), acts of violence, hallucinations of taste, smell or hearing. Unreal feelings. Memory disturbance. Time disturbance. Fear, anxiety, distorted perception. Impaired consciousness	Adolescent and adult	Mins to hours	Immediate no awareness

Generalised epilepsy usually has genetic influence (eg. low threshold). Focal and partial epilepsy is probably due to a damaged brain area. For further information on the International Classification of Epileptic Seizures (ICES), refer to *Epilepsia* 1981, **22**, 489–501

Therapeutic drug monitoring

Drug	Plasma levels 'Optimum'	Plasma levels 'Toxic'	Half-life	Peak plasma concs	Sample time	Sample frequency	Other checks	Comments
Phenytoin *TDM essential	40–80micromol/L (10–20mg/l) upper end for partial seizures < 20mmol unlikely to work	> 80micromol/L	20–40 hrs (up to 140 at higher levels)	3–12 hrs dependent on total daily dose	Aim for trough unless confirmation of toxicity required	Every 3–12 months for well stabilised patients	Folate, calcium (both with phenytoin)	Missed doses, changes in absorption, tablet or capsule brand can all markedly affect plasma concentrations
Phenobarbital *TDM useful	60–180micromol/L (10–30mg/l) dependent upon response	> 180micromol/L ↑ chance of stupor	50–160 hrs, with age	2–6 hrs	Long $1\frac{1}{2}$, so time not vital. Best to be consistent each time	Every 6/12 for well stabilised patients	Folate 6/12	Blood levels can also be useful as a measure of long-term compliance
Carbamazepine *TDM fairly useful	20–50micromol/L (4–12mg/l) 20–40 for GTC+polytherapy, 30–50 for monotherapy	> 50micromol/L	5/38 hrs	2.5–24 hrs (mean 6H) – less if taken with food	Aim for trough level unless side-effects suspected	Every six months for well stabilised patients	FBC in initial stages of treatment. Thyroid?	Plasma levels only of real use for anticonvulsant action. Are of limited use (eg. toxic) in affective disorders
Sodium valproate/valproic acid *TDM unproven	300–700mmol/l (50–100meq/ml proposed care in elderly	> 700mmol/L – but few side-effects or correlation proved	6–20 hrs. longer in liver disease+ polytherapy	E/C tabs 2–4 hrs. Sol. Tabs+syrup; 1–3 hrs	Short $t\frac{1}{2}$ so need great care interpreting. Only serial levels are accurate	On request	LFT for 6/12 +Plasma amylase if in abdominal pain	Levels may be of some use where control is poor or if toxicity suspected. Hepatotoxicity may be dose related

and careful supervision initially will guard against major problems, eg. liver toxicity.

Prescribing points:

❖ Twice daily dosage is possible, especially with sustained release preparations.

❖ Plasma level monitoring is of very limited use.

❖ Measure LFTs early in therapy.

Topiramate (Topamax®)

Topiramate is now licensed as monotherapy for partial seizures, with or without secondary generalisation. No plasma levels are required and twice daily dosing is appropriate. There is a multiple mode of action, which may explain its effect in resistant epilepsy and severity of side-effects, eg. ataxia, dizziness and somnolence. These can be minimised by slower dose titration.

❖ Monotherapy target dose is 100mg/d, optimum being 200–400mg/d in a few.

❖ Start at 25mg/d for the first week, then increase by 25–50mg/d every 1–2 weeks.

❖ BD dosage recommended.

Benzodiazepines

Clobazam (Frisium®)

Use as an adjunct therapy is well known but tolerance can develop and so low doses (eg. 10–20mg/d) and drug-free periods may minimise this.

Prescribing point:

❖ Low or intermittent dosage can help maintain response.

Clonazepam (Rivotril®)

A benzodiazepine with marked anticonvulsant properties with usefulness limited by tolerance and sedation.

Diazepam

This is occasionally useful orally as an adjunct and in short-term therapy, although studies on diazepam are limited. Use in status epilepticus is well established (see *1.15.2*).

Adjunct therapy/others

A drug licensed for add-on therapy may be used as monotherapy as long as it was started as adjunct therapy.

Acetazolamide (Diamox®)

A potent anticonvulsant, used rarely for absence seizures, premenstrual epilepsy, in children and as an adjunct to carbamazepine in refractory epilepsy.

Prescribing point:

❖ Rapid tolerance and long-term side-effects render it of limited use.

Ethosuximide (Zarontin®)

A poorly studied drug useful in absence seizures but with a high side-effect profile, eg. gastric upset at higher dose.

Prescribing point:

❖ Has largely now been replaced by sodium valproate so reserve for valproate-resistant cases.

Gabapentin (Neurontin®)

An anticonvulsant licensed as add-on therapy in drug-resistant partial seizures, with a reduction of 50% or more of partial seizures in 25–33% patients. Most patients need doses of 1200mg/d or more and there is a strong dose:response relationship. It may act by enhancing GABA (the brains major inhibitory neuro-transmitter) turnover but this is not established. It has a low order of toxicity, uncomplicated kinetics, no clinically important interactions and blood levels are not necessary.

Prescribing points:

❖ A TDS dosage is recommended with no more than 12 hrs between doses.

❖ 1200mg/d is probably the minimum effective maintenance dose.

Levetiracetam (Keppra®)

This is licensed as add-on for partial seizures, with or without secondary generalisation. A BD dose is necessary.

Prescribing points:

❖ Initial somnolence can be minimised by starting at a lower dose.

Piracetam (Nootropil®)

Piracetam is a GABA derivative licensed in the UK for myoclonus, especially of cortical origin and up to 70% may become seizure-free if they can swallow enough of it.

Tiagabine (Gabitril®)

This is licensed as add-on for partial seizures, with or without secondary generalisation. It has a short half-life and so a BD to QDS dose is necessary.

Vigabatrin (Sabril®)

Vigabatrin is licensed as adjunctive treatment in resistant epilepsies, particularly complex partial seizures.

Prescribing points:

❖ Due to irreversible ocular changes eg. loss of field and contrast, use only where there is no alternative.

❖ Do baseline and six-monthly peripheral field examination.

Barbiturates

Phenobarbital (phenobarbitone)

A long-established drug useful in GTC and other seizures. Concerns about cognitive/psychomotor impairment and dependence have limited its use.

Prescribing point:

❖ Plasma level monitoring useful on a regular basis.

Primidone (Mysotine®)

Metabolised mainly to phenobarbital, primidone should be available in the UK until 2006.

Unlicensed/further information

Clomethiazole (Heminevrin®)

Use in refractory cases, particularly children, can be successful if used by specialists.

1.15.1. Anticonvulsant withdrawal

All anticonvulsants have side-effects (eg. cognitive impairment, disturbed behaviour

etc), especially when taken for long periods and even when therapeutic ranges are adhered to. They should be discontinued when no longer needed. About 70% of patients enter a prolonged remission. Relapse rates for children are about 20%, adults 45–50%. Little advice is usually given to adults on anticonvulsant discontinuation and so many stop on their own initiative. Withdrawal of anticonvulsants can also lead to emergence of seizures and psychiatric morbidity, particularly depression and anxiety. A concentration of fits during or in the first few months after withdrawal suggests that at least some are provoked by drug withdrawal. Other withdrawal effects such as anxiety, agitation and insomnia are a problem but only occur with the barbiturates and benzodiazepines. Unless withdrawing due to acute adverse effects, there is more to lose by discontinuing too fast so follow these principles:

● Each decrement should be undertaken at intervals of no less than five or six weeks

● Reduce stepwise over up to a year, with slower dose decrements during the final stages

● Examples include **carbamazepine** (200mg decrements to 1000mg/d, 100mg decrements to 100mg/d, 50mg, zero), **diazepam** (10mg decrements to 30mg/d, 5mg decrements to 15mg/d, 2mg decrements to zero), **phenobarbital** (60mg decrements to 180mg/d, 30mg decrements to 30mg/d, 15mg, 7.5mg, zero), **phenytoin** (20micromol/l stages to 40micromol/l [minimum step 50mg/d], 10micromol/l stages to 10micromol/l, 5micromol/l, zero), **primidone** (250mg decrements to 750mg/d, 125mg decrements to 125mg/d, then 62.5mg, 25mg, 12.5mg, zero) and **valproate** (500mg decrements to 1000mg/d, 100mg decrements to zero).

Favourable withdrawal factors:

● short duration of epilepsy
● no cerebral disorder

- normal EEG (or at least no gross abnormalities), persistently so before and after discontinuation
- few seizures documented
- history of non-compliance without relapse (in which case withdrawal should be encouraged)
- medication below therapeutic levels at time of discontinuation
- more than two years since last seizure, especially in children
- primary generalised seizures
- childhood onset (after the age of one).

Main risk factors for seizure recurrence on withdrawal

- longer duration of treatment or illness, eg. more than 30 months
- number of seizures before fits controlled, eg. more than 100 before control is achieved
- type of seizure, eg. complex partial, tonic-clonic (grand mal) or combinations of seizures are more likely to relapse than simple partial seizures
- number of drugs/time required for seizure control, eg. if fits are controlled by the drug of first choice, relapse rates are much less than where more drugs have to be tried or where polypharmacy is needed
- abnormal EEG, eg. 'Class 4' is highest risk
- adult/late onset
- underlying cerebral disorder (eg. mental retardation)
- withdrawal in less than 6 months.

1.15.2. Status epilepticus

Status epilepticus is where multiple seizures occur without complete recovery between them. To prevent permanent brain damage, first line therapy must be to use anticonvulsants (eg. rectal diazepam) and support with oxygen and a glucose drip if possible. The American Epilepsy Foundation has produced a very useful statement, review and guidelines for the treatment of status epilepticus.

BNF listed

Amylobarbital

Specialist use only, as this can be a highly toxic drug by injection.

Clonazepam (Rivotril®)

Slow IV injection (possibly followed by an infusion) may be useful in refractory cases not responsive to diazepam, if used with care in specialist centres.

Diazepam (inc Stesolid®, Rec-tubes®)

0.15–0.25mg/kg (ie. 10–30mg) given as a slow IV injection over 5 minutes or rectal administration (eg. rectal tubes) is first choice treatment. Note that injection rates above 5mg/minute IV are associated with respiratory depression.

Prescribing points:

❖ Use as first choice therapy.
❖ Rectal absorption is rapid, second only to IV absorption, and peaks at about 10 minutes.

Fosphenytoin (Pro-Epanutin®)

A pro-drug converted to phenytoin, it is better tolerated than phenytoin by IM injection and can be given more rapidly.

Prescribing points:

❖ It takes about 15 minutes to be converted to phenytoin so is less useful as sole initial treatment.

Lorazepam (Ativan®)

Lorazepam injection is taking over from diazepam injection as first choice in some areas, due to a longer duration of action (about 2 hours), shorter elimination half-life, no active metabolites and possibly less respiratory depression.

Phenytoin (Epanutin®)

Phenytoin injection is second choice therapy in the UK after the benzodiazepines, used as 10–15mg/kg intravenously over 15 minutes (not exceeding 50mg/minute) in 0.9% saline for recurrent or persistent seizures.

Prescribing points:

❖ Not effective intramuscularly.

❖ Extreme care needed due to the risk of hypotension and cardiac dysrhythmias.

1.16 Insomnia

Insomnia is usually a symptom of an illness, not an illness itself, and any underlying problems (eg. environment, stress, pain etc) should always be treated first or as well. The principles of sleep hygiene should be discussed and any corrected before prescribing hypnotics. Avoiding psychological dependence is important.

Principles of sleep hygiene

Before prescribing a hypnotic, it is important to ensure "sleep hygiene" is good:
1. Avoid excessive use of caffeine, alcohol or nicotine, especially within 3–4 hours of going to bed. A hot milky (decaffeinated) drink at bedtime may promote sleep.
2. Do not stay in bed for more than about an hour if not asleep, but watching TV can have an alerting effect.
3. Avoid daytime naps or periods of inactivity.
4. A warm bath or exercise a few hours before bedtime may promote sleep.
5. Avoid engaging in strenuous exercise or mental activity near bedtime (except sex, which aids sleep in men, apparently).
6. Make sure that the bed and bedroom is comfortable and avoid extremes of noise, temperature and humidity.
7. Establish a regular routine of a time to go to bed. The most vital thing is to get up at the same time each morning, *regardless* of the time spent asleep.
8. Carbohydrate helps sleep, but not a big meal within 2 hours of going to bed. Sugar and some vitamin supplements may inhibit sleep.

Role of drugs

Assuming sleep hygiene is good, any hypnotics should always be used on an 'as needed' basis (although this is easier said than done) as tolerance may develop to the sedative effects within 2–3 weeks

(especially with the benzodiazepines). Short-term use for short-term reasons is usually without problem and can be very useful and comforting for the patient. Longer-term use needs the risk:benefit analysis to be considered extremely carefully.

Predicting hypnotic dependence risk

Factor	Score
Benzodiazepine hypnotic used	3
Dose higher than *BNF* mean	2
Duration of treatment > 3 months	2
Dependent personality	2
Short elimination half-life drug	2
Tolerance or dose escalation	2
Total	
Score:	
No dependence, abrupt withdrawal possible = 0	
Some dependence risk, withdraw over two weeks recommended = 1–4	
Strong dependence risk, withdraw over 4–12 weeks = 5–8	
High risk of dependence, withdraw gradually plus support programme = 8–13	

If considering withdrawing a hypnotic, work out the risk factor score for that patient, then check for guidance on withdrawal.

BNF listed

Benzodiazepines

A meta-analysis of major benzodiazepine studies shows a significant effect on improved sleep latency and duration but an increased risk of RTAs and fractures, especially if combined with alcohol.

Loprazolam

An intermediate-acting benzodiazepine, with a half-life of 7–15 hours.

Lormetazepam

An intermediate-acting benzodiazepine marketed as a hypnotic.

Nitrazepam

A longer-acting benzodiazepine (half-life of 18–36 hours) similar to diazepam which has active metabolites and was promoted as a long-acting hypnotic.

Prescribing point:

❖ Stable plasma levels can be attained in 5 days and so use should be avoided in the elderly.

Temazepam

A shorter-acting benzodiazepine (half-life 5–11 hours, which may be longer in the elderly) which was the most widely prescribed hypnotic in the UK. It has an abuse potential.

Prescribing points:

❖ Now a widely misused drug.
❖ Now a controlled drug.

The Z hypnotics

Zaleplon (Sonata®)

Zaleplon hits benzodiazepine-1 receptors and has a very rapid peak (1 hour) and short half-life (1 hour). It can even be taken as late as 3 hours before someone would expect to get up as there are fewer hangover effects than there would be from not having slept.

Prescribing point:

❖ Should be taken half an hour before wishing to go to sleep, because if you're still awake after an hour it won't help much.
❖ No rebound insomnia reported.

Zolpidem (Stilnoct®)

Zolpidem, apart from having one of the worst trade names ever devised, also hits benzodiazepine-1 receptors. It is indicated for the short–term treatment of insomnia. It has a rapid onset (15 minutes) and a short (4 hrs) duration of action, very low residual psychomotor effects and seems to have a low incidence of side-effects. Anecdotally it helps with jet-lag by forcing sleep when you need it.

Zopiclone (Zimovane®)

This non-benzodiazepine hypnotic has a low incidence of side-effects and hangover effect than benzodiazepines. It acts on a binding site at, or close to, the benzodiazepine receptor complex. Treatment duration is recommended for up to 28 days, but is frequently used for longer.

❖ Withdrawal effects and abuse have been reported occasionally.
❖ There may be an increased risk of RTAs especially if combined with alcohol.
❖ An initial metallic taste in the mouth may be unpleasant.

Others

Chloral betaine (Welldorm®)

An hypnotic and sedative with properties similar to the barbiturates. Relatively safe in the elderly as the half-life is not significantly lengthened. An abuse potential exists.

Clomethiazole (Heminevrin®)

This is a sedative-hypnotic with anticonvulsant properties. Its onset of action is rapid and not prolonged, even in the elderly, although they may be more sensitive to it. Dependence and abuse has been reported but is not considered too important if the patient is not dependence prone.

Prescribing points:

❖ Useful in the elderly.
❖ Unsafe in overdose.

Promethazine/ other antihistamines

These may be useful occasionally as drugs with a low abuse potential, although abuse of diphenhydramine has been reported. Promethazine has a relatively long half-life but has been linked with cognitive decline in the elderly.

Unlicensed/further information

Alcohol

Alcohol causes sedation, increases slow wave sleep and reduces and disrupts REM sleep, the diuretic effect is counter-productive and overdose is serious. Rebound arousal can occur with higher doses when blood concentrations reach zero, leading to awakening. Alcohol is not recommended for routine medical use although it is used widely as self-medication and, unlike chloral, is available in a number of palatable formulations (eg. Adnams, Woodfordes).

Melatonin

Melatonin may improve sleep patterns in people with disturbed circadian rhythms although the published data is patchy.

Other sedative drugs at night

Other sedative drugs the patient may already be taking, especially phenothia-zines and antidepressants such as mirta-zapine, may be prescribed as a single dose at night. In longer-term therapy most can be given this way. It is also important to avoid the use of 'stimu-lating' drugs at night, eg. anticholinergics such as procyclidine, MAOIs etc. Tricyclics are toxic in overdose and may disrupt REM sleep.

Phenothiazines

Promazine at 25–100mg has been used and can be fairly sedative with a low abuse potential, but risks the side-effects of the phenothiazines.

1.17   Mania and hypomania — see also bipolar disorder (*1.9*) and rapid-cycling bipolar disorder (*1.26*)

Symptoms

Hypomania is the more common and milder form of mania where there is an abnormal elation of mood alternating with irritability, great energy, inability to concentrate, flight of ideas (rapid changing of the subject with some connections), insomnia etc. Obsessive preoccupation with some idea, activity or desire may occur. The main presenting symptoms are thus an euphoric and labile mood (irritable, angry, grandiose), bright or untidy appear-ance, low sleep requirement, increased drive and energy, reduced insight, pres-sure of speech, flight of ideas, expansive thought, and an overactive and intrusive manner.

Role of drugs

Hypomania or mania represents a parti-cular moment/part of a bipolar (or rarely unipolar) illness. (See bipolar mood disorder *1.9* for maintenance strategies.) Hypomania requires specific long-term treatment for the bipolar component (ie. lithium, valproate etc) and non-specific shorter-term treatments (eg. antipsycho-tics/neuroleptics, benzodiazepines) for insomnia, agitation, hyperactivity etc. One study showed that a night of sleep depriva-tion is likely to escalate any manic patient to a higher degree of mania and so hypnotic/sedative use can be considered appropriate, or even essential.

In the longer-term, relapse can be minimised or prevented by prophylactic therapy, eg. lithium or valproate and so the patient must be encouraged to continue these drugs long-term. Any co-morbid substance misuse should be tackled at the same time as recovery from mania is poorer with substance misuse. The main treatment goals should be to discontinue any manicogenic agents (eg. antidepressants — see *5.7* for list), start non-specific calming measures (eg. benzo-diazepines, antipsychotics) and consider mood stabilisers, especially valproate.

BNF listed

Antipsychotics/neuroleptics (see also olanzapine below)

Antipsychotics are frequently used to help long-term control of recurrent hypomania, as well as use in the acute situation. Evidence that hypomania is a hyper-dopaminergic state (and treatable long-term with dopamine blocking drugs) is controversial with some evidence that many antipsychotics have little effect on relapse rates other than by behavioural

control. Although technically not licensed (although it was specifically licensed in USA in 2003), **risperidone** has also been studied and shown effective as an adjunct in mania, as has **quetiapine**.
Prescribing points:

❖ May not be needed long-term.

Carbamazepine (Tegretol®)

Carbamazepine is an effective alternative to lithium in the maintenance therapy of bipolar (manic-depressive) disorders. See main entry under bipolar disorder (*1.9*).

Lithium (Camcolit®, Priadel® etc)

Lithium remains the treatment of choice for maintenance or prophylactic therapy of bipolar (manic-depressive) conditions and can assist in acute treatment. Lithium is effective in acute mania/hypomania and serum levels of 0.8–1.2mmol/l may be necessary in the short-term for a therapeutic effect and reduced once mood is normalised. There may be a reduced antimanic response to lithium if the person has had 12 previous manic episodes. See main entry under bipolar disorder (*1.9*).
Prescribing points:

❖ Short-term use of lithium has particular problems (see bipolar) and so long-term treatment should usually be implemented.

Olanzapine (Zyprexa®)

Olanzapine is licensed for moderate to severe manic episodes. Several studies have shown a superior response to placebo in mania, starting at 15mg/d. Long-term side-effects such as weight gain need to be considered if prescribing is continued into the maintenance phase.
Prescribing points:

❖ The IM injection might be useful.

Quetiapine (Seroquel®)

Quetiapine is now licensed for mono-therapy (and combined with mood stabilisers) in mania. The recommended dose of 600mg/d can be reached over 5 days (in-patients) or longer in out-patients, due to the risk of postural hypotension.

Valproate semisodlum (Depakote®)

Valproate semisodium is now an established anti-manic agent, being at least as effective as antipsychotics (but with many less side-effects) in the acute phase. It may be a highly effective drug in lithium and carbamazepine non-responders, acute mania, hypomania and prophylaxis. The doses used should be around 20mg/kg/d (1000–2000mg/d) initially, then reduced for longer-term maintenance. The rapid and relatively well-tolerated antimanic effect often allows transition to maintenance without the need for neuroleptics.
Prescribing points:

❖ Expensive but better tolerated at high doses than sodium valproate, although there is probably little advantage of Depakote for maintenance.
❖ Depakote® also has an SPC with clear dosage guidance eg. with loading dose.

Combinations

Lithium+carbamazepine

This combination is used by specialists in resistant cases. Occasional neurotoxic reactions have been reported, but mostly these have occurred in patients with pre-existing brain damage. An additive anti-thyroid effect can occur, lowering T4 and free T4 levels.

Unlicensed/further information

Benzodiazepines

Short-term use of medium or high doses of benzodiazepines can be used as adjuvants to other therapies in acute phases of hypo-mania to control acute symptoms (see 'Psychiatric emergency' — *1.24*). In the long-term, they can (rarely) have disinhibiting effects.

Useless

Antidepressants

Antidepressants can exacerbate mania and lead to rapid-cycling, although there is still some (inappropriate) use in mania.

1.18 Movement disorders (drug–induced)

1.18.1 Akathisia

Akathisia is a sadly under-rated side-effect of the neuroleptics/antipsychotics, eg. it occurs in up to 36% of schizophrenics and mainly presents as an uncontrolled physical restlessness with an unpleasant feeling of being unable to keep still, rocking whilst standing and crossing and uncrossing legs whilst sitting. If confused with agitation it can easily result in an inappropriate increase in antipsychotic dose. Switching antipsychotics to one less likely to cause akathisia eg. an atypical, is the best option if possible.

Unlicensed/further information

Anticholinergics (antimuscarinics)

Drugs such as procyclidine may be useful if the akathisia forms part of a Parkinsonian side-effect profile, where one drug will treat both conditions.

Beta-blockers

Propranolol (30–80mg/d) can produce a dramatic and persistent improvement, particularly if the akathisia is not connected with Parkinsonian side-effects. It may take up to three months to act in chronic cases.

Clonazepam (Rivotril®)

0.5–3mg/d has been used for neuroleptic-induced akathisia.

Cyproheptadine (Periactin®)

A recent trial has shown 16mg/d could be rapidly effective.

1.18.2 Parkinsonian or extra-pyramidal side-effects

Drug-induced extra-pyramidal or Parkinsonian side-effects include akinesia, rigidity and coarse tremor, but not pill-rolling. It can take a few weeks to occur and may remit spontaneously. Antipsychotics are the most common cause of EPSE (see *5.8.1* for a full list).

BNF listed

Anticholinergics (antimuscarinics)

There is little, if any, clinically significant difference between the agents in this group. With antipsychotic-induced side-effects, few patients need them regularly long-term, rather as 'when required' (eg. often only for a couple of days after a depot to match peak blood levels). Indeed, most patients may be able to continue without them. They are probably best prescribed only for overt symptoms and then discontinued gradually after three months, reinstated only if symptoms reappear. A gradual attempt should be made to reduce the dose or discontinue the drug every three to six months. They may be detrimental to positive symptoms of schizophrenia in the acute phase, but probably not during stable phases. However, if patients desire them, anticholinergics may facilitate compliance with antipsychotics, although ensuring doses do not escalate is important.

There is an abuse potential, possibly due to an alleged euphorant effect or as an attempt to self-medicate. Anticholinergics may exacerbate tardive dyskinesia and adversely effect memory (especially visual). The drugs in this class are:

Benzhexol/trihexyphenidyl (Artane®)

This anticholinergic also has some smooth muscle relaxing effects. Abuse has been reported with doses of up to 100mg/d taken.

Prescribing points:

❖ Avoid night doses, which can cause insomnia.
❖ Try dose reduction every three months.

Procyclidine (Kemadrin®)

An anticholinergic similar to benzhexol/trihexyphenidyl. Abuse has been reported but another study was unable to show a euphorant effect.

Prescribing points:

❖ Avoid night doses, which can cause insomnia.

❖ Try dose reduction every three months.

Orphenadrine (Disipal®)

Another similar anticholinergic, but reports of higher death rates than expected in overdose should limit use.

1.18.3 Tardive dyskinesia

Symptoms

Tardive dyskinesia is generally seen as repetitive, involuntary and purposeless movements of the tongue, neck and jaw. TD can be consciously suppressed by the sufferer for limited periods but reappears when distracted and worsens during periods of stress. There is a clear association between antipsychotic drug use and TD, but there is now evidence that non-drug treated schizophrenic populations have virtually the same incidence of TD as treated populations, suggesting TD to be a late-onset symptom of schizophrenia rather than a drug side-effect as such. The incidence may be up to 30–40% in long-term schizophrenics, although figures of 10–20% seem more likely.

Treatment strategies

1. Consider switching to another antipsychotic eg. quetiaplne, olanzapine, risperidone or clozapine.
2. Reduce dose or withdraw the antipsychotic. Beware of relapse and, since TD is not necessarily progressive or drug-related, it may be possible to reintroduce the antipsychotic again in the short-term or at reduced doses. Drug 'holidays' seem detrimental.
3. Withdraw or reduce any anticholinergic drugs if possible—these can exacerbate TD, although are not a risk factor as such.
4. Keep drug use down in the long-term to minimum effective doses.
5. Do not increase the dose or add another antipsychotic—this does not work in the long-term as it merely blocks any excess dopamine activity initially. It may, however, be useful in the short-term and can be useful for that, eg. special occasions.
6. Adjuncts such as tetrabenazine (licensed), benzodiazepines, buspirone and calcium-channel blockers have been used.

BNF Listed

Tetrabenazine (Xenazine®)

Tetrabenazine is licensed in UK for TD. Since TD is often a fluctuating condition, short-term and rescue/special occasion use is appropriate.

Prescribing points:

❖ Start at 12.5mg/d, titrating up to 25–75mg/d.

Unlicensed/further information

Calcium-channel blockers

Diltiazem, verapamil and nifedipine (probably most effective) have been used for TD in the elderly. The mechanism of action is unknown and use by non-specialists can not be recommended.

Clonazepam (Rivotril®)

This specific GABA agonist may decrease TD symptoms by up to 35%, although a Cochrane review was unimpressed with the evidence.

Sodium valproate/valproic acid (Epilim® etc)

There is growing evidence that valproate is useful in TD but use by non-specialists can not be recommended.

Vitamin E/other vitamins

Vitamin E may be useful soon after the onset of tardive dyskinesia, although the majority of studies have shown it ineffective. Pyridoxine has also been used as a preventative measure.

1.19   Narcolepsy

Narcolepsy is a distinct neurological disorder of excessive sleepiness and abnormalities in REM sleep, with a strong genetic linkage. The incidence ranges from 1 in 1000 to 10,000 in Europe, and being rare is an often-missed diagnosis. About 70% of sufferers also experience cataplexy (sudden temporary episodes of paralysis with loss of muscle tone) during the day.

Role of drugs

Modafinil, stimulants and/or tricyclics have some effect in a few people and the risk of side-effects is usually outweighed by the risk of vehicle and workplace accidents.

BNF listed

Dexamfetamine (Dexadrine®) CD

5–50mg/d can be a highly effective treatment. Although not immune from problems of chronic stimulant ingestion, many can take dexamfetamine for decades without apparent adverse consequences.

Prescribing point:

❖ If tolerance develops, drug holidays may be necessary eg. one week off.

Modafinil (Provigil®)

Modafinil is not a stimulant but promotes wakefulness in patients with excessive daytime sleepiness associated with narcolepsy. It has a low abuse potential, and no tolerance, rebound or withdrawal syndromes.

Prescribing points:

❖ 200–400mg/d appears optimum with 600mg/d the maximum.

❖ Although not a stimulant, it is a banned substance by the Olympic and Athletics bodies.

Unlicensed/further information

Antidepressants

Imipramine can be effective in narcolepsy, particularly in stimulant-resistant or intolerant patients. Clomipramine at 10–25mg/d has been considered effective and may have the most specific effect on cataplexy, but side-effects and rebound are a major constraint. Fluoxetine may be as effective, with fewer side-effects.

Methylphenidate (Ritalin®) CD

2.5–5mg bd (up to 10–60mg/d) has been used (see also dexamfetamine above) and may improve performance and waking. Tolerance can be a problem, with drug holidays helpful.

1.20   Neuroleptic malignant syndrome (NMS)

Symptoms

NMS is a rare but potentially fatal idiosyncratic dose-independent adverse drug reaction resulting in a sudden loss in control of body temperature during drug therapy. Symptoms include hyperthermia or fever, muscle rigidity and autonomic instability, with labile blood pressure, raised temperature and severe Parkinsonian symptoms being early indicators. NMS can be fatal in a short time (eg. 24–72 hrs) due to renal and respiratory failure. The incidence is unknown but it may possibly occur in around 0.2–1% of all patients given neuroleptics. Features progress over 24 to 72 hours and subside over 5–10 days (oral drugs) or 10–21 days (depots). Death rates are reported to be 14% for oral and 38% for depot antipsychotics. Anaesthetists see a similar syndrome as malignant hyperthermia.

Causes

NMS is mostly precipitated by the use of therapeutic or high doses of neuroleptics, particularly phenothiazines and high potency drugs. It usually occurs within the first 4–11 days after initiation, or alteration of dosages, of antipsychotic/neuroleptic therapy. See *5.9* for a full list of drug-related causes.

Rechallenge with neuroleptics may show a high recurrence rate so if neuroleptics are needed again, seek expert advice. Depot injections are contraindicated.

Risk factors include a previous history, agitation or overactivity, dehydration and rapid changing of doses of higher-potency antipsychotics.

Role of drugs

NMS is potentially life-threatening and treatment should be immediate and intensive. The main management strategies are to **stop all drugs immediately**, use symptomatic measures to **keep the body temperature down**, eg. using ice packs and **refer to the nearest casualty or intensive care unit as quickly as possible**.

The main treatment strategies are:

1. Immediate withdrawal of drugs, particularly antipsychotics, lithium and antidepressants.

2. Correct any dehydration and hyperpyrexia, eg. using ice packs, rehydration and sedation with benzodiazepines if necessary.
3. Measure WCC, U&E, LFT and CK.
4. Drug treatment of acute symptoms is usually essential. Dantrolene or bromocriptine are probably most useful so refer to your local A&E immediately.

BNF mentioned

The *BNF* mentions **bromocriptine** and **dantrolene** as drugs that have been tried in NMS (as has amantadine). The first two are hospital specialist use only. IV dantrolene (a directly-acting skeletal muscle relaxant licensed for malignant hyperthermia) has been used successfully by specialists and is probably the treatment of choice. It reduces body temperature in 2–24 hours but muscular rigidity may take 4–16 days and has been shown to reduce the duration and mortality of NMS.

Unlicensed/further information

Lorazepam

IV lorazepam has been used by specialists as a second line treatment if dantrolene/bromocriptine fail.

1.21 Obsessive-compulsive disorder (OCD)

Symptoms

A person with OCD has a striking lack of adaptability to new situations, rigid views, an inflexible approach to problems, lacks imagination, becomes immersed in trivial detail, lacks a sense of humour and enjoyment, may become indecisive, judgemental and moralistic and shows little emotion, but with underlying feelings of anger and resentment.

Role of drugs

Several major meta-analyses of the good trials show clomipramine and the SSRIs as a class to be clearly superior to placebo in obsessive-compulsive symptoms. Dosage needs to be high (eg. 250–300mg/d clomipramine or 60–80mg/d fluoxetine) and response is slow (allow 2–3 months for full

response). An element of depression does not seem necessary for improvement in obsessive-compulsive symptoms with antidepressants. Other therapies, eg. psychotherapy also help. Relapse is common on drug discontinuation.

BNF listed

Clomipramine (Anafranil®)

This tricyclic is the most widely used for OCD. Of the 11 double-blind, cross-over studies published, 10 show clomipramine clearly superior to placebo.

Prescribing points:

❖ Doses of 250–300mg/d may be needed for full effect, but need specialist care, eg. plasma level monitoring to avoid cardiotoxicity.

Fluoxetine (Prozac®)

Several studies have shown a positive effect at 60–80mg/d, but may take 8 weeks to reach an optimal effect.

Fluvoxamine (Faverin®)

A clinical effect can start to be seen in 4–6 weeks, but a therapeutic window has been noted, with doses above 200mg/d reversing the effect.

Paroxetine (Seroxat®)

Studies have shown an effect, starting at 20mg/d, and increasing by 10mg/d per week to 40–60mg/d.

Sertraline (Lustral®)

Sertraline is now licensed for OCD in children and adults, with acute and relapse prevention effects shown in a variety of studies. CSM warnings about SSRI use in under-18s do *not* apply to OCD.

Prescribing points:

❖ Dose in children is 25–50mg/d (6–12 years old). The adult dose should be used for older children but do not increase doses after less than a week.

Unlicensed/further information

Antidepressants (other)

Tricyclics (other than clomipramine), citalopram and venlafaxine have been studied and shown to be superior to placebo.

Antipsychotics

Risperidone, quetiapine and olanzapine have been used successfully to augment SSRIs in resistant cases.

Prescribing points:

❖ Make sure you've done high-dose SSRI/clomipramine for an adequate duration first, before considering a case is resistant and adding an antipsychotic.

1.22 Panic disorder

Symptoms

Panic disorder usually presents as sudden attacks of anxiety, where physical symptoms predominate, peak within 10 minutes and with an associated fear of serious consequences, eg. heart attack. Panic attacks need to include four of the following: palpitations, abdominal distress/nausea, numbness/tingling, inability to breath or shortness of breath, choking, sweating, chest pains, dizziness, depersonalisation, flushes/chills, fear of dying and trembling/shaking. The lifetime prevalence is up to 3.5%, frequently with a family history.

Role of drugs

In general, short–term benefits may be gained with drug therapy but relapse is common (30–75%) within 6–12 months of stopping drugs and so continued treatment may be necessary in some patients. Placebo responders tend to show an early but temporary remission. Benzodiazepines have a quicker onset but obvious problems eg. dependence potential and tolerance, and so are useful for short-term management. SSRIs are as effective as tricyclics, but with a slower onset and some initial exacerbation.

BNF listed

Benzodiazepines

Benzodiazepines are active more quickly than the tricyclic antidepressants and so are useful in patients needing immediate relief, although claims for the effectiveness of the benzodiazepines have been strongly challenged. There is some evidence that people with panic disorder have abnormal benzodiazepine receptors. Clonazepam at 1–2mg/d probably has the best balance between benefit and tolerability.

Prescribing point:

❖ The *BNF* urges great caution in prescribing benzodiazepines. It is best to transfer to an SSRI or tricyclic in due course if possible.

Citalopram (Cipramil®)

Citalopram is now licensed for panic, with or without agoraphobia. Start with 10mg/d for the first week, then increase to 20mg/d. A faster response compared to other SSRIs has been shown, as has relapse prevention over a year.

Prescribing points:

❖ There is little to be gained from going above 40mg/d.

❖ A starter pack with 10mg tablets is available, so use a slow dose titration (perhaps even starting at 5mg/d) to minimise initial exacerbation.

Escitalopram (Cipralex®)

Escitalopram is also licensed for panic, with or without agoraphobia. Start with 5mg/d for the first week, then increase to a maximum of 20mg/d.

Paroxetine (Seroxat®)

Paroxetine is now licensed for panic, with or without agoraphobia, and for relapse prevention. Start with 10mg/d for the first week, then increase by 10mg/d each week to 40mg/d.

Tricyclic antidepressants

Imipramine is effective (*vs* placebo) in all studies using doses above 150mg/d, lofepramine a useful second line as it has fewer anticholinergic side-effects. **Clomipramine** has been effective in two studies at less than 100mg/d (*Arch Gen Psych* 1988, **45**, 453–9) and may have a biphasic response, with symptoms worsening over 12 weeks before improving.

Prescribing point:

❖ Initial jitteriness is a common problem with many tricyclics and so it is usually necessary to start at a low tricyclic dose (10–25mg/d), and warn patients that they may feel more jittery and anxious initially.

Unlicensed/further information

Other SSRIs

Fluoxetine has been shown to be effective when initial doses are kept very low (2.5–5mg/d) then increased. Higher doses can produce anxiety and over-stimulation. Fluvoxamine has also been shown to be effective and may have a similar biphasic response to the tricyclics, but abrupt withdrawal can produce a discontinuation syndrome.

MAOIs

Phenelzine at 45–90mg/d may be at least as effective as imipramine in patients with panic attacks as part of depressive syndrome but MAOIs are generally considered third line for SSRI-resistant cases.

Mirtazapine (Zispin®)

Some recent studies have suggested a rapid response is possible to standard doses.

Venlafaxine (Efexor®)

One trial has shown an effect at a mean dose of 50mg/d.

1.23 Post-traumatic stress disorder (PTSD)

PTSD may be quite common yet often unrecognised and may lead to significant morbidity and mortality. Indeed, lifetime prevalence in the community may be as high as 1–9%.

Role of drugs

Drug treatment is still relatively poorly researched but there is an almost total lack of response to placebo drugs in chronic PTSD, and only drugs with an effect on the serotonin system seem to work. Positive (eg. nightmares) symptoms seem to respond better than negative (withdrawal, avoidance) symptoms. Higher doses for longer durations eg. longer than 5 weeks, seem necessary for a response.

BNF Listed

Paroxetine (Seroxat®)

Paroxetine is licensed at a starting dose of 20mg/d, increasing gradually to 50mg/d if necessary.

Prescribing points:

❖ Allow 12 weeks for full response.

Sertraline (Lustral®)

Sertraline is licensed in the UK for PTSD, but oddly may only be effective in women. A mean dose of 150mg/d is superior to placebo, particularly for the psychological symptoms eg. anger, anhedonia and numbing. A relapse prevention effect has also been shown.

Prescribing points:

❖ Allow 12 weeks for full response.

Unlicensed/further information

Antipsychotics

Some antipsychotics, particularly atypicals such as risperidone, olanzapine and quetiapine have been used as adjuncts, although have been ineffective in RCTs as monotherapy.

Benzodiazepines

A potent antiarrousal effect can be useful but care is needed with potential abuse and disinhibition.

SSRIs

Two studies have shown fluoxetine (up to 60mg/d) to ameliorate PTSD, particularly avoidant symptoms, but don't increase doses too quickly.

Tricyclics

Amitriptyline and imipramine have been shown to produce a modest and clinically meaningful effect. The main feature is that doses of 300mg/d for at least 8 weeks (higher than UK SPC limits) are needed. Lower doses show no effect.

1.24 Psychiatric emergency (acute) — see also mania/hypomania (*1.17*) and psychosis/schizophrenia (*1.25*)

Cautions:

Violent patients (usually either schizophrenic, hypomanic or substance abusers) present a risk to themselves and others and swift, safe and effective treatment is needed. In an acute psychiatric emergency, the GP will frequently be referring on to psychiatric specialists but may be called upon to act in the interim to control a dangerous situation. Use of rapid, safe and effective treatment is essential, with no heroic use of inappropriate, obsolete or dangerous drugs. There are enough accidental deaths reported already. The main factors to consider are:

Routes: IV administration is generally much quicker than IM but carries additional dangers, so IM, oral liquids or oral dispersible tablet use should generally be preferred for rapid action.

Doses: There really is no need to use very high doses as most respond to combinations of drugs at standard doses.

Complications of high dose neuroleptic use in acute psychiatric emergency include extrapyramidal symptoms (Parkinsonian effects), local bruising, pain or extravasation (common, in up to 30% patients), respiratory complications (2%), cardiovascular complications (3%) and acute hypotension. Sudden (unexplained) death may occur, often within 2–3 minutes of injection, and in very many cases *toxic* blood concentrations are present, indicating over-dosage.

BNF listed

Drugs in this section are licensed for emergency, short-term or adjunct therapy of acute psychosis, mania, anxiety or exacerbations of chronic psychosis, violent or impulsive behaviour, psychomotor agitation and excitement or violent or dangerously impulsive behaviour. You are advised to see the UK SPC of the drug if in any doubt. See particularly **haloperidol** plus **diazepam** or **lorazepam** (perhaps followed by **Clopixol Acuphase**®) for a safe and effective first choice therapy.

Chlorpromazine (Largactil®)

Chlorpromazine injection should only be given by deep intramuscular injection.

Prescribing points:

❖ IM injection is 2–4 times as potent on a mg for mg basis as oral chlorpromazine.

❖ Great care/avoid in the elderly as haloperidol is a safer alternative.

Diazepam

The recommended dose of diazepam is 10mg IM or rectal, repeated after not less than 4 hours.

Prescribing points:

❖ See also combinations with haloperidol for additional information.

❖ Rectal tubules are quicker than IM, peaking in 10 minutes.

Haloperidol (Haldol®, Serenace®)

Haloperidol is a relatively safe drug to use at *BNF* doses (up to 18mg/d by IM injection), especially with diazepam.

Prescribing point:

❖ See also combinations with diazepam or lorazepam.

Lorazepam (Ativan®)

Lorazepam is usually given orally or by the IV route into a larger vein, diluted 50:50 with water or normal saline pre-injection.

Prescribing points:

❖ May be useful in combination with haloperidol. See combinations.

❖ Lower doses are usually needed in renal and hepatic impairment and the elderly.

Methotrimeprazine/ levomepromazine (Nozinan®)

This is licensed as a more sedative alternative to chlorpromazine.

Olanzapine injection (Zyprexa IM®)

Plasma levels peak at 1 hour and a rapid effect in APE has been shown, especially if combined with benzodiazepine. Olanzapine Velotabs®, whilst an attractive alternative, give peak levels at the same time as ordinary tablets (ie. 4 hours) and so do not provide a rapidly-acting alternative to the injection.

Trifluoperazine (Stelazine®)

This is licensed as an adjunct therapy.

Zuclopenthixol acetate (Clopixol-Acuphase®)

Clopixol Acuphase® can be given at a dose of 50–150mg stat, then repeated after 2–3 days (maximum every 1–2 days) after the first injection. The maximum cumulative dose is 400mg per 'course'; 4 injections or 2 weeks, whichever comes first. The maximum single dose in the elderly is 100mg. Care is needed with Acuphase to avoid it being given into a vein of a struggling or overactive patient.

Prescribing points:

❖ Very useful in the sub-acute situation and may be used by GPs, usually under advice from a specialist.

❖ Onset is within a few hours and lasts for about up to two days.

❖ Ensure no confusion with Clopixol® (oil-based) depot.

Combinations

Patients receiving only a single drug in an emergency at first are more likely to need further injections. The only major UK study showed that the combination of a neuroleptic and a sedative was favoured by ward staff as being the most effective combination in the acute situation.

Antipsychotic+benzodiazepine

(particularly haloperidol plus diazepam or lorazepam)

This combination is recommended widely as first choice therapy in acute psychiatric emergency. The drugs act synergistically, reducing the amount of each drug (but particularly the antipsychotic) required. The effect is rapid and predictable and the patient less likely to require a second injection. 10mg IM/IV of both haloperidol and diazepam for a 'drug-naive' patient is recommended, with up to 20mg of each for previously antipsychotic-treated patients. Risperidone plus lorazepam (both orally) has been shown to be as effective as haloperidol plus lorazepam (both as IM) but with fewer complications.

Prescribing points:

❖ This is a reliable, effective, predictable and safe combination at the doses noted.

❖ Rectal diazepam is an alternative to IV/IM.

❖ Risperidone 'Quicklets' and liquid peak plasma level after 90 mins and offer an alternative to injections.

1.25   Psychosis and schizophrenia

Symptoms

Schizophrenia is a neurodevelopmental disorder, with symptoms first developing usually in the mid to late teens. Schneider's 'First Rank symptoms' are often quoted, and include hearing thoughts spoken aloud, 'third person' hallucinations, hallucinations in the form of a commentary, somatic hallucinations, thought withdrawal or insertion, thought broadcasting, delusional perceptions and feelings experienced as made or influenced by external agents. These are also called the 'positive' symptoms. 'Negative' symptoms include apathy, withdrawal and depression and may be exacerbated by some older antipsychotics. Schizophrenics most frequently have a lack of insight, auditory hallucinations, ideas of reference, suspiciousness, flatness of affect, voices speaking to the patient, delusional mood, delusions of persecution and hearing their own thoughts spoken aloud.

Role of drugs

Many symptoms seem related to excess dopamine activity in the mesolimbic system and antipsychotics all have some dopamine-blocking activity, although other receptor systems may be involved. Neuroleptics or antipsychotics are thus the mainstay in the drug treatment of schizophrenic illnesses. Their two main actions and uses are for:

1. **Acute phase:** an immediate calming effect, useful in relieving patient distress and in the acute situation. There

appears no advantage of using high doses, eg. above 12mg/d haloperidol for eliminating or reducing the intensity of psychotic experiences, the onset usually being delayed by one or two weeks from the start of full-dose treatment in the acute phase.

2. **Relapse prevention:** in people diagnosed as chronic schizophrenics, over three years about 80% will relapse on no antipsychotic, 50% on oral antipsychotics (although this figure may be lower with the atypicals) and only 20% on depots. They may also help by reducing the vulnerability to adverse life events. If antipsychotics are stopped, schizophrenics may not relapse for 2–6 months, often feeling better before the relapse occurs. The risk factors for relapse of schizophrenia include the antipsychotics used (atypical relapse is lower than with typicals), duration of untreated psychosis (the longer and more insidious the untreated stage, the lower the chances of good response) and concurrent substance misuse (reduces response).

Relapse (and the consequential deterioration) is a major problem and can be minimised by:

(a) using drugs the person is happiest taking eg. optimal doses or the drug with the least unacceptable side effects.

(b) reducing or managing any concurrent substance misuse.

NICE Guidance on the use of newer (atypical) antipsychotic drugs for the treatment of schizophrenia (June 2002)

1.1 "The choice of antipsychotic drug should be made jointly by the individual and the clinician..." based on informed discussion of relative benefits and side-effects

1.2 Recommended that "...amisulpride, olanzapine, quetiapine, risperidone and zotepine are considered in the choice of first-line treatments for ... newly diagnosed schizophrenia."

1.3 Atypicals should be considered as options for people "currently receiving typical antipsychotic drugs who, despite adequate symptom control, are experiencing unacceptable side-effects" and those in relapse with previous poor management or unacceptable side-effects with typicals

1.4 It is "...not recommended" ...to... "change to one of the oral atypicals"...if the patient is ... "currently achieving good control ... without unacceptable side-effects" from typicals

1.5 In "treatment-resistant schizophrenia (TRS), clozapine should be introduced at the earliest opportunity" ie. 2 antipsychotics (at least one atypical) for 6–8 weeks

1.6 "...depot preparations should be prescribed when appropriate"

1.7 "Where more than one atypical ... is considered appropriate, the drug with the lowest purchase price ... should be prescribed"

1.8 "When full discussion ... is not possible" (eg. in acute episode) "oral atypical drugs should be considered as the treatment options of choice because of the lower risk of EPS"

1.9 Antipsychotics should be "part of a comprehensive package of care", and monitoring is important when switching drugs

1.10 "Atypical and typical" drugs "should not be prescribed concurrently except for short periods" during changeovers

---

The term **"atypical"** is a marketing term used to describe new antipsychotics. It may be better to consider antipsychotics as being on a spectrum, from 'typical' (eg. chlorpromazine) through haloperidol, to sulpiride in the middle, then risperidone (Risperdal®), olanzapine (Zyprexa®) and quetiapine (Seroquel®) nearer the clozapine (Clozaril®) 'atypical' end.

BNF listed

Antipsychotics probably largely exert their effect via blockade of dopamine-2 (D2) receptors but D2 blockade usually also produces Parkinsonian side-effects. They are not addictive and do not generally produce withdrawal effects (see *1.32*).

Phenothiazines

Chlorpromazine (Largactil®)

The prototype phenothiazine, chlorpromazine, has a wide range of effects on many systems. It is quite sedative and hypoten-sive. It is used for a wide range of psychotic conditions but use in the elderly is problematical.

Prescribing point:

❖ Great care needed in the elderly.

Fluphenazine (Moditen®)

An oral preparation is available but this is usually used as a depot (see under depots).

Methotrimeprazine/levomepromazine (Nozinan®)

A phenothiazine related to promethazine, methotrimeprazine/levomepromazine also has strong sedative effects and is thus referred to by some patients by the name 'Noddy-land' in this respect.

Pericyazine (Neulactil®)

A piperidine phenothiazine similar to thioridazine, with marked sedative and hypotensive side-effects.

Perphenazine (Fentazin®)

A piperazine phenothiazine with a relatively short half-life (8–12 hours).

Promazine

A phenothiazine closely related to chlor-promazine. Often used in the elderly and in alcoholics as a non-dependence prone hypnotic, although the potential for side-effects in these groups should not be ignored.

Thioridazine (Melleril®)

Due to QTc prolongation concerns, thiori-dazine is now only approved for resistant schizophrenia. There is a published association with sudden unexplained death in psychiatric in-patients.

Prescribing point:

❖ Requires baseline ECG and serum potassium, and repeated regularly throughout treatment.

Trifluoperazine (Stelazine®)

A long-established piperazine phenothia-zine widely used as an antipsychotic and sometimes claimed to have 'activating' effects at low doses.

Butyrophenones

Benperidol (Anquil®)

A standard butyrophenone, marketed originally as specific for anti-social forms of sexual behaviour, but the only controlled study showed no significant effect on behaviour and responses to sexual stimuli.

Prescribing point:

❖ Expensive and of no specific use in anti-social sexual behaviour.

Haloperidol (Serenace®, Haldol®)

Prototype butyrophenone for the treat-ment of acute and chronic psychosis. Doses over 12mg/d may have **no** advan-tage in acute schizophrenia and, indeed, a 63% dose reduction in chronic treatment resistant schizophrenics on high dose haloperidol resulted in improvement of symptoms and side-effects, further improved by intensive behaviour therapy. See also haloperidol decanoate.

Prescribing point:

❖ Doses above 12–20mg/d have no additional *antipsychotic* activity.

First-episode or early-onset schizophrenia

There is growing evidence that early intervention with antipsychotics for prodromal symptoms of schizophrenia may:

● Allow lower doses to be used (and hence reduce adverse experiences)
● Minimise deterioration, harm and stigma
● Improve long-term outcomes and reduce concurrent substance misuse

There are unfortunately no clear prodromal symptoms and no way of treating these without treating some false-positives.

The principles of pharmacotherapy in this group are:

● Start low and go slow (with slow discontinuation as well)
● Consider patient preference (eg. weight gain and EPSE must not be trivialised as they make the person look "odd" to their peers)
● Maintain therapy and explain that the relapse rates are very high, and that discon-tinuation will almost inevitably lead to relapse (eg. in a 53pt RCT, 78% relapsed within one year and 96% within 2 years of stopping; Gitlin *et al*, *Am J Psych* 2001, **158**, 1835-42)

The best evidence base is available for:

● Risperidone (at least 7 good published trials) — start at 0.25–0.5mg/d and gradu-ally increase to about 2mg/d (depending on response and tolerability) as there is probably little advantage of higher doses over the first 8 weeks
● Olanzapine (some studies) and quetiapine (awaiting publication)

Thioxanthenes

Flupentixol (Depixol®)

See under depots. An oral preparation is also available.

Zuclopenthixol (Clopixol®)

A slow onset and long half-life make longer-term therapy well tolerated and hence established. See zuclopenthixol acetate (Acuphase®) and decanoate (Clopixol®) for use in acute and chronic illness.

Diphenylbutylpiperidines
Fluspirilene (Redeptin®)

See depots.

Pimozide (Orap®)

Pimozide is a pure dopamine antagonist effective against a wide range of 'positive' symptoms.

Prescribing point:

❖ CSM has warned about potential cardio-toxic effects (see 3.2.1, where there is a list of CSM requirements).

Benzamides

Amisulpride (Solian®)

Amisulpride is a specific D2 and D3 receptor blocker, related to sulpiride (but listed as atypical) and shown to be as effective as a selection of other antipsychotics. EPSEs are dose-dependent and sedation is minimal.

Sulpiride (Dolmatil®, Sulpor®, Sulpitil®)

A specific D2 receptor blocker antipsychotic well established in the UK. The incidence of extra-pyramidal side-effects is much reduced, making it a useful drug.

Atypicals or second generation

Aripiprazole (Abilify®)

Aripiprazole may be available later in 2004 and a true novel antipsychotic in that it is a dopamine regulator, by acting as a partial dopamine agonist at low dose and antago-nist at higher dose. It stimulates dopamine receptors up to about 30% but blocks anything above this. It has a low incidence

of standard antipsychotic side-effects eg. EPSE, weight gain etc.

Prescribing points:

❖ 15mg/d seems the optimal dose.

❖ Use with other dopamine-blocking anti-psychotics is probably counter-productive.

Clozapine (Clozaril®, Denzapine®, Zaponex®)

Clozapine is the prototype potent atypical antipsychotic indicated only for treatment-resistant schizophrenic patients. Treat-ment can only be initiated by consultant psychiatrists, supplied by hospital pharma-cies (for the first year) and to registered patients. Prescribing by GPs is possible in patients with stable haematological profiles after one year of treatment. It is generally considered that a third of resistant schizo-phrenics improve dramatically on clozapine (anecdotally particularly younger adults with early-onset illness), a third derive significant benefit and a third do not respond. Suicide rates are also reduced with clozapine, a unique effect in schizo-phrenia.

The main problem is that clozapine usually causes a reversible neutropenia in 3% of patients which may lead to a fatal agranulocytosis in about 1% of patients. Onset of this problem occurs usually around 8–10 weeks. Full blood counts are thus taken weekly for the first eighteen weeks, then fortnightly until one year, then four-weekly for the remaining duration of treatment. These have to be satisfactory for the next supply of drug to be made — 'No bloods, no drugs' being the main message, causing much hassle for patients, pharmacies, doctors and CPNs.

Clozapine had previously only been licensed for initiation in hospital, but can now be started in the community, with strict monitoring. Rare, but definite, risks in the first month include hypotension and tachycardia, with cardiac collapse in 1 in 3000. Pulse (testing for heart failure or myocarditis), temperature (for NMS) and BP (standing and sitting) must be moni-tored at least every 2 days for the first fort-night. If asked to advise, any sustained rise in BP, pulse or temperature (2 successive measurements) should be reported to the patient's Consultant (SPC recommendation) and a reduced dose or (temporary) discontinuation is often indicated.

Despite a relatively high direct cost, it can be a very cost-effective treatment for resistant schizophrenia, cost savings resulting almost exclusively from reduced costs of hospitalisation.

Prescribing points:

❖ Consultant Psychiatrist initiation only, although this can now be as an outpatient (see above).

❖ During initiation, the patient should be monitored regularly for the risk of hypotension and cardiac problems.

❖ Clozapine interacts with many drugs which can enhance the chances of a blood dyscrasia, eg. **carbamazepine, antibiotics** etc, so great care is needed in additional prescribing (see *Chapter 4.2.3* for the list).

❖ The risk of seizures rises above 600mg/d — valproate is the best prophylactic anticonvulsant cover.

❖ If you have any doubts, your local (mental health) hospital pharmacy will have full records and can also advise on treatment options.

Olanzapine (Zyprexa®)

Olanzapine is licensed for the treatment of schizophrenia and for relapse prevention and is now a standard atypical for a wide range of psychotic symptoms (albeit licensed only for schizophrenia). It blocks a wide variety of dopamine, serotonin and other receptors. The starting dose is 10mg/d, the range 5–20mg/d, although 15–20mg/d should only be used if needed (although it is the average dose used). A significant effect on positive (eg. hallucinations, delusions) and negative (eg. apathy, withdrawal) symptoms has been shown. The main side-effects are somnolence and weight gain, with occasional dizziness, postural hypotension and transient anticholinergic effects.

Prescribing points:

❖ 10mg/d should be the standard dose.

❖ Often used for a variety of other indications, for which there may be less of an evidence-base than for schizophrenia.

❖ Weight gain is a common side-effect; weigh (baseline), warn (patient) and watch (early intervention being better than trying to reverse it once it's happened) is the best strategy.

Quetiapine (Seroquel®)

Quetiapine is licensed for schizophrenia and relapse prevention. It has a very low incidence of EPSEs, raised prolactin and related side-effects. Doses of 300–450mg/d (range 150–750mg/d) are quoted as the most effective. Doses need to be increased gradually over several days initially due to infrequent initial hypotension.

Prescribing point:

❖ A starter pack is available for initial dose titration (see also *BNF*).

Risperidone (Risperdal®)

Risperidone is licensed for acute and chronic psychosis and has specific D2 and 5-HT2 receptor blocking effects. It has become a standard atypical due to the relative incidence of side-effects eg. few EPSEs at the optimum dose of 4–6mg/d. The $D2:5HT_2$ balance is the claimed reason the drug has less EPSEs. If this is true, use with other antipsychotics will negate this effect. A recent robust study has shown a significantly superior relapse prevention effect compared to haloperidol, and several other studies that improved cognitive functioning can occur. Dose titration over 3 days is recommended. A long-acting injection is available (Risperdal Consta® — see depot and long-acting injections).

Prescribing points:

❖ Doses above 6mg/d appear to have little antipsychotic advantage.

❖ A slower dose titration (over weeks rather than days) may help in antipsychotic-naïve patients (see separate box) and the elderly.

❖ Quick-dissolving tablets (Risperdal Quicklets®) are available, as well as a syrup.

❖ Risperdal Consta® releases risperidone for two weeks about 3–4 weeks after an injection, so needs additional care (see depots/long-acting injections).

Sertindole (Serdolect®)

Sertindole has become available again after concerns of QTc prolongation proved unfounded. It is currently undergoing post-marketing research, but should a patient of yours be prescribed sertindole, prescribing other drugs that might prolong the QT interval (see *3.2*) or inhibit the 2D6 enzyme (see *4.2.7*) are contraindicated.

Zotepine (Zoleptil®)

Zotepine is a little used atypical, with some data showing efficacy, but nothing outstanding.

Prescribing points:

❖ The risk of seizures rises sharply at doses of 300mg/d or more.

❖ Start at 25mg TDS and titrate up every 4 days (to minimise hypotension) to a maximum of 300mg/d.

❖ An ECG is recommended pre-treatment in people with CHD, at risk of hypokalaemia or taking other drugs known to prolong the QTc interval.

Depot and long-acting injections

Depot administration of antipsychotics is widely used throughout Europe, with up to 60% of schizophrenics receiving them. The major advantage is assured compliance, with associated and proven reduction in relapses, re-hospitalisation and severity of relapse. For example, after 36 months, only 20% of (drug) untreated schizophrenics will remain in remission and only 50% of those treated with oral neuroleptics. Conversely, about 80% given depots will remain in remission. Bioavailability problems are also reduced (some people metabolise antipsychotics extensively on the first-pass). By being sure of doses received, depots **should** be able to facilitate better downward titration of doses to reduce the incidence of side-effects. The major disadvantages include the impossibility of altering a dose if side-effects develop (eg. dystonia, NMS), patients seeing depot administration as "being controlled", having no control over their treatment or, worse still, as being a punishment. Many patients and families/carers are insufficiently educated about the pros and cons of depot administration. Used properly they can lead to reduced relapses, low side-effects and stable therapeutic effects. It should not be enough just to prevent relapse. The debate over the use of depots has been opened out with the first atypical depot/long-acting injection.

Flupentixol decanoate (Depixol®)

The most widely prescribed depot in the UK, flupentixol is a dopamine specific thioxanthene antipsychotic with potentially activating effects at low dose.

Prescribing point:

❖ Can be given weekly but fortnightly is usually more appropriate.

Fluphenazine decanoate (Modecate® plus generics)

A potent phenothiazine which can be given up to four-weekly as a depot.

Fluspirilene (Redeptin®)

This diphenylbutylpiperidine is available only on a named-patient basis as a water-based microcrystalline injection.

Prescribing point:

❖ Often leads to tissue damage where the fluspirilene precipitates out in the muscle.

Haloperidol decanoate (Haldol Decanoate®)

A longer-acting depot. A 4-week interval between injections is possible but this risks giving too high a dose and exposing the patient to quite severe Parkinsonian side-effects.

Prescribing points:
* ❖ Dose titration can be difficult.
* ❖ Probably best reserved for chronic relapsing schizophrenics known to be responsive to haloperidol.

Pipothiazine palmitate (Piportil®)

A piperidine phenothiazine marketed in the UK as the palmitate, giving a 4-week dosage interval. Fluphenazine decanoate also gives this release characteristic.

Risperidone (Risperdal Consta®)

Risperdal Consta is the risperidone molecule in synthetic and absorbable polymer microspheres suspended in water. There is no significant drug release for 3–4 weeks after injection, then risperidone is released between 4 and 7 weeks (see graph below). The injection must be kept at 2–8°C — once above this for more than 15 minutes it must be used within 7 days.

Prescribing points:
* ❖ Oral cover may be needed for at least the first three weeks (and possibly for several weeks longer) before the first dose starts to release risperidone, then tapered gradually.
* ❖ Care with dose increases is needed as it will be three injections before the outcome of the first or increased dose is clear.
* ❖ Elimination is complete 7–8 weeks after the last dose so beware of additive side-effects if switching from Consta®.
* ❖ May be optimally effective for patients responding to oral risperidone first.

Risperidone release from Consta®

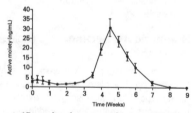

(Reproduced courtesy of Janssen-Cilag)

Zuclopenthixol decanoate (Clopixol®)

Established UK depot antipsychotic. It has also been used in high dose in aggression, particularly in patients with learning disabilities and forensic patients.

Zuclopenthixol acetate (Clopixol-Acuphase®)

50–150mg as a single dose has provided a rapid and effective reduction in acute psychotic symptoms in many patients over about 78 hours. It has taken over from barbiturates and phenothiazines in many acute psychiatric services as a drug of choice in acute psychiatric emergency. The peak blood level of zuclopenthixol is at about 32 hours after a 100mg dose.

Combinations

Despite widespread use, there is only one RCT of combined antipsychotics (clozapine+sulpiride). Other antipsychotics such as amisulpride, risperidone, olanzapine and quetiapine have been used with clozapine to try to enhance it's efficacy in resistant schizophrenia.

Unlicensed/further information

Benzodiazepines

Benzodiazepines have no antipsychotic effect but may reduce a patient's anxiety, tension and insomnia in the short-term. They are probably most useful in psychotic agitation. A disinhibiting effect can occur rarely and so care is needed if benzodiazepines are used in the short-term.

Others

A great many other drugs have been tried as adjuncts, including galantamine (to improve negative symptoms), celecoxib (as an adjunct to risperidone), omega-3 fatty acids (which may be effective but since you reek of fish, double-blind trials are virtually impossible) and SSRIs.

1.26 Rapid-cycling bipolar disorder — see also bipolar mood disorder (*1.9*) mania/hypomania (*1.17*) and depression (*1.12*)

Rapid-cycling bipolar disorder is a subclass of bipolar mood disorder, where four or more mood episodes occur in one year. Although it is a relatively uncommon (eg. 5–15% of all bipolars seen at mood disorder clinics) and often transient condition, the clinical significance of the subgroup is that rapid-cycling is a major risk factor for suicide and is difficult to manage.

Role of drugs

Stopping any antidepressants or other contributory drugs (see *5.7* for a list) has to be first-line treatment. Carbamazepine, valproate and lithium (although many may be lithium non-responders) are the first-line monotherapy options. If ineffective, they may then be used in combination. Levothyroxine and nimodipine may be effective in some patients not responsive to first-line drugs.

BNF listed

Carbamazepine (Tegretol®)

Several studies have shown a long-term response rate ranging from 20% to 70%. Doubt has, however, been raised about long-term efficacy as many people seem to lose the therapeutic response over several years.

Lithium (Camcolit®, Priadel®)

Although around 80% of rapid-cyclers are lithium non-responsive, lithium undoubtedly has some effect, probably by reducing the intensity of relapses rather than the actual number. Poor compliance with lithium (particularly if intermittent eg. frequent abrupt stopping), may complicate treatment by inducing relapse.

Combinations

Combinations of carbamazepine, valproate and lithium have been used, with some synergy reported. Low-dose levothyroxine (see below) with lithium or a tricyclic may be particularly effective.

Unlicensed/further information

Lamotrigine (Lamictal®)

One large and prospective study in rapid-cycling disorder showed lamotrigine was well-tolerated and useful in some rapid-cyclers. The optimum dose appears to be 50–200mg/d.

Levothyroxine/thyroxine/liothyronine

Levothyroxine has efficacy in some people at 0.1–0.5mg/d (or liothyronine 140–400mcg/d) for rapid-cycling mania.

Valproate (Epilim® etc)

Open studies have found a significant effect, with up to 83% showing a good response.

Useless

Antidepressants

See introduction, which notes that antidepressants can exacerbate the cycling frequency.

1.27 Seasonal affective disorder (SAD)

Seasonal affective disorder is a recurrent affective disorder (predominantly major depression, but can include mania or hypomania) with a characteristic seasonal pattern of relationship to a season, usually autumn or winter, for two years at least and with full remission at a characteristic time of the year. Atypical depressive features include hypersomnia, increased appetite and weight and carbohydrate cravings. Theories for the cause include excess melatonin secretion (which is suppressed by bright light), delayed circadian rhythms (early morning bright light bringing this forward), reduced amplitude of circadian rhythms and dysfunction of the serotonin system.

Role of drugs

Whilst bright light phototherapy is well established, SSRIs and moclobemide may have some effectiveness, although the data is relatively sparse.

Unlicensed/further information

Beta-blockers

Some trials have indicated that pre-sunrise propranolol may help, via a short-term short-acting beta-blocker-induced truncation of nocturnal melatonin secretion early in the morning but not in the evening.

Moclobemide (Manerix®)

Moclobemide 400mg/d for SAD was superior to placebo in a 34-patient trial.

SSRIs

Fluoxetine and other SSRIs may produce clinically useful improvements in SAD symptoms, eg. fluoxetine at 20mg/d.

1.28   Self-injurious behaviour (SIB)

Self–injurious behaviour includes head-banging, biting, cutting etc. It occurs in some patients with learning disabilities and others who seem to derive some reward from self-harm.

Unlicensed/further information

Antipsychotics

There is now data showing that risperidone (and possibly low-dose olanzapine) may be useful over the long-term in developmentally disabled in-patients. Chlorpromazine and haloperidol were the most frequently prescribed, with the atypicals now used, although evidence for their efficacy is suggestive rather than conclusive and risks side-effects.

Naltrexone (Nalorex®)

25–100mg/d orally has been shown to reduce self-injurious behaviour in small studies but larger studies have been less hopeful. The rationale is that SIB may induce the production of endogenous opiates in the person's brain, producing a powerful reward strategy. When using naltrexone to block the effect of these endorphins, the SIB may get worse over the first few days or weeks (as the person strives to damage themselves further to gain the same reward) but then improves (as the person learns that the activity now hurts rather than being rewarding and stops it). There is some evidence of raised opioid peptide activity in autism, fragile-X syndrome and other learning disabilities.

1.29   Serotonin syndrome

Serotonin syndrome (SS) is a condition caused by drug-induced serotonin hyperstimulation. It probably goes largely unreported as symptoms are usually mild and difficult to diagnose, although it can be severe, with deaths reported. Onset is usually within a few hours of drug/dosechanges and usually resolves in 24 hours.

"Sternbach's Diagnostic Criteria" include physical symptoms (at least three of: mental state changes such as confusion, agitation/restlessness, sweating, diarrhoea, fever, hyperreflexia, tachycardia, myoclonus, lack of co-ordination, shivering, tremor), with other causes excluded (eg. infection, metabolic, substance abuse or withdrawal) and no concurrent antipsychotic dose changes.

Serotonin syndrome is usually caused by any combination of antidepressants and/or related drugs such as dextromethorphan, tramadol and levodopa (see *5.13* for sample list).

Role of drugs

First-line treatment should be to discontinue identifiable serotonergic drugs (including over-the-counter sympathomimetics), then provide symptomatic support, eg. cooling blankets etc. More severe cases require major supportive measures.

Unlicensed/further information

Benzodiazepines

Lorazepam by slow IV injection has been used in hospitals.

Cyproheptadine (Periactin®)

Cyproheptadine is a non-specific 5-HT blocker and 4–8mg orally repeated every 2–4 hours has been claimed to be the best antiserotonergic drug strategy, with case reports of rapid success.

Mirtazapine (Zispin®)

Mirtazapine has been proposed as a possible treatment as it blocks 5-HT$_2$ and 5-HT$_3$ receptors.

1.30 Social phobia (social anxiety disorder) — see also anxiety disorder (*1.6*).

Social phobia is relatively common, with sufferers fearing public ridicule, scrutiny and negative evaluation and fear making a public mistake, embarrassment or criticism. Public speaking, social gatherings, writing under supervision or eating and drinking in public are commonly avoided. It is a serious and disabling anxiety disorder associated with marked reduction in quality of life but underdiagnosed, with less than 5% receiving a diagnosis.

Role of drugs

Drugs and behavioural approaches are commonly used. SSRIs are clearly superior to placebo and are emerging as the gold standard drug therapy, with another SSRI or moclobemide second line and MAOIs and benzodiazepines third. Length of treatment should be at least 12 weeks. Combined drugs and psychological treatments does not generally provide better results than psychological therapies alone.

BNF listed

Paroxetine (Seroxat®)

Several studies show paroxetine to be superior to placebo, eg. at 20–50mg/d

reducing symptoms and avoidance, with 40mg/d the optimum dose, although with high drop-out rates exist.

Prescribing points:

❖ Lack of response at 8 weeks does not predict long-term lack of response and so a minimum of 12 weeks treatment is necessary.

Unlicensed/further information

Benzodiazepines

The BDZs have a rapid onset, good tolerability and the option of a flexible dose, but cause sedation, incoordination and long-term use is probably not advisable.

Beta-blockers

There is no evidence for efficacy, except perhaps in people where short-term management of tremor is essential, eg. musicians.

Moclobemide (Manerix®)

Moclobemide, building up to 600mg/d over two weeks and maintaining for twelve weeks, may produce a therapeutic effect.

SSRIs (other than paroxetine)

Citalopram 40mg/d appears well-tolerated and effective (75% response) as moclobemide. **Sertraline** (up to 200mg/d) was more effective than placebo in a well designed flexible-dose trial, although **fluoxetine** was ineffective in one large RCT.

1.31 Tourette's syndrome (Gilles de la Tourette)

Symptoms

The main diagnostic symptoms include multiple tics, vocal tics (grunts and snarls, including obscenities), stereotyped movements (jumping and dancing), overactivity, learning difficulties and emotional problems. This hereditary disorder occurs in 1–5 per 10,000 population, is more common in males and has an onset at 5–6 yrs.

Role of drugs

Pharmacotherapy may be useful to help control some of the more distressing symptoms.

BNF listed

Haloperidol (Serenace®, Haldol®)

Haloperidol 0.5–20mg/d has been the drug of choice, but side-effects may be limiting. The depot has also been used.

Unlicensed/further information

Clonidine (Catapres®, Dixarit®)

Clonidine has been used and may be as effective as haloperidol in some patients.

Lorazepam (Ativan®)

Lorazepam 1.5–10mg/d has been used as adjuvant therapy.

Risperidone (Risperdal®)

There are now several studies showing a significant effect at a mean dose of 2.5mg/d and it appears at least as effective as the standard drugs, as well as being better tolerated than haloperidol.

Combinations

Naltrexone+codeine

Sequential use of naltrexone (100–300mg/d) and codeine phosphate (15–120mg/d) proved effective in two cases.

Others

Other drugs tried include cannabinoids (popular with sufferers, who claim an 82% success rate), SSRIs, methylphenidate, nicotine (as patches or gum), pergolide and selegiline.

1.32 Caffeinism

Caffeine consumption at 250–500mg/d is regarded as moderate use. Caffeinism is estimated to start at a consumption of between 600mg and 750mg/d, with above 1000mg/d well into the toxic range. Caffeine dependence displays features of a typical psychoactive substance dependence, ie. withdrawal, continued use despite caffeine-induced problems, tolerance and persistent desire or unsuccessful attempts to cut down or control use. Positive effects of moderate amounts include increased alertness and vigilance and reduced fatigue.

Caffeine withdrawal is a DSM-IV diagnosis and thus should be taken seriously. Sudden withdrawal can produce headaches (52%), rebound drowsiness, fatigue/lethargy and depression, with many other effects reported.

Intake can be calculated thus:

Source	Caffeine Content	
	per 100ml	per container
Brewed coffee	55–85mg	140–210mg/mug
Instant coffee	35–45mg	85–110mg/mug
Decaffeinated coffee	2mg	5mg/mug
Cocoa	3mg	7mg/mug
Brewed tea	25–55mg	55–140mg/mug
Coca Cola	11mg	36mg/can
Pepsi Cola	7mg	22mg/can
Milk chocolate		22mg/100g
Hedex Seltzer		60mg/sachet
Aqua Ban		100mg/tablet
A mug is taken as being 250ml		

Symptoms of caffeinism (acute or chronic):

Adverse-effects of low to moderate doses: Diuresis, increased gastric secretion, fine tremor, increased skeletal muscle stamina, mild anxiety, negative mood, palpitations, nervousness.

Side-effects of high doses: chronic insomnia, persistent anxiety, restlessness, tension, irritability, agitation, tremulousness, panic, poor concentration, confusion, disorientation, paranoia, delirium, tremor, muscle twitching and tension, convulsions, vertigo, dizziness, tinnitus, auditory and visual hallucinations, facial flushing, hyperthermia, hypertension, nausea, vomiting, abdominal discomfort, headaches, tachypnoea and disturbed sleep.

Adverse consequences: There is some contradictory evidence about the effect of caffeine on people with mental health problems. Clearly, high doses can cause significant effects. Acute high doses (10mg/kg) significantly increase arousal and have a psychotogenic effect in schizophrenics. Schizophrenics often have higher caffeine intakes and average intake should be routinely monitored as it can exacerbate schizophrenia. Ward studies have shown that '*chronic caffeine use created clinically significant levels of anxiety and tension that could be reduced by decreasing caffeine*

consumption'. Caffeinism can present as anxiety neurosis, precipitate or exacerbate psychosis and make these more resistant to drug treatment, especially antipsychotics. The clinical signs of affective diseases can be modified. 150mg of caffeine at bedtime has been shown to have a marked effect on sleep latency, total sleep time and reduced sleep efficacy and REM periods.

Conversely, there are reports of lack of correlation between caffeine consumption and anxiety and depression, with no changes when a ward moved to decaffeinated products and little difference in behaviours between caffeinated and decaffeinated periods. Withdrawal of caffeine from a group of severely retarded and highly disturbed patients produced no improvement in sleep patterns, but reintroduction was accompanied by a highly significant increase in ward disturbances, which may explain the contradictions in evidence.

Methods of caffeine reduction:

1. Recognition of the problems of excess (> 750mg/d) caffeine and the likely benefits of reduction.
2. Identification of all current caffeine sources and pattern of consumption.
3. Gradual reduction, eg. making weaker drinks, taken less often, increasing use of caffeine-free equivalent drinks, particularly at 'usual' drinking times of the day, mixing caffeine and decaffeinated coffee to give a lower strength drink.
4. Limited use of analgesia (caffeine-free, of course) for withdrawal headaches.
5. Setting a target for consumption, which will not need to be complete abstinence, eg. caffeine drinks only at set times in the day, eg. on rising etc.

Causes:

Patients may drink large quantities of tea and coffee to relieve thirst/dry mouth caused by tricyclic and phenothiazine side-effects. Heavy caffeine drinking is often part of the culture of in-patient settings, nursing homes and other residential premises, especially in the evening.

1.33 Tolerance, dependence and addiction

A MORI poll carried out in 1991 showed that 78% of the people interviewed agreed with the statement that 'antidepressants are addictive'. The recent publicity around 'Seroxat' in the media has only served to reinforce this misconception, but is quite rightly a serious concern for many people. This section includes the way the author's service discusses the topic with service users and carers and allows them to make up their own minds.

For a drug to be addictive, or produce dependence, it must have at least four main features. It must produce:

1. Desire or craving, ie. the person must crave another dose of the drug when the previous one is wearing, or has worn, off.
2. Withdrawal symptoms, ie. a specific set of symptoms which start when the drug wears off and which disappear when the next dose is taken.
3. Tolerance, ie. the person gets used to the effect, which can be the therapeutic effect or side-effects.
4. An immediate effect ie. do people receive a reinforcement when they take it. In addition, a drug needs to have some reward ie. the person knows they have had a dose.

If we list some drugs which effect the brain and look at these features we can see some differences: Generally speaking, the known drugs of abuse can produce craving, withdrawal symptoms and tolerance to their desired actions and are taken for their immediate effect. Most prescribed drugs do not cause craving, have no significant withdrawal symptoms and no tolerance to the therapeutic effects are seen. Furthermore, as you can see from the right hand column, all are helping to correct a known chemical imbalance in the brain.

	Does the drug produce:			
Drug or Craving	**Craving or desire**	**Dependence? ie. a specific withdrawal syndrome**	**Tolerance? ie. need more to get the same effect**	**An immediate effect?**
Alcohol	Yes	Yes eg. DTs	Yes	Yes
Caffeine	Yes	Yes eg. headaches	Yes	Yes
Smoking/nicotine	Yes	Yes	Yes	Yes
Amphetamines	Yes	Yes	Yes	Yes
Heroin etc.	Yes	Yes eg. cold turkey	Yes	Yes
Gambling	Yes	Yes	Yes	Yes
Cannabis	Yes	No, except high doses for prolonged periods	Yes	Yes
Hypnotics	Sometimes (for sleep)	Sometimes eg. 'rebound' insomnia	Sometimes	Yes
Benzodiazepines	Sometimes but usually not with appropriate use	Sometimes	Sometimes	Sometimes
Antidepressants	No	With some drugs sometimes, if abrupt	Possibly in about 5–10% cases	No
Neuroleptics	No	Not usually — can happen with phenothiazines	No	Sometimes

A few antidepressants, antipsychotics/ neuroleptics and benzodiazepines may produce some discontinuation effects if stopped abruptly, argueably more an 'adjustment reaction' than withdrawal (see *Chapter 2.2.2, section 13*). Gradual stopping usually solves the problem. Stopping lithium quickly can also be a problem (see *1.9*).

2.
Selecting psychotropic drugs and dosage

2.1 Comparative information

Table 2.1.1: Hypnotics — relative side-effects

Drug	Usual night dose mg/d	Adult max. dose mg/d	>Elderly max dose mg/d	Half-life (hours)		G/I upset	Hang-over	Depen-dence potential
				adult	elderly			
Shorter-acting benzodiazipines								
Loprazolam	1	2	1	7–15	20	○	●	●
Lormetazepam	1	1.5+	<Ad	10	14	○	●	●
Temazepam	10–20	40	20	5–11	14+	○	●	●●
Longer-acting benzodiazipines (potential for accumulation)								
Flunitrazepam*	1	2	1	35	35	○	●●	●
Flurazepam*	15	30	15+	47–95	?	○	●●●	●●
Nitrazepam	5	10	5	18–36	40+	○	●●●	●
Chloral and derivatives								
Chloral betane	707	5 tabs	<Ad?	7–10	Same	●●●	●	●
Triclofos	1 g	2 g	1 g	?	?	●	?	?
Other hypnotics								
Clomethiazole	N/A#	2caps#	Same	4–5	Same	○	●	●●
Promethazine	25	50	–	?	?	○	○	○
Zaleplon	10	10	5	2	3	○	○	○
Zolpidem	5	(10)	10	2(2–5)	Longer	○	○	○
Zopiclone	7.5	7.5	<Ad	35–6	8	●	●	●

Side-effects:
●●● = marked effect
●● = moderate effect
● = mild effect

○ = little or nothing
? = no information available

\# = indicated for severe insomnia in the elderly only
 * = Black-listed in UK

Table 2.1.2: Anxiolytics — relative doses and side-effects

Drug	Average dose mg/ day	Adult max dose mg/d	Elderly max dose mg/d	Half-life(hrs) adult (+range)	elderly	Drowsi-ness	Depen-dence potential
Shorter-acting benzodilazipines (minimal accumulation)							
Alprazolam*	1	3	0.75	14(6–20)	Longer	••	••
Bromazepam*	9	18–60	< Ad	16(9–20)	?	••	••
Lorazepam	4	4	< Ad	12(8–25)	Same	•••	•••
Oxazepam	30	120	80	8(5–15)	Same	•••	••
Longer-acting benzodiazipines (potential for accumulation)							
Chlordiazepoxide	30	100	< 50	12(6–30)	Longer	•••	••
Clobazam*	30	60	20	18(9–77)	Longer	•	••
Clorazepate*	15	15?	< Ad	PD	Longer	•••	••
Diazepam	6	30	15	32(21–50)	Longer	•••	••
Beta-blockers							
Oxprenolol	80	80	80	4#(3–6)	Same	•	o
Propranolol	80	120	–	2#(1–2)	Same	•	o
Other anxiolytics							
Buspirone	30	45	45	7(2–11)	Same	o	o

Side-effects:

••• = marked effect   o = little or nothing
•• = moderate effect   ? = no information available
• = mild effect

Adult max dose = Maximum adult dose, most only recommended for up to four weeks at this dose
Elderly max dose = Maximum elderly dose, most only recommend that half the adult dose should be adequate
PD = pro-drug metabolised to desmethyldiazepam (long-half-life)
# = pharmacological action longer than suggested by the half-life
* = Black-listed in UK

Table 2.1.3: Antidepressants — relative side-effects

Drug	Adult max dose mg/d (SPC)	Elderly max dose mg/d (SPC)	Relative side-effects (most are dose-related)					
			Anticho-linergic	Cardiac	Nausea	Seda-tion	Toxicity in over-dose	Procon-vulsant poten-tial
Tricyclics								
Amitriptyline	200	75	•••	•••	••	•••	•••	••
Clomipramine	250	75	•••	••	••	••	•	••
Dothiepin/ dosulepin	150	75	••	••	o	•••	•••	••
Doxepin	300	< Ad	•	••	•	••	••	••
Imipramine	300	50	••	••	••	•	•••	••
Lofepramine	210	< Ad	••	•	•	•	o	o
Maprotiline	150	75	••	••	••	•	•••	•••
Nortriptyline	150	50	••	•	••	•	••	•
Trimipramine	300	< Ad	•••	••	•	••	••	•
SSRIs (Selective serotonin reuptake inhibitors)								
Citalopram	60	40	o	o	••	o	o	o
Escitalopram	20	< 20	o	o	••	o	o	o
Fluoxetine	(20)	(80)	o	o	••	o	o	o
Fluvoxamine	300	300	•	o	•••	•	o	o
Paroxetine	50	40	o	o	••	o	o	o
Sertraline	200	200	o	o	••	o	o	o
MAOIs (Mono-amine oxidase inhibitors)								
Isocarboxazid	60	< Ad	••	••	••	o	••	o
Phenelzine	90	(90)	•	•	••	o	••	o
Tranylcypromine	CA30	(30)	•	•	••	•	•••	o
Others								
Flupentixol	3	2	••	o	o	•	•	?
Mianserin	90+	< Ad	•	o	o	•••	o	o
Mirtazapine	45	45	o	o	o	••	o	o
Moclobemide	600	600	•	o	•	o	o	o
Reboxetine	12	NR	•	•	•	o	o	o
Trazodone	600	≡300	•	•	•••	••	•	o
Tryptophan	6 g	6 g	o	o	•	••	•	o
Venlafaxine	375	375	o	••	••	•	••	•

Side-effects:

••• = marked effect   o = little or nothing
•• = moderate effect   ? = no information available
• = mild effect   CA = Care

Table 2.1.4 Antipsychotics/neuroleptics – relative side-effects

Drugs	Adult max dose mg/d (SPC)	Elderly max dose mg/d (SPC)	Relative side-effects at average dose					
			Anti-cholin-ergic	Cardiac	ESPE	Hypo-tension	Sedation	Minor O/D
Typicals — phenothiazines								
Chlorpromazine	1000	< Ad	•••	••	••	•••	•••	•••
Levomepromazine	1000	NR	•••	•••	••	•••	•••	?
Promazine	800	< Ad	••	••	•	••	••	••
Thioridazine	600	< Ad	••	•••	•	••	••	••
Pericyazine	(300)	< Ad	•	••	•	••	•••	••
Fluphenazine	CA20	CA10	••	••	•••	•	••	••
Perphenazine	24	< Ad	•	••	•••	•	••	••
Trifluoperazine	–	< Ad	o	••	•••	•	•	••
Typicals — others, more dopamine specific								
Amisulpride	1200	1200	o	o	•	o	o	o
Flupentixol	18	< Ad	••	o	••	o	•	•
Haloperidol	30	30	•	••	•••	•	•	•
Pimozide	20	< Ad	•	•••	••	••	•	•
Sulpiride	2400	2400	•	o	•	o	•	•
Zuclopenthixol	150	< Ad	••	•	•••	•	••	••
Second generation/Atypicals								
Aripiprazole	30	TBA	o	o	o	o	o	o
Clozapine	900	(900)	•••	•••	o	•	•••	?
Olanzapine	20	20	•	o	o	o	••	o
Quetiapine	750	< Ad	•	•	o	•	•	?
Risperidone	(16)	4	o	o	•	•	•?	?
Sertindole	20	(20)	o	••	o	••	o	o
Zotepine	300	150	••	••	•	••	•	?
Depot and long-acting injections (max dose per week)								
Fluphenazine	50	< Ad	••	•	•••	•	••	•
Flupenthixol	400	< Ad	•••	o	••	o	•	•
Haloperidol	75	< Ad	•	•	•••	•	••	?
Pipothiazine	50	< Ad	••	••	••	•	•	?
Risperidone	25	12.5	o	o	•	•	•	?
Zuclopenthixol	600	< Ad	••	•	•••	•	••	?

Side-effects:
••• = marked effect
•• = moderate effect
• = mild effect

o = little or nothing
? = no information available

2.2   Switching or discontinuing psychotropics

Switching psychotropics can be surprisingly difficult. A variety of methods (varying in rate, overlap, gap and complexity) can be used. These are summarised in the graphs and comments shown.

Switch 1: drug-free interval

(discontinue first drug, leave drug-free interval, introduce second drug):

Advantages:

1. Minimises combined side-effects.
2. Minimal interaction potential.
3. Side-effects from the second drug are less likely to be confused with discontinuation effects from first drug (eg. as in SSRIs).
4. Low medication error potential.

Disadvantages:

1. Delays desired relief of symptoms or side-effects.
2. Fear of relapse during gap and changeover (probably rare if stable and gap not prolonged).
3. Early relapse might be seen as lack of efficacy of second drug.

Switch 2: No interval

(stop first drug, start second immediately)

Advantages:

1. Easy.
2. Low potential for drug error.
3. Appropriate where an acute, severe reaction to a drug has occurred.

Disadvantages:

1. May raise unrealistic expectations from patient of a rapid improvement on the second drug.
2. Combined ADRs may occur, albeit short-lived.
3. Potential for drug interactions if the first drug has a long half-life.
4. Rapid discontinuation may produce withdrawal effects from the first drug, which might be interpreted as side-effects of the second.

Switching psychotropics

1. Drug-free interval (safest)

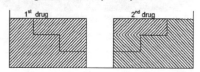

2. No interval (generally preferred)

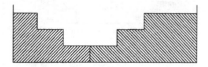

3. Partial overlap (usually OK)

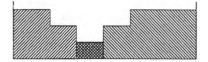

4. Full overlap (risks NMS or serotonin syndrome and combined ADRs)

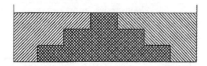

5. Avoid (switch never completed, resulting in polypharmacy)

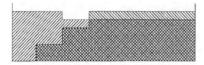

Switch 3: Partial overlap

(Add new drug, either at standard dose or quickly titrated upwards, while slowly tapering the first drug)

Advantages:

1. Useful for side-effects of first drug but there is a higher relapse risk.
2. No sudden changes occur, which might destabilise the patient.
3. Useful for high potency antipsychotics (eg. haloperidol) to an atypical, and from a low potency drug where cholinergic rebound may occur. Either way, anticholinergic cover can be retained for several weeks.

Disadvantages:

1. If taper is too quick, two drugs may be given at sub-therapeutic doses.
2. Combined ADRs will/may occur.
3. Potential for drug interactions, especially with antidepressants.
4. Potential for medication errors if not planned fully in advance — involve carers and patient if patient is at home.
5. High potential for multiple drugs if the switch is never completed, eg. if discharged and message not passed on, or the patient improves and there is a reluctance to discontinue the first drug (see Switch 5) and possibly destabilise the patient

Switch 4: Full overlap

(add new drug to therapeutic dose and then slowly taper previous drug)

Advantages:

1. Safest if relapse prevention of greatest concern.
2. Low risk of discontinuation effects of the first drug.
3. Slow taper is possible and is better for drugs with high anticholinergic activity.

Disadvantages:

1. Combined ADRs may occur.
2. Highest potential for drug interactions.
3. Potential for medication errors if not planned and completed fully.
4. High potential for polypharmacy if switch never completed, eg. if discharged and message not passed on, or patient improves and there is a reluctance to discontinue the first drug and possibly destabilise the patient.

2.2.1 Switching antipsychotics/ neuroleptics — dose equivalents

Switching an antipsychotic may need to be carried out for a number of reasons, eg. side-effects, poor response etc. Switching risks relapse and is usually best done under the supervision of a psychiatrist as not all antipsychotics are equally effective, or have the same side-effects, in a given patient, but the table on *page 68* may be useful. The dose(s) of each drug within this section is approximately equivalent in **antipsychotic** potency to others under the same heading (eg. perphenazine 24mg/d is equivalent to chlorpromazine 300mg/d and to flupentixol 60mg 2/52). Inter-patient variability, differing half-lives and conflicting data means that the figures can never be exact and should be interpreted using your own pharmacological experience, bearing in mind the *BNF* limits for drug doses (especially since many of these have been reduced recently).

Antipsychotics displace ligands from dopamine receptors at a rate that correlates with their antipsychotic potency and so *roughly equivalent* antipsychotic doses can be calculated. Sedation and anxiety may not be directly related to dopamine blockade. It is important to note that **antipsychotic equivalence** is specifically quoted here and the doses quoted are as accurate as data allows but to avoid any confusion you *must* also consider the following:

1. *Antipsychotic* equivalence should not be confused with *sedative* equivalence, eg. haloperidol has a relatively low sedative effect and, indeed, there is evidence that there is no extra antipsychotic effect from haloperidol doses above 12mg/d.
2. With some drugs there may not be a linear relationship between dose and antipsychotic effect, and some may have a therapeutic window.
3. Dose frequency with depots may be important as the first-pass effect may reduce the effective doses of oral preparations.

Drug	mg/d (+range)
Typicals-phenothiazines	
Chlorpromazine	100mg (= 250mg rectally, 25–50mg IM)
Fluphenazine	2mg (1.25–5mg)
Pericyazine	24mg
Perphenazine	8mg (7–15mg)
Levomepromazine	NK
Promazine	100mg (50–200mg)
Thioridazine	100mg (75–104mg)
Trifluoperazine	5mg (2–8mg)
Typicals-dopamine specific	
Benperidol	2mg
Haloperidol	3–5mg (1.5–5mg)
Flupentixol	2mg
Zuclopenthixol	25mg (25–50) up to 150mg/d
Amisulpride	100mg (40–150mg)
Pimozide	2mg (1–3) (long $t_{\frac{1}{2}}$)
Sulpiride	200mg (200–333mg)
Second generation/atypicals	
Aripiprazole	NA
Clozapine	50–100mg (30–150mg)
Olanzapine	NA
Quetiapine	NA
Risperidone	0.5–1mg
Sertindole	NA
Zotepine	NA
Depot	**mg/week**
Risperidone Consta	NA
Fluphenazine	5mg (1–12.5mg)
Pipothiazine	10mg (10–12.5mg)
Haloperidol	15mg (5–25mg)
Flupentixol	10mg (10–20mg)
Zuclopenthixol	100mg (40–100mg)
Fluspirilene	2mg (NE)

4. If using a 'broad-spectrum' drug (eg. chlorpromazine) and converting to a receptor-selective drug (eg. flupentixol, sulpiride etc as dopamine D2-selective), the use of straight conversion tables may not be appropriate and may result in enhanced side-effects.

5. Differing half-lives may complicate the calculations.

6. These equivalent doses are not necessarily equivalent in terms of maximum doses in the *BNF*/UK SPC.

You should always **check your answer against *BNF*/UK SPC limits** to ensure an inappropriately high dose is not inadvertently considered.

Before switching to atypical antipsychotics

1. Warn about possible ADRs (eg. weight gain, short-term sedation, implications of reduced prolactin levels).
2. Need for adequate trial and need to complete switch.
3. Agree how to define success or failure, and the chances thereof.
4. Warn that the new drug isn't perfect — you're swapping one set of side-effects for another.

Assessing response:

1. For all drugs, aim for a minimum of 3 months at full therapeutic dosage.
2. Be cautious of any significant gains (eg. reduced side-effects) within 6/52 of the last drug stopping — receptor effects may outlast plasma levels and a gradual loss of side-effects may be interpreted as improvement.
3. Raised prolactin levels may take over 3/12 to resolve, so women need to be warned about this, and to ensure they have adequate contraceptive cover.
4. If positive changes occur, warn the patient not to risk relapse by 'over doing it'.
5. Initial response followed by worsening of positive symptoms — check worsening is not actually improvement (eg. hidden symptoms now surfacing), try to restabilise and aim for 12/52 at full dose.

Advice on specific switches

1. Phenothiazine to phenothiazine:
Get dose equivalent right, then switches 2 or 3 are probably reasonable.

2. Phenothiazine to specific D2-blocker:
Get dose equivalent as best as possible, then switches 2 or 3 are probably OK but beware of cholinergic rebound (nausea, vomiting, restlessness, anxiety, insomnia,

Switching antipsychotics

From \ To	Pheno-thiazines	D2 blockers	Typical depots	Aripiprazole	Clozapine	Olanzapine	Risperidone	Consta	Quetiapine
Phenothiazines	RT (1)	RT (2)	RT (3)	RT (4, 16)	Care (5, 16)	NOP (6, 16)	RT (7)	RT (8)	RT (9, 16)
D2 blockers	RT (10)	RT (11)	RT (3)	RT (4, 16)	Care (5, 16)	NOP (6, 16)	RT (7)	RT (8)	RT (9, 16)
Typical depots	RT (12)	RT (12)	RT (12)	RT (4, 12, 16)	Care (5, 12, 16)	RT (6, 12, 16)	RT (7, 12)	RT (8, 12)	RT (9, 12, 16)
Aripiprazole	RT (4)	RT (4)	RT (4)		Care (4)	RT (4)	RT (4)	RT (4)	NOP (4)
Clozapine	Care (5)	Care (5)	Care (5)	RT (4)		Care (6)	RT (5)	RT (8)	RT (9)
Olanzapine	NOP (13)	NOP (13)	NOP (13)	RT (4, 13)	Care (5, 13)		RT (7, 13)	RT (8, 13)	NOP (9, 13)
Risperidone	RT (14)	RT (14)	RT (14)	RT (4, 14, 16)	Care (5, 14, 16)	NOP (6, 14, 16)		RT (8, 14)	NOP (9, 14, 16)
Risperdal Consta	RT (8)	RT (8)	RT (8)	RT (8, 16)	Care (8, 16)	RT (8, 16)	RT (8)		RT (8, 16)
Quetiapine	NOP (15)	NOP (15)	NOP (15)	RT (4, 15)	Care (5, 15)	NOP (6, 15)	RT (7, 15)	RT (8, 15)	

NOP = no obvious problems

RT = read text

Care = Great care needed, also read text

fatigue, GI distress) and stronger D2-blockade leading to additional EPSE.

3. Phenothiazine/D2-blocker to depot typical:
Studies have shown this is usually straight forward, remembering that typical depots' peak plasma level (see box) and so reduce doses accordingly. Beware of additive EPSEs.

4. Anything to aripiprazole:
Aripiprazole binds only relatively weakly to dopamine receptors, and so the clinical effect of aripiprazole will only start as the previous antipsychotic clears from the system, which would be gradually over several weeks or even months. Warn women about possible normalisation of prolactin and need for adequate oral con-traception if necessary. In one switching study outcomes and side effects were similar for abrupt, double-cross-taper and abrupt start and gradual discontinuation.

5. Anything to clozapine:
Initiation is Consultant Psychiatrist only. Care would be needed with the increased risk of dyscrasias with phenothiazines and delayed clearance of depots (especially Consta). Generally accepted that switch 2 is usually appropriate.

6. Switching to olanzapine:
Risperidone to olanzapine: one study in stable but still symptomatic schizophrenic out-patients showed switch 4 was the most successful; limited overlap switch 3 was best for elderly or frail patients and switch 2 had the poorest outcomes (mostly sleep-related problems). Prolactin warning (see 16).

7. Various to risperidone:
Hypotension may occur so gradually dose titrate over at least 3/7 to 4mg/d (or longer if possible). One study recommended switch 3 (limited overlap) as better than abrupt switches.

8. Various to/from Risperdal Consta:
Remember the 4–6 week delay before plasma levels start reaching therapeutic levels, so cover may be needed from oral medication in the interim. Consta may have the best chance of success if the person has been shown to respond to oral risperidone first.

Typical depot to Consta: Start Consta one week before the last fortnightly injection, and be prepared for additional oral cover.

Oral risperidone to Consta: Continue risperidone for 3–4 weeks, then gradually discontinue in weeks 4–5.

Consta to others: The last dose of Consta will finally stop releasing risperi-done about 6 weeks later, so wait, then introduce the new drug gradually from about day 42.

9. Anything to quetiapine:
Warn women about possible normalisation of prolactin (see 16) and need for adequate oral contraception if necessary.

Phenothiazine to quetiapine: switch 3 may be OK, but be aware of additional initial postural hypotension, so a slightly slower dose titration or additional monitoring might be prudent.

D2-blocker to quetiapine: switch 2 or 3 should be tolerable, as receptor blockade

Comparison of depots Long-acting injections

	Peak (days)	Usual frequency	Main duration	Depot half-life	Time to steady state from first dose
Flupenthixol	7–10	2/52	2–4/52	7/7	10–12/52
Fluphenazine	1–2	2–4/52	3–4/52	14/7	6–12/52
Fluspirilene	1–2	1/52	1/52	7/7	5–6/52
Halopendol	3–9	4/52	4/52	21–28/7	10–12/52
Pipothiazine	9–10	4/52	4/52	21–28/7	8–12/52
Zuclopenthixol	4–9	2/52	2–4/52	7/7	10–12/52
Risperidone	35	2/52	2–3/52	?	12/52

with quetiapine is quite different to that of standard D2 blockers.

Typical depot to quetiapine: switch 2 should be tolerable, starting quetiapine when the next depot dose is due.

Aripiprazole to quetiapine: N/K

Clozapine to quetiapine: Switches 2, 3 or 4 should be tolerable, depending on the reason for switch. The two have been used together to help reduce weight gain.

Olanzapine to quetiapine: Any switch should be acceptable.

Risperidone to quetiapine: switch 2 or 3 should be tolerable.

10. D2-blockers to phenothiazines: Switches 2 or 3 should be considered first.

11. D2-blocker to D2-blocker: Consider switches 1–3 first, bearing in mind the potential for NMS and additional EPSE. Prolactin warning (see 16).

12. Depot typicals to others: Stop depot and introduce the next drug when the next depot dose would be due, remembering that a slow decay in depot plasma levels may occur so beware of adding a new drug too quickly. Depots are occasionally given more often than strictly necessary.

Typical depot to typical depot: not usually a problem, with a direct switch often possible.

13. Olanzapine to anything: No apparent problems with stopping olanzapine suddenly, so any switch should be tolerable.

14. Risperidone to anything: There are no obvious problems with stopping or switching risperidone (eg. interactions, except potential for NMS, prolactin warning (see 16) and additive EPSE if switching to a phenothiazine or D2-blocker) so switches 2 or 3 should be OK.

15. Quetiapine to anything: Few obvious problems with stopping or switching quetiapine (except perhaps NMS) so switches 2 or 3 should be OK.

16. Prolactin warning: Warn women about the possibility that raised prolactin (particularly with D2-blockers) may be causing amenorrhoea, and normalisation of prolactin with the new drug may occur. Adequate oral contraception may thus be needed.

2.2.1.2 Discontinuing antipsychotics
Withdrawal symptoms (eg. tardive psychosis, dyskinesias etc) have been reported upon abrupt discontinuation eg. cholinergic rebound-headache, restlessness, diarrhoea, nausea and vomiting. With gradual withdrawal, the risk of relapse is lower.

2.2.1.3 Long-term issues
With improvements in insight, increased psychosocial support and monitoring will be needed to reduce the risk of post-psychotic depression and self-harm.

2.2.2 Switching benzodiazepines

Switching benzodiazepines may be advantageous for a variety of reasons, eg. to a drug with a different half-life pre-discontinuation. While there is broad agreement in the literature about equivalent doses, clonazepam has a wide variety of reported equivalences and particular care is needed with this drug. Interpatient variability and differing half-lives means the figures can never be exact and should be interpreted using your own pharmaceutical knowledge.

BENZODIAZEPINES	
See note in introduction re: half lives	
Diazepam	5mg (all routes)
Alprazolam	0.5mg
Bromazepam	3mg
Chlordiazepoxide	15mg +/– 5mg
Clobazam	10mg
Clonazepam	0.5mg (0.25–4)
Clorazepate	7.5mg
Flunitrazepam	0.5mg
Flurazepam	7.5mg–15mg
Loprazolam	0.5–1mg
Lorazepam	0.5–1mg at ≤4mg/d 2mg at ≥5mg/d
Lormetazepam	0.5–1mg
Nitrazepam	5mg
Oxazepam	15mg
Temazepam	10mg

2.2.3 Switching antidepressants

Switching from one antidepressant to another, either for reasons of side-effects or lack of efficacy, can be surprisingly problematical. It is often necessary to leave gaps of drug-free days, eg. the 14-day gap after stopping an MAOI before starting another antidepressant is well known. However, other problems may occur and the prescriber must be aware of these to avoid unnecessary adverse events.

Factors that must be considered before choosing a switch regimen:

1. **Speed** at which the switch is needed, eg. with less urgency a more cautious regimen can be used. Since many drugs are used in combination, faster switches can obviously be made, but additional monitoring is recommended.
2. Current dose of the first drug (higher dose will cause more problems).
3. Individual drugs and their neurotransmitter effects, kinetics etc.
4. Individuals susceptibility to (additive) side-effects.

Main problems:

1. Cholinergic rebound, eg. headache, restlessness, diarrhoea, nausea and vomiting from withdrawal of drugs affecting acetylcholine eg. tricyclics.
2. Antidepressant withdrawal or discontinuation symptoms (see 13).
3. Serotonin Syndrome for drugs affecting serotonin (see *Chapter 1.12*).
4. Interaction between the two drugs, eg. altered drug levels from altered metabolism (see *Chapter 4.3*).

How to use the tables (Pages 74–75)

❖ Look down the vertical column headed 'from' and find the drug or drug group that the patient is currently taking.
❖ Follow that line along until you come to the column of the drug to which you wish to change.
❖ The details there give the current known information. For further details look up the reference number quoted.

Example: Changing from tranylcypromine to a tricyclic requires a 14-day drug-free gap (*Reference 9*) but changing from a tricyclic to tranylcypromine only requires a 7-day drug-free gap (*Reference 9*).

1. MAOI→MAOI:

Different MAOIs may interact with each other and deaths have been reported (see *Chapter 4.3.4*). A two-week gap is recommended especially if the MAOI is changed to tranylcypromine. The UK SPC for **tranylcypromine** recommends leaving at least a seven-day gap after stopping other antidepressants, then starting tranylcypromine at half the usual dosage for one week. If changing from tranylcypromine to another antidepressant, a two-week drug-free gap is recommended.

2. SSRI→tricyclic:

Fluoxetine, paroxetine and fluvoxamine (but not citalopram or sertraline at standard doses) can double or triple tricyclic antidepressant levels by P450 enzyme inhibition and so care is needed. Running both drugs together over a change-over period is not advised unless the drugs are chosen carefully and specific care is taken. Ideally 'drop-and-stop' before starting the next drug is recommended.

Factors which must be considered before choosing a switch-regimen:
● Speed
● SSRI dose, eg. doses above standard
● Tricyclic — interactions vary
● P450 status of the patient — not routinely detectable but be aware of severe reactions
● Individual susceptibility to tricyclic and SSRI side-effects.

Potential problems
● Cholinergic rebound (see *introduction*)
● TCA/SSRI discontinuation symptoms (see *13*)
● Serotonin syndrome (see *1.12*)
● Increased tricyclic levels from decreased metabolism (see *4.3*).

Suggested switch regimens

Tricyclic→fluoxetine, paroxetine or fluvoxamine — taper tricyclic to no more than 20mg/d, start SSRI at usual dose and discontinue tricyclic over the next 5–7 days, with careful observation. Be wary of serotonin syndrome, raised tricyclic levels, cholinergic rebound or tricyclic withdrawal.

Tricyclic→citalopram or sertraline — Taper tricyclic to around 50mg/d, start SSRI at standard dose and discontinue tricyclic over next 5–7 days. Be wary of cholinergic rebound, serotonin syndrome and tricyclic withdrawal.

Fluoxetine→tricyclic — Stop fluoxetine, wait several days for peak levels to fall, then add tricyclic cautiously at low dose and build up slowly. Care is needed for up to four weeks. Be wary of serotonin syndrome (especially with clomipramine, for example) and higher tricyclic levels via CYP2D6 inhibition.

Paroxetine→tricyclic — Taper paroxetine dose to about 10mg/d, and introduce tricyclic at low dose. After several days, withdraw paroxetine and increase tricyclic dose to therapeutic levels. Be wary of paroxetine withdrawal, serotonin syndrome (especially with clomipramine) and higher tricyclic levels via CYP2D6 inhibition.

Fluvoxamine→tricyclic — As paroxetine. Be wary of fluvoxamine withdrawal (rare), serotonin syndrome (especially with eg. clomipramine) and higher tricyclic levels via enzyme inhibition.

Citalopram/sertraline→tricyclic — If necessary, reduce to standard doses of citalopram (20mg/d) or sertraline (50mg/d), then stop the SSRI and introduce the tricyclic, titrating the dose upwards. Few problems should be seen but be wary of SSRI withdrawal (rare), serotonin syndrome (especially with, eg. clomipramine) and higher tricyclic levels via CYP2D6 inhibition

3. Trazodone →others:

Trazodone and fluoxetine have been used together with only a few reports of enhanced sedation. A gradual switch with observation would seem adequate. There is no information on changing from trazodone to any of the SSRIs at present but assuming a similar situation would be sensible until more data is available. See also 5.

4. Tricyclic →tricyclic:

No significant problem reported. A gradual switch is recommended.

5. SSRI →SSRI:

Any combination of SSRIs could in theory predispose to the serotonin syndrome (see The Serotonin Syndrome box (*page 21*) in *1.12*). In a report of a 'therapeutic substitution', 54 patients were abruptly swapped from fluoxetine to sertraline. 34 swapped successfully and 20 failed, including 10 with intolerable adverse effects (nervousness, jitters, nausea and headache, suggestive of a serotonin-like syndrome) and 2 with lack of efficacy. Thus initial careful observation and a gentle change-over is needed. A washout period would further minimise the possibility of problems. Rapid changing from **fluoxetine** to **paroxetine** has caused insomnia, nausea, dry mouth, nervousness and tremor.

6. Mianserin:

The only recommendation for **mianserin** is a 2-week washout period when changing to or from MAOIs.

7. MAOIs →SSRIs:

The time to wait between starting an MAOI and stopping an SSRI varies depending upon the respective SSRI. The *BNF* recommends a two-week gap from the SSRIs before an MAOI is started but this appears only to be strictly correct for paroxetine. The UK SPC for tranylcypromine recommends leaving at least a seven-day gap after stopping other antidepressants, then starting tranylcypromine at half the usual dosage for one week.

Citalopram→MAOI — 7-day gap (manufacturers' information).

Fluvoxamine→MAOI — Isocarboxazid/ phenelzine may be started 4–5 days after stopping fluvoxamine or 7 days for tranylcypromine.

Table 2.2.3.1: Switching antidepressants

From \ To	MAOIs		Tricyclics	SSRIs				
	Hydra-zines	Tranyl-cypro-mine		Citalo-pram/escitalo-pram	Fluvox-amine	Fluox-etine	Sertra-line	Parox-etine
MAOIS Hydra-zines	$14/7^1$	$14/7^1$	$7–14/7^9$	$14/7^7$	$14/7^7$	$14/7^7$	$14/7^7$	$14/7^7$
MAOIS Tranyl-cypro-mine	$14/7^1$		$14/7^9$	$14/7^7$	$14/7^7$	$14/7^7$	$14/7^7$	$14/7^7$
Tricyclics	$7/7^9$	$7/7^9$	NSPR^4	Care^2	Great Care^2	Great Care^2	Care^2	Great Care^2
Citalopram/ escitalopram	$7/7^7$	$7/7^7$	Care^2		SSP^5	SSP^5	SSP^5	SSP^5
Fluvoxamine	$4/7^7$	$7–14/7^7$	Great care^2	SSP^5		SSP^5	SSR^5	SSR^5
Fluoxetine	$5/52^7$	$5/52^7$	Great care for $28/7^2$	SSP^5	SSP^5		SSP^5	SSP^5
Sertraline	$7/7^7$	$7–14/7^7$	Care^2	SSP^5	SSP^5	SSP^5		SSP^5
Paroxetine	$14/7^7$	$14/7^7$	Great care^2	SSP^5	SSP^5	SSP^5	SSP^5	
Trazodone Nefazodone	$7/7^{6,7}$	$7/7^{6,7}$	OP^{13}	Care^{3,6}	Care^{3,6}	Care^{3,6}	Care^{3,6}	Care^{3,6}
Tryptophan	$14/7^{10}$ or care	$7–14/7^{10}$ or care	NSPR	Care^{11}	Care^{11}	Care^{11}	Care^{11}	Care^{11}
Moclobemide	NSPR^7	NSPR^7	OP^{15}	NSPR^8	NSPR^8	$2/52^8$	NSPR^8	NSPR^8
Venlafaxine	$7/7^{16}$	$7/7^{16}$	NSPR^{16}	Care^{16}	Care^{16}	Care^{16}	Care^{16}	Care^{16}
Mirtazapine	$7/7^7$	$7/7^7$	NSPR^{12}	NSPR^{12}	NSPR^{12}	NSPR^{12}	NSPR^{12}	NSPR^{12}
Mianserin	$14/7^1$	$14/7^1$	NSPR	NSPR	NSPR	NSPR	NSPR	NSPR
Reboxetine	$1/52^{17}$	$1/52^{17}$	NSPR^{17}	NSPR^{17}	NSPR^{17}	NSPR^{17}	NSPR^{17}	NSPR^{17}
Just plain stopping:^{17}	Over $4/52^{17}$	Over $4/52^{73}$	Over $4/52^{17}$	Over $4/52^{17}$	Over $4/52^{17}$	Reduce to 20mg/d, then stop^{17}	Over $4/52^{17}$	Over $4/52^{17}$ or longer

NSPR = No significant problems reported, careful cross-taper
OP   = Occasional problems
SSP = Serotonin Syndrome possible (see ref 5)
NB: Patients with bipolar mood disorders should be monitored closely for manic epi-
    sodes following discontinuation or change of any antidepressant medication (*J Clin
    Psych* 1985, **5**, 342–3)

From \ To	Trazo-done[16] Nefa-zodone	Trypto-phan	Moclo-bemide	Venla-faxine[16]	Mirtaza-pine	Mianserin	Reboxe-tine
M A O I S — Hydra-zines	14/7[6,7]	14/7[10] or care	1/7[7] with care	14/7[16]	2/52[7]	14/7[1]	2/52
M A O I S — Tranyl-cypro-mine	14/7[6,7]	1/7[10]	7/7[1,7] with care	14/7[16]	2/52[7]	14/7[1]	2/52
Tricyclics	NSPR	NSPR[10]	NSPR[15]	Variable[16]	NSPR[12]	NSPR	NSPR
Citalopram/ escitalopram	Care[3,6]	Care[11]	7/7[14]	Care[16]	NSPR[12]	NSPR	NSPR
Fluvoxamine	Care[6]	Care[11]	4–5/7[14]	Care[16]	NSPR[12]	NSPR	NSPR
Fluoxetine	Care[6]	Care[11]	4–45/7[14]	Care[16]	NSPR[12]	NSPR	NSPR
Sertraline	Care[6]	Care[11]	4–13/7[14]	Care[16]	NSPR[12]	NSPR	NSPR
Paroxetine	Care[6]	Care[11]	4–5/7[14]	Care[16]	NSPR[12]	NSPR	NSPR
Trazodone Nefazodone	Care[16]	NSPR	NSPR	Care[16]	NSPR[12]	NSPR	NSPR
Tryptophan	NSPR		NSPR	NSPR	NSPR[12]	NSPR	NSPR
Moclobemide	NSPR[6,8]	NSPR		NSPR	NSPR[12]	NSPR	NSPR
Venlafaxine	Care[16]	NSPR[16]	NSPR[16]		NSPR[16]	NSPR[16]	NSPR
Mirtazapine	NSPR[12]	NSPR[12]	NSPR[12]	NSPR[12]		NSPR[12]	NSPR
Mianserin	NSPR	NSPR	NSPR	NSPR	NSPR[12]		NSPR
Reboxetine	NSPR[17]	NSPR[17]	NSPR[17]	NSPR[17]	NSPR[17]	NSPR[17]	
Just plain stopping:	Over 4/52[17]	Over 4/52[17]	Over 4/52[17]	Over 4/52[17] or longer	Over 4/52[17]	Over 4/52[17]	Over 4/52[17]

NSPR = No significant problems reported, careful cross-taper
OP = Occasional problems
SSP = Serotonin Syndrome possible (see ref 5)
NB: Patients with bipolar mood disorders should be monitored closely for manic episodes following discontinuation or change of any antidepressant medication (*J Clin Psych* 1985, **5**, 342–43)

Paroxetine →MAOI — Two-week gap (manufacturers' information).

Fluoxetine →MAOI — Several reported interactions exist (eg. serotonin syndrome) so allow at least a 5-week gap.

Sertraline →MAOI — A one-week gap should elapse before starting an MAOI as a serotonin syndrome has been reported.

Trazodone →MAOI — Less than a one-week gap risks increased side-effects, eg. sedation, postural hypotension etc.

Moclobemide →MAOI — Moclobemide has a half-life of 1–4hrs and so stopping moclobemide one day and starting the next antidepressant the next day is adequate.

Mirtazapine →MAOI — A 2-week washout period is recommended.

MAOI →SSRIs — A 2-week gap (*Drug & Ther Bull* 1990, **28**(9), 334; *BNF*) has been recommended but longer may be safer as a severe serotonin syndrome has been reported even with a two-week gap.

MAOI →trazodone — The UK SPC recommends a 2-week gap after stopping trazodone before MAOIs.

MAOI →moclobemide — The usual 10–14-day gap does not need to be left between stopping an **MAOI** and starting **moclobemide**, provided MAOI dietary restrictions are maintained for 10–14-days. Abrupt swapping of MAOIs has resulted in deaths and careful observation is essential.

MAOI →mirtazapine — A 2-week washout period is recommended.

8. Moclobemide →SSRIs:

Lilly recommend that normal MAOI procedures be observed after **moclobemide**, and so a 2-week gap after stopping moclobemide before starting fluoxetine is stated. This appears overcautious as Roche recommend that when changing to an SSRI only an 8–12-hour gap is needed.

9. MAOI →tricyclic:

MAOIs and tricyclics have been used together uneventfully (see combinations in depression in *1.12*) but have also interacted (see MAOI interactions, *4.3.4*).

MAOIs →tricyclic — A 10–14-day gap is often recommended (isocarboxazid '1–2 weeks') particularly if imipramine, clomipramine or tranylcypromine are involved. Use of initial low doses of the tricyclic is essential.

Tricyclic →MAOI — A one-week gap is recommended (*BNF*) and is advisable particularly if imipramine, clomipramine or tranylcypromine are involved. Using initial low doses of the MAOI is essential.

10. Tryptophan →MAOIs:

Some toxicity has been reported with high dose **tryptophan** and **MAOIs** and so care would seem **advisable. See also** *reference 1.*

11. Tryptophan →SSRIs:

Cases of agitation and nausea have occurred with **tryptophan** and **fluoxetine** and may occur with other SSRIs and so it would be prudent to observe for this. The possibility of a serotonergic syndrome developing should not be ignored.

12. Mirtazapine →others:

Apart from MAOIs (class warning), it is possible to switch to and from mirtazapine without tapering or gaps.

13. Trazodone →tricyclics:

Isolated cases of hypomania and serotonin syndrome have been reported.

14. SSRIs →moclobemide:

Citalopram/escitalopram →moclobemide — a 7-day gap is recommended.

Fluoxetine →moclobemide — a gap of 3-weeks with carefully monitoring should be adequate.

Fluvoxamine →moclobemide — a 3–5-day gap is recommended.

Paroxetine →moclobemide — a 5-day gap is recommended.

Sertraline →moclobemide — a 5–7-day gap is recommended.

15. Tricyclics →moclobemide:

Tricyclic →moclobemide: clomipramine needs a 7-day gap; for the others probably a 3–5-day gap would probably be adequate.

Moclobemide→tricyclic: abrupt switching has been reported to be problem-free so "drop-and-swap" followed by normal tricyclic dose titration should be safe.

16. Venlafaxine →others:

The manufacturers recommend a 14-day gap after stopping an MAOI before starting venlafaxine and a 7-day gap after venlafaxine before an MAOI is used. Wyeth quote that 5 times a tricyclics' half-life should be allowed as a washout time before starting venlafaxine. For some tricyclics this would require leaving a 2–3-week gap, an unnecessarily extended period. The company, however, have no evidence of any problems. There is little data with other drugs but beware of serotonin syndrome with serotonergic drugs such as SSRIs.

17. Discontinuing:

The *Drug and Therapeutics Bulletin* recommends that if antidepressants are used continually for more than two months, then withdrawal slowly over four weeks will minimise the chance of discontinuation reactions. Discontinuation reactions have been reported for many antidepressants, which are more an 'adjustment' reaction than indicative of dependence, which usually requires three of the following (see *1.33*):

● tolerance
● withdrawal symptoms
● use greater than needed
● inability to reduce doses
● excessive time taken procuring drug
● primacy of drug taking over other activities
● continued despite understanding of adverse effects.

Discontinuation symptoms have a number of characteristics, eg. start within 1–14-days of stopping, resolve within 24 hours of restarting the drug and are more common with longer courses or higher doses. They can occur even with missed doses.

Main withdrawal symptoms:
Tricyclics — cholinergic rebound, eg. headache, restlessness, diarrhoea, nausea and vomiting, flu, lethargy, abdominal cramps, sleep disturbance, movement disorders.
MAOIs — confusion, delirium, psychosis, hallucinations.
SSRIs and venlafaxine — dizziness, vertigo or light-headedness, nausea, fatigue, headache, electric shocks in the head, insomnia, abdominal cramps, chills, increased dreaming, agitation, volatility.

Individual drugs (SSRIs):
Citalopram — few published reports to date, even after rapid withdrawal.
Paroxetine — has been associated with more SSRI withdrawal reports than other SSRIs, as well as getting its own TV shows. Studies and case reports include fever, severe fatigue, headache, nausea, vomiting and agitation, and electrical shock-like sensations. A rapid drop in plasma levels on stopping may be the explanation. Symptoms, if occurring, tend to resolve in a few days or on reintroduction of paroxetine. The CSM and UK SPC recommend tapering of paroxetine if withdrawal symptoms occur, ie. stop, if problems occur then restart and taper over 12 weeks.

Fluoxetine — has a long half-life and withdrawal problems are very rare. There are a couple of cases of extreme dizziness and severe, dull, aching pain in the left arm after abrupt fluoxetine withdrawal, which remitted after reintroduction, but people usually interpret it as a mild dose of 'flu' and get over it without consequences.
Fluvoxamine — a slow withdrawal may be preferred.
Sertraline — withdrawal reactions are rare, eg. fatigue, cramps, insomnia etc, and electrical shock-like sensations.

Individual drugs (others):
Mirtazapine — a single case of withdrawal mania is just about all that has been reported.
Moclobemide — 'flu-like symptoms have been reported rarely.

Reboxetine: no withdrawal or discontinuation syndrome has been reported.

Tryptophan — many patients had their tryptophan stopped abruptly after it was withdrawn from the market without apparent serious withdrawal problems, other than recurrence of depression.

Venlafaxine — if used for more than six weeks, it should be withdrawn over at least a week as discontinuation effects within 1–3-days of abrupt withdrawal have included fatigue, headache, nausea, abdominal distension and congested sinuses (resolving within 12 hours of restarting). Venlafaxine may have a particular problem with discontinuation symptoms.

What to do about withdrawal symptoms:

● Test what the symptoms are with a small rechallenge of the antidepressant

— if the symptoms go, then it's the drug that is the culprit

● Use a dose reduction including half-tablet doses (or smaller portions of a tablet if the person is handy with a craft knife), sequentially diluted syrup (eg. with clomipramine, fluoxetine, paroxetine, citalopram — after every dose you take, replace it with some diluent, and the liquid becomes gradually more dilute), use syrup with oral syringes (allowing ever smaller doses).

● If someone is having real problems (and has good eyesight), then the Efexor XL capsule granules are about 0.6mg each and a slow dose reduction could in theory be managed.

● Transfer to fluoxetine, then make use of it's long half-life and gradually withdraw

● Tough it out (easier said than done).

2.3   Weight changes with psychotropic drugs

Importance

Weight gain is relatively common, a potential threat to health, lowers self-esteem, costs the person money to buy replacement clothes and the social embarrassment caused may lead to non-compliance as the person doesn't want to go out. The available data is difficult to compare due to the non-equivalence of collection and presentation, but prescribers must be aware of the potential for this side-effect, which is, not surprisingly, of *great importance* to patients.

2.3.1 Antipsychotics

The top ten league table for antipsychotic-induced weight gain goes roughly like this:
1. Perphenazine (worst)
2. Clozapine
3. Chlorpromazine
4. Olanzapine
5. Thioridazine
6. Quetiapine
7. Risperidone
8. Fluphenazine
9. Polypharmacy
10. Haloperidol (probably close to neutral)

Chlorpromazine appears to have the most potent appetite stimulating effect and up to 80% of people treated with it gain weight, although some don't. Weight gain is common with olanzapine, with up to 40% gaining significant amounts, and this is a major cause for people wanting to switch drugs. Most weight is gained in the first 6–12 months of treatment and then stabilises. Weight gain is unrelated to mental state and so is almost certainly drug-related, but only mildly dose-related. The mechanism is probably a drug-induced increase in appetite (carbohydrate craving), leading to increased food intake.

Management:
"WWW - Warn, weigh and watch"

Warn the patient it might happen, take a baseline weight (for accurate comparison and assessment) and watch to see what happens. If the pounds start to pile on, immediate dietetic advice is needed. Adjusting the dose may help, although only a major reduction is likely to help.

Appetite suppressants may exacerbate psychosis.

2.3.2 Antidepressants

Weight change in depression is well-documented but not well-recognised. Weight loss or gain can be part of the presenting symptoms. Although weight gain with antidepressants may be a reversal of a pre-treatment weight loss in some people (although heavier people are more likely to gain weight if they become depressed), the main mechanism is either a drug-induced appetite increase (carbohydrate craving) or **reduced metabolic rates**. It is not usually a major problem with the SSRIs but it definitely is with the tricyclics.

Tricyclic antidepressants

Weight gain with tricyclics is well known. It is often attributed to improved mood (hence increased appetite) but is more likely to be drug-induced carbohydrate craving via a central 5-HT blockade and a reduced metabolic rate, a double-whammy.

Amitriptyline is known to have marked effects, with one study showing an average of 2.25 kg gained over 6 months. Other studies have shown a similar effect for **imipramine** (eg. 46% of patients gaining between 1 kg and 6 kg) and **clomipramine** (22% of patients gaining an average of 1.1 kg over 8 months).

This is a **major** and much under-rated complaint of people taking therapeutic doses of tricyclics, leading to under-dosing and poor/sub-therapeutic compliance.

SSRIs

Fluoxetine-induced weight loss has been reported, probably via appetite suppression, with more obese patients tending to lose more weight and underweight people actually tending to gain weight. **Paroxetine** has a slight clinically insignificant weight loss potential. **Fluvoxamine** causes a non-significant weight loss. **Sertraline** may have a limited weight gain effect. No significant weight changes have been reported with **citalopram**. The SSRIs are thus an important alternative to

the tricyclics in this respect, although some recent data suggests slight weight loss may occur in the first year, then weight is gained after that.

MAOIs and RIMAs

With the MAOIs, weight gain may occur through a variety of central mechanisms. **Tranylcypromine** is least likely and **phenelzine** the most likely to cause weight gain. In one study with **moclobemide**, there was an overall mean 0.1 kg weight loss in all patients.

Other antidepressants

Slight weight loss seems to occur with **venlafaxine**. There are no reports of appetite changes with **trazodone**. Weight changes have not been reported with **reboxetine** (SPC). Increased appetite and weight gain has been reported in patients treated with **mirtazapine**, anecdotally patients get either little or no weight gain or, in a few cases, substantial carbohydrate craving.

Management

Weight gain with antidepressants is a much under-rated side-effect, leading to dissatisfaction with drug therapy, non-compliance and early relapse. Dose adjustment is possible but risks relapse (although only a major reduction is likely to help). It is best to warn/counsel the patient or alter drugs — the SSRIs are probably the most reliable antidepressants for a low weight change effect.

2.3.3 Lithium

Weight gain is reported to occur in between 11% and 65% of patients on lithium, with about a third claiming to feel more hungry and the majority gaining some weight. Increased thirst has been noted in 89% of lithium takers and strongly correlates with weight gain. Increased hunger/food intake has not been shown and so the predominant mechanism may thus be due to reduced metabolism or an increased intake of high-calorie drinks. Counselling in this area (eg. use plain/low-calorie beverages) along with normal sodium intake may be adequate.

2.3.4 Anticonvulsants

Carbamazepine
One study showed that 8% of patients gained over 5 kg (12lbs) with carbamazepine.

Gabapentin
Some weight gain has been reported in 5% of patients.

Lamotrigine
Weight gain is likely to be minimal.

Tiagabine
No effects have been reported.

Topiramate
Weight loss is not uncommon with topiramate and it has even been abused for this reason.

Valproate
Weight gain, probably attributable to increased appetite, is a recognised side effect and mentioned in the SPC. One study indicated that 20% of patients may gain more than 5 kg (12lbs) in weight.

2.3.5 Others
There are no problems with **acamprosate**, weight loss may, predictably, occur with **methylphenidate** and weight loss may also occur with **bupropion**, although a few people gain weight.

2.4   Sexual dysfunction with psychotropics

Sexual dysfunction of the three phases of sexual activity (desire, excitement/ erection and orgasm) is associated with some psychiatric illnesses, eg. reduced sexual desire/activity in schizophrenia, impotence and loss of libido in depression etc. Drug effects are thus difficult to identify. Many drugs, however, cause sexual problems and luckily this seems to be rapidly reversible on discontinuing treatment. These effects have been attributed to various receptor blocking effects.

The literature does not treat this issue systematically or with a great deal of respect, despite being of the greatest importance to patients, who are often unwilling to volunteer or talk about sexual matters or even realise that they could be drug-related. Such side-effects (and fear thereof) will increase the risk of non-compliance and hence early relapse of the psychiatric illness. With sexual dysfunction incidence rate of 45% in schizophrenics on typical antipsychotics (compared with only 61% people attending a sexual dysfunction clinic), one can see the problem. The incidence of sexual dysfunction with antidepressants (particularly the SSRIs and venlafaxine) can be as high as 60–70%.

Sexual functioning — stages, mechanisms and the effects of psychotropic drug therapies

State	Mechanisms	Drugs reported to enhance	Drugs that inhibit/cause problems	Management of problems
Libido or desire	Controlled by dopamine Facilitated by NA and 5-HT Prolactin *may* be inhibitory Testosterone (male) and estrogen and progesterone (female) essential	Stimulants (enhance dopamine) BDZs (indirectly, reduced anxiety) Bupropion Cannabis (some disinhibition) Moclobemide Mirtazapine (esp. in women) SSRIs (rare) Trazodone (but is sedative) Yohimbine	Anticholinergics Anticonvulsants (esp. barbiturates and phenytoin) Any sedating drug (indirect effect) Any drug increasing prolactin eg antipsychotics etc Lithium SSRIs/SNRIs (indirectly, via inhibition of arousal and orgasm)	Switch drugs (eg. if antidepressant, then switch to mirtazapine or moclobemide) and monitor outcome systematically
Arousal, erection or lubrication	Acetylcholine (facilitates) Adrenergic fibres Dopamine (for arousal) Nitric oxide (NO) — necessary for erection (broken down by PDEs)	*Nitric Oxide enhancers:* Alprostadil (injection only) Apomorphine (stimulates NO) Papaverine (injection only) Sildenafil and PDE inhibitors *Others:* Moclobemide (rare) Pentoxifylline Prostaglandins (erection without stimulation) Yohimbine	Anticholinergic drugs, eg. tricyclics and typical antipsychotics Antipsychotics causing hyperprolactinaemia (infertility, loss of libido, erectile dysfunction) Any drug causing hypotension (eg. typical antipsychotics, tricyclics) Any sedating drug (indirect) MAOIs (40% incidence) Reboxetine (5% incidence) SSRIs (inhibit NO production)	PDE5 inhibitors Switch drugs eg. to atypical, non-TCA/SSRI Withdraw drug (rapidly reversible)

Sexual functioning — stages, mechanisms and the effects of psychotropic drug therapies (Continued)

State	Mechanisms	Drugs reported to enhance	Drugs that inhibit/cause problems	Management of problems
Orgasm	Noradrenaline (facilitates) Serotonin (inhibits orgasm via $5HT_{2A}$ receptors)	Benzodiazepine withdrawal (rare) Cannabis Clomipramine and fluoxetine (rare reports of spontaneous orgasm) Moclobemide (rare)	Antipsychotics (eg. typicals) Beta-blockers Bupropion (reports) Gabapentin (cases) SSRIs, TCAs, SNRIs, MAOIs, trazodone (enhance the inhibitory activity of $5HT_{2A}$ receptors) — dose/plasma-level dependent (paroxetine > sertraline > fluoxetine > citalopram > fluvoxamine, although 8% men/partners prefer the effect)	Discontinue (gradually, beware of discontinuation effects) Dose adjust (reduce, omitting selected doses, ensure single daily dose eg. at night to give trough levels at peak sexual activity) Switch (eg. trazodone or mirtazapine) Wait for spontaneous resolution (occurs in less than third) Augmentation: many have been tried, few achieve much
Priapism	Alpha-1-adrenergic antagonism Duration > 4 hrs is a urological emergency (up to 50% become impotent as a result)	Antidepressants: trazodone (incidence may be up to 1 in 1000), isolated reports with SSRIs Antipsychotics eg. phenothiazines plus isolated cases with clozapine, haloperidol, olanzapine, quetiapine, risperidone, zuclopenthixol Other drugs include diazepam, gabapentin, phenytoin and buspirone		Early treatment (within 4–6 hours before local hypoxemia) Short-term (pain control, vigorous hydration, cold compress) and refer to A&E
Fertility		Clozapine may improve male fertility	Hyperprolactinaemia (esp. with typical antipsychotics) — may cause up to 50–90% women to become amenorrhoeic	Switch to antipsychotic with a lower effect on prolactin

3.
Psychotropics in problem areas

3.1 Breast-feeding

See also the *BNF* (Appendix 5).

	Lower risk	Moderate risk	High risk
Antipsychotics	Sulpiride[5]	Amisulpride[5] Flupentixol[4] Haloperidol[6] Loxapine[8] Phenothiazines (low dose only)[7] Zuclopenthixol[4]	Aripiprazole[2] Clozapine[3] Olanzapine[2] Phenothiazines[7] Quetiapine[2] Risperidone[1] Sertindole[2] Zotepine[2]
Antidepressants	Flupentixol LD[4] Moclobemide[16] Tricyclics (most)[12] Tryptophan[16]	Mianserin[16] Mirtazapine[11] St. John's wort[16] SSRIs[9] Trazodone[12]	Doxepin?[12] MAOIs[15] Maprotiline[12] Reboxetine[14] Venlafaxine[10]
Anxiolytics and hypnotics	Benzodiazepines LD[17] Chloral[21] Temazepam LD[17] Zolpidem[19]	Benzodiazepines[17] Beta-blockers[20] Clomethiazole[21]	Buspirone[18] Zaleplon[19] Zopiclone[19]
Anticonvulsants	Carbamazepine[22] Phenytoin[24] Valproate[23]	Acetazolamide[28] Benzodiazepines[17] Vigabatrin[27]	Barbituarates[25] Gabapentin[26] Lamotrigine?[26] Levetiracetam[27] Ethosuximide[28] Oxcarbazepine[22] Tiagabine[27] Topiramate[27]
Others		Anticholinergics[30] Disulfiram[31] Methadone[34]	Acamprosate[31] Anticholinesterases[29] Bupropion[36] Lithium[34] Memantine[29] Methylphenidate[34] Modafinil[33]

General Principals (*adapted from Maudsley Guidelines, 2003*)

1. All psychotropics pass into the milk, so no drugs are risk-free. The higher lipid content of the hind milk (second half of feed) makes it likely to have a higher drug concentration than the fore milk (first half).
2. Milk levels are usually around 1% of maternal plasma levels, but there have been few formal studies.
3. Drugs should be avoided if the infant is premature, or has renal, hepatic, cardiac or neurological impairment.
4. Avoid sedating drugs and those with long half-lives.
5. Since nearly all psychotropics can be taken as a once daily dose, this should be done as a single daily dose just before the infant's longest sleep period feed, minimising actual concentration and maximising clearance before the next feed.
6. If a mother was taking a drug during pregnancy, it will not usually be necessary to switch drugs during breast-feeding as the amount the infant is exposed to will be less than that exposed to *in utero*.
7. Adverse effects will often be dose related so use the minimum effective maternal dose.
8. Polypharmacy may lead to enhanced adverse effects in the infant.
9. Drug effects on the development of the infant's brain are not clear and so monitor biochemical and behavioural parameters, especially if any infant shows signs of possible psychotropic side-effects (eg. sedation, tremulousness, colic etc.), and then take appropriate action, eg. dose reduction, drug change, etc.

3.1.1 Antipsychotics

1. The UK SPC for **risperidone** states that women should not breast-feed.
2. The **olanzapine** SPC states that it should be avoided, although there are 5 case reports of low milk levels and no adverse effects. No human information is available for **quetiapine, aripiprazole** and

sertindole and the UK SPCs recommend avoiding. **Zotepine** should *not* be used as it is definitely excreted into the milk.
3. **Clozapine** is contraindicated in breast-feeding as animal studies suggest it is excreted into breast milk. This risks agranulocytosis and accumulation may occur, resulting in sedation.
4. 1–2% of the maternal **flupentixol** dose might reach the infant and thus is probably safe at lower dose (eg. <2mg/d). Higher doses of zuclopenthixol and flupentixol can produce drowsiness in the child.
5. A maternal **sulpiride** dose of 100mg/d is likely to give the child less than 1mg/d. No adverse effects have been reported at higher doses. There is no information available for **amisulpride**.
6. **Haloperidol** is excreted into breast milk but levels are probably low, although infant levels may be the same as adults and some element of delayed development has been detected and so the infant must be monitored carefully.
7. High doses of **phenothiazines** can produce drowsiness in the infant. Drowsiness and lethargy are possible with **chlorpromazine**, but not inevitable. With careful monitoring it should be safe. In the longer term, neonatal exposure to chlorpromazine was shown to have no effect on development up to 5 years of age. **Perphenazine** should be **avoided** as it may become 'trapped' in milk due to its physiochemical properties.
8. **Loxapine** should be avoided.

3.1.2 Antidepressants

9. Treatment with the **SSRIs citalopram, escitalopram, fluvoxamine, paroxetine** or **sertraline** seems to be compatible with breast-feeding although, given safer options, **fluoxetine** should probably best be avoided during lactation, unless also used during pregnancy. The limited data indicates that healthy full-term infants are unlikely to be harmed by SSRIs (McElhatton, *Prescriber* 1999, **10**, 101–17). An average of about 10% of a **fluoxetine** dose reaches the infant and this is considered to be low enough for

women to continue, with care, to breast-feed, with no developmental effects seen. Care with potential accumulation is needed, and 11 studies (n = 190) indicate that although about 10% of the adult dose reaches the infant, there are a few higher levels reported so be alert to possible toxicity. **Paroxetine** is found in milk but less than 1% of the daily dose would be expected to pass to the infant and so this would appear safe. **Fluvoxamine** daily intake by an infant is about 0.5% of the maternal dose and this is thought to be of acceptable risk. There is limited evidence that **sertraline** may be excreted into breast milk at only very low levels, even at higher doses, although some discontinuation reactions in infants have been reported. A small single-dose study has shown that **citalopram/escitalopram** is excreted into breast milk at about the same level as fluoxetine, and the infant might receive around 4–17mcg/kg/d, and no adverse effects were seen in the infants. With all the SSRIs, there are case reports of higher levels in a few infants and so one should remain alert for rare but possible toxic effects.

10. Some **venlafaxine** and metabolite have been detectable in breast-fed infant plasma (mean 6% adult dose). No acute adverse effects have been reported, but exposed infants should be monitored closely.

11. **Mirtazapine** is excreted only in small amounts in breast milk, but use cannot be actually formally recommended as such.

12. **Tricyclic antidepressants** should be used with care, but it does not seem warranted to recommend that breast-feeding should be discontinued completely, as significant tricyclic levels have not been detected in neonatal serum (**except** for doxepin and maprotiline). For **imipramine**, up to 0.1% of the maternal daily dose could appear in the milk. **Amitriptyline** levels were undetectable in the serum of a breast-fed infant whose mother was taking 75mg/d of amitriptyline for three weeks. Infant **nortriptyline** levels are not

detectable and adverse effects have not been reported. **Avoid doxepin**, however, as it has a longer-acting metabolite which may accumulate in breast-fed infants, causing severe drowsiness and respiratory depression (several severe cases reported). Avoid **maprotiline** as it has a long half-life and is present in milk in significant amounts. A tricyclic with a short half-life would appear to be the better tricyclic option, eg. imipramine, nortriptyline or trimipramine. Two studies with **dosulepin/dothiepin** in breast-feeding have shown no long-term effects on childhood development. A recent study has shown that **tricyclic** levels decrease during the third trimester and then rise rapidly immediately after birth (probably due to decreased metabolism) and so one needs to observe for toxic effects and adjust doses rapidly if needed. The general advice is to observe the child carefully for sedation and respiratory depression. A tricyclic with a short half-life for itself (and any active metabolites) would appear to be the better option. It has been recommended that amitriptyline and imipramine are the preferred tricyclic antidepressants.

13. 1% of a **trazodone** dose passes into the milk, which would seem of minimal importance, although drowsiness and poor feeding have been reported.

14. **Reboxetine** is excreted in milk in rats but no human data exists so the drug should be avoided (SPC).

15. Little data is available for the **MAOIs**. **Tranylcypromine** is excreted in breast milk but levels are not thought to be significant. Some views are that MAOI levels in milk are too small to affect the child but until more information is available, great care is needed.

16. **Moclobemide** is excreted unchanged in milk but at low levels and this would seem unlikely to produce adverse effects in the baby. Low levels of **mianserin** in milk have been reported, with infants showing no untoward effects. **Amoxapine** appears in human milk, but probably only at low levels. Although there

is a case of uneventful use, lack of toxicity data means **St. John's wort** should best be avoided in breast-feeding. There are no known problems with **tryptophan**.

3.1.3 Anxiolytics and hypnotics

17. The CSM has noted that since benzodiazepines are excreted in breast milk, they should not be given to lactating mothers (*Curr Prob* 1997, **23**, 10). Repeated doses of **long-acting benzodiazepines** can produce lethargy and weight loss but low and single doses are probably of low risk provided the infant is monitored for drowsiness. **Diazepam, oxazepam, lorazepam, lormetazepam, nitrazepam** and **flunitrazepam** have all been shown in breast milk. **Temazepam** levels have been reported to be below detection levels at doses of 10–20mg/d and no adverse effects have been seen. **Oxazepam** seems to be preferable to **diazepam** in lactating women but, as with all anxiolytic benzodiazepines, infants should be observed for signs of sedation and poor suckling.

18. **Buspirone** is contraindicated although there is no specific human data to show adverse effects.

19. **Zaleplon** is excreted in breast milk, and should not be administered to breastfeeding mothers, although the actual amount likely to be transferred may be very low eg. 0.02% of maternal dose. **Zopiclone** is contraindicated in breastfeeding as it is excreted in appreciable amounts (up to 50% of maternal levels). Single occasional doses of 7.5mg are probably of low risk as accumulation is unlikely. The AAPCD considers **zolpidem** compatible with breast-feeding, as it is found only in minute amounts in milk due to its low lipophilic properties and rapid onset and excretion. A low dose at bedtime and avoiding breast-feeding for the next few hours would minimise the small (unknown) potential effect on an infant.

20. The amounts of **beta-blockers** in milk are probably too small to effect the baby but could produce bradycardia and hypoglycaemia in high doses.

21. **Clomethiazole** is excreted in insignificant amounts and, although the sedative effects of this could be relevant, is unlikely to be harmful. **Chloral** is excreted in breast milk and may cause sedation, although only minimal sedation after large feeds has been reported. The AAPCD recommends that it can safely be used in lactating mothers and it is in routine use in Europe.

3.1.4 Anticonvulsants

All anticonvulsants are excreted into breast milk but at much lower levels than in maternal plasma and so "sub-therapeutic" doses only are received by the infant. Breast-feeding should be encouraged as bonding is especially important in epileptic mothers.

An extensive review (Hägg and Spigset, *Drug Safety* 2000, **22**, 425–40) of anticonvulsant use during lactation concluded that:

● **Carbamazepine, valproate** and **phenytoin** are compatible
● **Ethosuximide, phenobarbital** and **primidone** should be regarded as potentially unsafe and close clinical monitoring of the infant is recommended
● Data on the newer drugs is too sparse for reliable recommendations
● Occasional or short-term treatment with **benzodiazepines** could be considered as compatible with breast-feeding, although maternal diazepam treatment has caused sedation in suckling infants after short-term use.

22. **Carbamazepine** has been classified by the AAPCD as compatible with breastfeeding, as levels have been found to be relatively low but this is based on case reports in epilepsy, with only two so far when used as a mood stabiliser. The infant is likely to receive a maximum of 10% of an appropriate therapeutic dose of carbamazepine for an infant with epilepsy (UK SPC). The mother should be informed of the potential signs of hepatic dysfunction and CNS effects. **Oxcarbazepine** is excreted into breast milk and it is contraindicated in UK.

23. **Valproate** has been classified by the AAPCD as compatible with breast-feeding, based on case reports in epilepsy. Valproate appears in breast milk, with infant plasma levels ranging from 12% of maternal plasma levels. Care and counselling is needed for higher doses, and there is the risk of haematological effects.

24. Small quantities of **phenytoin** are excreted in breast milk, peaking at 3 hours, and have been considered clinically safe.

25. Larger doses of **phenobarbital** and **primidone** may accumulate in breast milk. This may cause unacceptable drowsiness and lead to the need to stop or at least reduce breast-feeding.

26. **Lamotrigine** passes into breast milk, and with a slow elimination in the newborn, concentrations in the infant may reach levels at which pharmacological effects can be expected. This is probably of low risk provided all remain alert to the potential for life-threatening rashes. **Gabapentin** crosses into breast milk, but there are no reports of infant plasma levels.

27. **Vigabatrin** ingestion via milk is small but the information is contradictory. **Topiramate** and **tiagabine** are not recommended as no human information is currently available. Animal studies indicate **levetiracetam** is excreted into breast milk and so breast-feeding is not recommended.

28. **Ethosuximide** is excreted in insignificant amounts with infant levels subtherapeutic and without apparent effect. Monitor plasma levels if possible. Very low doses of **acetazolamide** were transferred by breast-feeding in one reported case.

3.1.5 Others

29. There is no information available on **donepezil, galantamine** and **rivastigmine** so should not be used in breast-feeding mothers (UK SPC). **Memantine** is probably excreted in breast milk.

30. There is no data on **anticholinergics** in breast milk.

31. No information is available to date on **disulfiram** in breast milk and so use must be with great caution. There is the possibility of interactions with paediatric medicines (eg. alcohol-containing gripe mixtures, see *4.7.1*). The UK SPC for **acamprosate** states that use in breast-feeding is a contraindication, although there is no human data available.

32. **Lithium** has been classified by the AAPCD as contraindicated in breast-feeding, although this recommendation is based on limited evidence. Lithium is present in milk in concentrations of 33–50% of the mother's plasma levels, which can produce side-effects occasionally in the baby. The toxicity risks are probably small provided maternal levels are moderate (eg. less than about 0.8mmol/l) and well-controlled. Dehydration in the infant can also increase the problems. Reduce maternal lithium or breast-feeding if hypotonia or lethargy develop, or infection or dehydration make the child more susceptible to lithium toxic effects. With careful monitoring of the infant (considering poorer renal excretion and fluid balance/electrolytes) and education of the mother, use of lower doses may be valuable as the risk of relapse on stopping is high.

33. **Modafinil** is contraindicated in breast-feeding (MI).

34. No information is available for **methylphenidate** (UK SPC) so do not use.

35. **Methadone** at maintenance doses reduces the risk of poor quality street drugs being used and has been used successfully in breast-feeding. Maternal doses of up to 20mg/d have been recommended as safe for healthy infants. The conclusion from a 12-mother study was that breast-feeding should not be discouraged in women on a methadone maintenance programme. Stopping opiates is also dangerous as withdrawal reactions can damage the foetus more than methadone, but the amount received via the milk is unlikely to be sufficient to prevent withdrawal in the infant.

36. **Bupropion** and metabolites accumulate in breast milk at higher levels than plasma, although one report indicated that bupropion was not detectable in the infant's plasma.

3.2 Cardiovascular disease

	Lower risk	Moderate risk	High risk
Antipsychotics	Amisulpride[5] Flupentixol[4] Olanzapine[2] Quetiapine[2] Risperidone[1] Sulpiride[5] Zuclopenthixol[4]	Aripiprazole[2] Haloperidol[6] Loxapine[8] Phenothiazines[7] Risperidone[1]	Clozapine[3] Pimozide[8] Sertindole[2] Thioridazine[7] Zotepine[2]
Antidepressants	Mianserin[16] Mirtazapine[11] SSRIs[9] Trazodone[13] Tryptophan[16]	MAOIs[15] Moclobemide[16] Reboxetine[14] Venlafaxine[10]	Tricyclics (especially dothiepin/dosulepin)[12]
Anxiolytics + hypnotics	Benzodiazepines[17] Buspirone[18] Zaleplon[19] Zolpidem[19] Zopiclone[19]	Beta-blockers[20] Chloral[21] Clomethiazole[21]	
Anticonvulsants	Benzodiazepines[17] Gabapentin[26] Lamotrigine[26] Tiagabine[27] Topiramate[27] Valproate[23] Vigabatrin[27]	Barbiturates[25] Carbamazepine[22] Oxcarbazepine[22] Paraldehyde[28] Phenytoin[2]	Fosphenytoin[24]
Others	Acamprosate[31]	Anticholinergics[30] Anticholinesterases[29] Bupropion[36] Dexamfetamine[34] Lithium[32] Memantine[29] Modafinil[33]	Disulfiram[31]

General Principals (*adapted from Maudsley Guidelines, 2003*)

1. Polypharmacy should be avoided where possible, particularly with drugs likely to effect cardiac rate and electrolyte balance.
2. Awareness of QT prolongation is increasing, and so care is essential. A QTc prolonged to about 450ms is considered of some concern, and above about 500ms to be at risk of leading to Torsade de Pointes, which may be fatal.
3. Avoid drugs specifically contraindicated eg. thioridazine, pimozide etc.
4. Start low and go slow is, as ever, good advice. Avoid rapid dose escalation.
5. Specific guidance
   - **Angina** — avoid drugs that may exacerbate postural hypotension and cause tachycardia
   - **Arrhythmias** — SSRIs, sulpiride, risperidone and olanzapine appear lowest risks

- **Heart failure (HF)** — avoid drugs causing postural hypotension and care with lithium and diuretics (see *4.4*)
- **Hypertension** — only use drugs causing postural hypotension with care as erratic compliance could be problematic, and avoid high-dose venlafaxine, clozapine and tricyclics
- **Myocardial infarction (MI)** — SSRIs, mirtazapine, haloperidol, flupentixol and sulpiride appear safest
- **QT prolongation** — many antipsychotics may lengthen the QT interval with a class IA antiarrhythmic effect eg. thioridazine, pimozide, sertindole and haloperidol, with no association with risperidone, olanzapine and quetiapine.

3.2.1 Antipsychotics

1. **Risperidone** should be used with caution due to orthostatic hypotension and increase in heart rate. It is best to introduce it slowly over several weeks.
2. Postural hypotension has been seen infrequently with **olanzapine** so monitor bp in the over 65s. Olanzapine may raise fasting triglyceride levels. Triglycerides are a significant risk factor for exacerbation of CHD, and so needs care. The SPC for **quetiapine** recommends caution with drugs known to prolong the QTc interval, particularly important in those patients with cardiovascular disease or conditions predisposing to hypotension. **Zotepine** causes a dose-related QTc interval prolongation and should be avoided. **Aripiprazole** may cause postural hypotension so use with care in known CV disease or hypotension. **Sertindole** should be avoided due to a documented QT prolongation effect.
3. **Clozapine** has cardiac side-effects, eg. tachycardia and postural hypotension (particularly early in treatment) and recent studies indicate cardiac abnormalities may occur in up to 20% patients. Clozapine has also been associated with potentially fatal myocarditis and cardiomyopathy in physically healthy young adults. The CSM (*Curr Prob Pharmacovig* 2002, **28**, 8) has recommended:

- Avoid clozapine if cardiomyopathy has occurred
- Exclude severe heart disease before starting
- Myocarditis most commonly occurs in the first 2 months so be alert to this, especially if persistent tachycardia at rest is seen
- Refer any ECG changes to a cardiologist
- Discontinue as soon as possible if cardiomyopathy or myocarditis is suspected
- Regular ECG monitoring, especially at higher doses, may be very valuable.

4. Cardiac disease is a UK SPC precaution for **flupentixol** and **zuclopenthixol**.
5. No changes in ECG status have been reported in short and long-term studies of **amisulpride**. There are no specific problems reported with **sulpiride** (SPC).
6. **Haloperidol** risks occasional arrhythmias so restrict high dosages to non-responders. A prolonged QT-interval has been reported although it may be no greater risk than thioridazine (Hennessy *et al, BMJ* 2002, **325**, 1070–72).
7. Some ECG abnormalities have been reported with **phenothiazines** eg. tachycardia, T-wave abnormalities, ST depression, QT prolongation and right bundle branch block but these are mostly reversible and asymptomatic. **Thioridazine** is, however, now contraindicated in patients with a history of cardiac arrhythmias or at risk of problems, dose-related increase in risk of lengthened QT-interval has been reported, detectable at doses as low as 10mg/d (n = 596, Reilly *et al, Lancet* 2000, **355**, 1048–52). **Levomepromazine** causes orthostatic hypotension, which can on occasion be prolonged and profound.
8. With **pimozide**, the UK CSM has had many reports of serious or fatal cardiac reactions to pimozide. They recommend:

- start at 2–4mg/d, increase by 2–4mg/d weekly, maximum 20mg/d
- pre-treatment ECG. Contraindicate if prolonged QT interval or history of arrhythmia noted

- annual ECG and review carefully if QT interval is lengthened
- avoid concurrent treatment with other antipsychotics, tricyclics and other QT interval-prolonging drugs (eg. antimalarials, anti-arrhythmics, astemizole, diuretics etc).

3.2.2 Antidepressants

Depressed patients are at greater risk of myocardial infarction and vice versa. During the first six months post-infarction, patients who become depressed (and this is particularly difficult to detect) have a five-fold increase in mortality, and are less likely to follow recommendations to reduce cardiac risk during recovery from a myocardial infarction. Treatment of depression in this vulnerable group is thus of singular importance as whilst antidepressants in cardiac disease have risks, so does *not* using them.

9. **SSRIs** are generally considered safer to use in cardiac diseases, but care is needed with drug interactions. **Sertraline** has been shown not to increase cardiac events in depressed patients with unstable angina or recent MI and may even reduce post-MI deaths by about 10% (Glassman *et al*, *JAMA* 2002, **288**, 701–9). **Fluoxetine** up to 60mg/day may have no significant adverse cardiac effects in patients with pre-existing CHF, conduction disease and/ or ventricular arrhythmia. **Citalopram/ escitalopram** have no significant reported effects on blood pressure, cardiac conduction nor heart rate.

10. **Venlafaxine** has been associated with a dose-dependent increase in blood pressure (13% incidence at above 300mg/d) and heart rate. Caution is required for patients with pre-existing cardiovascular disease and recent myocardial infarction. Blood pressure monitoring at doses above 200mg/d is recommended as the effect is dose-related.

11. Hypertension, hypotension and tachycardia have been reported with **mirtazapine**, but only rarely, and mirtazapine would seem relatively safe.

12. A recent study has indicated that the chances of developing IHD is significantly raised in people who have *ever* received a **tricyclic** (even when adjusting for other factors), especially dosulepin (Hippisley-Cox *et al*, *BMJ* 2001, **323**, 666– 69). Tricyclics also produce orthostatic hypotension (and hence occasional myocardial infarction), have antiarrhythmic actions (quinidine-like) in high dose and antimuscarinic actions (raising heart rate). Tricyclics should thus only be used with caution in patients with ischaemic heart disease and/or ventricular arrhythmia. SSRIs are generally considered safer in angina, arrhythmias (tricyclics are contraindicated if severe), heart failure, hypertension and myocardial infarction.

13. Rare problems have been reported with **trazodone** but is generally considered of low risk.

14. **Reboxetine** increased baseline heart rate in 20% of patients in short-term trials. Orthostatic hypotension occurs with increasing frequency at higher doses.

15. The **MAOIs** are all contraindicated in severe cardiac disease.

16. Mild hypertension and tachycardia have been reported with **moclobemide** so monitoring bp may be useful. Hypertension with tyramine in patients with pre-existing labile hypertension has also occurred rarely and so caution in cardiac disease would be sensible. There are no apparent problems with **mianserin** and **tryptophan**. In one small study, **St. John's wort** was reported not to effect heart rate.

3.2.3 Anxiolytics and hypnotics

17. **Benzodiazepines** are relatively safe but contraindicated in acute pulmonary insufficiency.

18. **Buspirone** may have some cardiac effects, eg. rare cases of hypertension and tachycardia.

19. There are no apparent problems with **zaleplon, zolpidem** and **zopiclone**.

20. The use of **beta-blockers** would depend upon the nature of the cardiac disease.

21. **Clomethiazole** is contraindicated in acute pulmonary insufficiency and should be used with care in chronic pulmonary insufficiency. **Chloral** is contraindicated in severe cardiac disease.

3.2.4 Anticonvulsants

22. Cardiovascular effects from **carbamazepine** are uncommon but cardiac conduction changes, hypertension and atrioventricular block have been reported. Patients on **oxcarbazepine** with cardiac insufficiency and secondary heart failure should have regular weight measurements to determine the occurrence of fluid retention (SPC).

23. There are some reports of cardiac effects with **valproate**, but no specific cautions.

24. **Phenytoin** is a useful third-line treatment in cardiac arrhythmias but is contraindicated in sinus bradycardia, sinoatrial block, 2nd and 3rd degree A-V block and Adams-Stokes syndrome. Severe cardiovascular ADRs have been reported with **fosphenytoin** IV, including asystole, VF and cardiac arrest, mostly within 30 mins of an injection. The CSM thus recommend careful monitoring during and for half an hour post-infusion, and dose reduction should hypotension occur (*Curr Prob Pharmacovigilance* 2000, **26**[May], 1).

25. **IV barbiturates** can cause hypotension.

26. ECG monitoring is recommended in **lamotrigine** overdose. There is no evidence of any problems with **gabapentin** in cardiac disease.

27. There is no evidence to date of cardiac adverse effects from **vigabatrin**. No significant changes in ECG, blood pressure or heart rate have been noted in initial clinical trials with **topiramate** and **tiagabine**.

28. There have been reports of hypotension and tachycardia in young children given IV **paraldehyde**.

3.2.5 Others

29. **Anticholinesterases** may cause bradycardia so care is needed with the use of donepezil in patients with sick sinus syndrome or other conduction conditions. There have been rare reports with **donepezil** (eg. heart block, *Curr Prob Pharmacovig* 1999, **25**, 7), **rivastigmine** (syncope and angina pectoris, although a very large study was unable to show any adverse ECG effects) and **galantamine** (syncope and severe bradycardia). There is little data on **memantine** so use in CV disease should only be with caution.

30. **Anticholinergics** should be used with caution, particularly in those with a tendency to tachycardia. Sinus bradycardia has been reported.

31. **Disulfiram** is contraindicated in the presence of cardiac failure, coronary artery disease, previous history of CVA and hypertension. The Antabuse-alcohol reaction can cause cardiac arrest even in healthy adults. There are no known problems with **acamprosate**.

32. **Lithium** rarely causes clinical problems at lower dose although cardiovascular disease is a UK SPC contraindication. Benign cardiovascular side-effects may occur in 20–30% patients, the main problems being T-wave flattening, ventricular ectopics and congestive myopathy. However, an 827-patient study considered that lithium does not pose a significant risk. A pre-treatment ECG is very useful, especially in elderly people.

33. **Modafinil** is contraindicated in severe hypertension and arrhythmia and should be used with caution in patients with concurrent heart disease. Monitor heart rate and blood pressure if used in moderate hypertension.

34. The manufacturers caution to monitor bp in hypertensive patients treated with **methylphenidate**.

35. There is little evidence of developing hypertension with **dexamfetamine** although regular bp testing has been recommended.

36. **Bupropion** may cause small rises in supine blood pressure, but tends not to cause significant conduction complications. Infrequent occurrences of orthostatic hypotension, tachycardia, stroke and vasodilation have been reported with bupropion.

3.3 Diabetes

	Lower risk	Moderate risk	High risk
Antipsychotics	Amisulpride[5] Aripiprazole[2] Butyrophenones[6] Loxapine[8] Risperidone[1] Sulpiride[5] Thioxanthenes[4]	Clozapine[3] Phenothiazines[7] Quetiapine[2] Sertindole[2] Zotepine[12]	Olanzapine?[2]
Antidepressants	Moclobemide[16] Reboxetine[14] SSRIs[9] Trazodone[13] Tryptophan[16] Venlafaxine[10]	Fluoxetine[9] Mianserin[16] Mirtazapine[11] Tricyclics[12]	MAOIs[15]
Anxiolytics and hypnotics	Benzodiazepines[17] Buspirone[18] Chloral[21] Clomethiazole[21] Zaleplon[19] Zolpidem[19] Zopiclone[19]	Beta-blockers[20]	
Anticonvulsants	Acetazolamide[28] Barbiturates[25] Benzodiazepines[17] Carbamazepine[22] Ethosuximide[28] Gabapentin[26] Oxcarbazepine[22] Vigabatrin[27]	Phenytoin[24] Tiagabine[27] Topiramate?[27] Valproate[23]	
Others	Acamprosate[31] Anticholinergics[30] Anticholinesterases[29] Lithium[32] Memantine[29] Methylphenidate[22] Modafinil[33]	Bupropion[34] Disulfiram[31]	

3.3.1 Antipsychotics

There is a increased risk of diabetes and elevated glucose levels with all antipsychotics, but especially some atypicals eg. clozapine, olanzapine and possibly quetiapine, but not risperidone (Sernyak *et al, Am J Psych* 2002, **159**, 561–66).

1. There is no evidence of any effects with **risperidone** on blood biochemistry and is probably the atypical least likely to exacerbate or cause diabetes.

2. The incidence of diabetes with **olanzapine** is about 1 in 1000 (PMS, CSM warning: *Curr Prob* 2002, **28**, 3). It may need insulin to manage and may severely exacerbate diabetic control. One study showed that olanzapine (mean 14mg/d) produced fasting triglyceride levels raised by a mean of 60mg/dL (37%), which needs care since triglycerides are a risk factor for precipitation or exacerbation of diabetes, and there are many case reports. There is a slightly increased risk of diabetes with **quetiapine** and **sertindole**. Occasional hypo- and hyperglycaemia has been reported with **zotepine** (MI). There are no apparent problems with **aripiprazole**.

3. Elevated insulin levels have been shown with **clozapine**, and a dose-related effect noted, indicating a probable influence on insulin secretion. One study showed a non-significant increase in the number of people having or developing type 2 diabetes mellitus and/or impaired glucose tolerance on clozapine compared to depot antipsychotics. Additional glucose monitoring is thus **strongly indicated** in diabetics on clozapine. In addition, a study has indicated that patients on clozapine experience significant weight gain and lipid abnormalities (eg. raised serum triglycerides) and have an increased risk (52% over 5 years) of hyperglycaemia and of diagnosed diabetes mellitus (37% over 5 years).

4. Lack of relationship has been shown between serum levels of **zuclopenthixol** (n = 9) and plasma insulin. The UK SPC for **flupenthixol** notes that control of diabetes may be impaired.

5. There are no apparent problems with **sulpiride** and **amisulpride**.

6. There are no apparent problems with **haloperidol**.

7. One study showed **chlorpromazine** to have no significant effects on blood sugar levels but some reports of problems exist.

8. There are no apparent problems with **pimozide** nor **loxapine**.

3.3.2 Antidepressants

Depression in diabetics may be as common as 27% and sertraline has been recommended as the drug of choice, with the SSRIs generally preferred to tricyclics and MAOIs. SSRIs may decrease serum glucose levels by up to 30% and cause anorexia, and may enable diabetics to control hunger and eating better, via their serotonergic effects, unlike the tricyclics, which often have an appetite-raising effect.

9. There are no major reported problems with **paroxetine, citalopram, escitalopram, fluvoxamine** and **sertraline**. Diabetics may become hypoglycaemic during fluoxetine treatment. **Fluoxetine** side-effects, eg. tremor, nausea, sweating and anxiety may also be mistaken for hypoglycaemia. Most problems have been reported with the more common non-insulin dependent diabetes mellitus (NIDDM, type 2 disease, adult-onset) rather than the insulin dependent form (IDDM, type 1 disease, juvenile-onset). If fluoxetine is used, advise the patient about this effect, possible loss of hypoglycaemia awareness and regularly check serum glucose levels.

10. There is no published evidence of problems with **venlafaxine**.

11. The manufacturers of **mirtazapine** recommend care although there are no reports of problems and this is purely a 'class labelling' precaution.

12. **Tricyclics** may adversely affect diabetic control as they increase serum glucose levels by up to 150%, increase carbohydrate craving and reduce metabolic rate but are generally considered safe unless the diabetes is very brittle.

13. There are no apparent problems with **trazodone**.

14. There are no apparent problems with **reboxetine**.

15. **MAOIs** may decrease serum glucose levels by up to 35% due to a direct influence on gluconeogenesis. Diabetes is a UK SPC precaution for eg. isocarboxazid.

16. There is a case of **mianserin** dose-related hyperglycaemia in a non-diabetic woman. **Moclobemide** 600mg/d did not modify the effect of glibenclamide on plasma glucose and insulin levels in healthy individuals.

3.3.3 Anxiolytics and hypnotics

17. There is a case of a diabetic presenting with a reduction in insulin requirements after discontinuing **clonazepam**.
18. There are no apparent problems with **buspirone**.
19. There are no apparent problems with **zaleplon, zolpidem** and **zopiclone**.
20. **Propranolol** may prolong the hypoglycaemic response to insulin and may effect hypoglycaemic episodes.
21. There are no apparent problems with **clomethiazole** or **chloral**.

3.3.4 Anticonvulsants

22. There are rare reported problems with **carbamazepine** but no apparent problems with **oxcarbazepine**.
23. **Valproate** may give false positives in urine tests for diabetes. Epilim liquid is sugar-free, unlike the syrup.
24. Hypoglycaemia has been reported with **phenytoin** and glucose metabolism can be affected.
25. There are no apparent problems with the **barbiturates**.

26. There are no apparent problems with **lamotrigine**. Blood glucose fluctuations have been reported with **gabapentin** (UK SPC).
27. No information is available on **topiramate** and **tiagabine**.
28. There are no apparent problems with **ethosuximide**.

3.3.5 Others

29. There are no apparent problems with **donepezil, galantamine** nor **memantine**, but diabetes mellitus is a precaution for **rivastigmine**.
30. There are no known problems with the **anticholinergics**.
31. The UK SPC for **disulfiram** recommends caution in diabetes mellitus. There are no apparent problems with **acamprosate**.
32. There are no problems with **lithium** in diabetes but polydipsia and polyuria can occur. Lithium may also increase insulin secretion.
33. There are no apparent problems with **methylphenidate**. A transient loss of appetite may occur. There are no apparent problems with **modafinil**.
34. Animal studies suggest some risks with **bupropion**, and hyper- and hypoglycaemia have been reported so use with caution in type II diabetics.

3.4 Epilepsy

	Lower risk	Moderate risk	High risk
Antipsychotics	Amisulpride[5] Haloperidol[6] Pimozide[8] Quetiapine[2] Risperidone?[1] Sulpiride[5] Zuclopenthixol[4]	Aripiprazole[2] Olanzapine[2] Phenothiazines (most)[7] Sertindole[2]	Chlorpromazine[7] Clozapine[3] Loxapine[8] Zotepine[2]
Antidepressants	MAOIs[15] Moclobemide?[16] Reboxetine[14] SSRIs[9] Tryptophan[16]	Mianserin[16] Mirtazapine[13] Trazodone[13] Tricyclics (most)[12] Venlafaxine[10]	Maprotiline[12]
Anxiolytics and hypnotics	Benzodiazepines[17] Beta-blockers[20] Chloral[21] Clomethiazole[21] Zaleplon[19] Zolpidem[19] Zopiclone[19]	Buspirone[18]	
Others	Acamprosate[24] Anticholinergics[23] Modafinil[26]	Disulfiram[24] Anticholinesterases[22] Lithium[25] Memantine[29] Methylphenidate[26]	Bupropion[27]

General principals

1. Keep the daily dose as low as possible — epileptogenic effects may be dose-related.
2. Take extra care with risk factors including head trauma, previous seizure history and concomitant (or withdrawing from) drugs (especially antipsychotics).
3. Use lowest risk drugs unless essential.
4. Introduce and withdraw drugs slowly. Anticonvulsant cover may be appropriate.
5. Dose changes should be small and gentle.
6. Avoid antipsychotics with higher antihistaminic, sedative and antiadrenergic effects, which may lower the seizure threshold.

3.4.1 Antipsychotics

1. There is little information about (nor evidence of problems with) **risperidone**.
2. The SPCs for **olanzapine** and **quetiapine** state that they should be used cautiously with patients with a history of seizures, although the incidence of seizures during quetiapine trials was equivalent to placebo (MI). There is no evidence of an increased risk with **aripiprazole**. **Sertindole** should be used with caution. **Zotepine** has an established dose-related pro-convulsive effect. It should not be used in patients with a

personal or family history of epilepsy. The risk of seizures is dose-related and rises above 300mg/d.

3. **Clozapine** can cause seizures, the risk rising steeply at doses above 600mg/d, and EEG changes may occur in 75% patients. Many centres use valproate as routine anticonvulsant cover at higher doses of clozapine.

4. **Zuclopenthixol** may have only mild to moderate effects, with few reports, and may be one of the drugs of choice.

5. There are no know problems with **amisulpride**. **Sulpiride** may be a reasonable choice, although care is recommended in patients with unstable epilepsy.

6. **Haloperidol** may have only mild to moderate effects and have a low risk of problems.

7. **Sedative phenothiazines** (eg. **chlorpromazine** and **promazine**) seem to have the worst epileptogenic reputation.

8. **Pimozide** may have a low risk. **Loxapine** lowers the seizure threshold and can cause convulsions even at normal doses, so avoid it.

3.4.2 Antidepressants

9. Serotonin function is unlikely to be of major importance in the genesis of seizures and so **SSRIs** are unlikely to lower the seizure threshold. **Fluvoxamine** has a low pro-convulsive effect but there have been some CSM reports of fits. **Fluoxetine** has a probable seizure incidence of 0.2%, similar to other antidepressants. **Paroxetine** does not interact with anticonvulsants and appears to have a minimal potential for producing seizures at antidepressant doses. With **sertraline**, seizures occurred in early clinical trials at a similar frequency to placebo and only in people with a history of seizures (MI). **Citalopram** has not been reported to interact with anticonvulsants or cause seizures.

10. Seizures have been reported in 0.26% of patients treated with **venlafaxine** during clinical trials and so a slow introduction and withdrawal is recommended.

11. Only one grand mal seizure has been reported in a patient with a history of seizures receiving **mirtazapine** at a high dose of 80mg/d during a trial. Care and monitoring would thus be standard.

12. All **tricyclics** seem to lower the seizure threshold, with **amitriptyline** and **maprotiline** probably the most proconvulsive antidepressants. **Doxepin** may be the safest based on current evidence. A slow rate of introduction reduces the risk.

13. The UK SPC for **trazodone** includes care in epilepsy, and to avoid abrupt changes in dose.

14. **Reboxetine** may be particularly useful in epilepsy as the spontaneous incidence of seizures is equivalent to placebo, with no seizures (even minor) in overdose and minimal interaction potential.

15. **MAOIs** are probably relatively safe based on current evidence. A slow rate of introduction reduces any risk. Care is needed with interactions.

16. There have been no reports of problems with **moclobemide** nor **tryptophan** to date. **Mianserin** is often quoted as being relatively safe and it is at least no worse than the tricyclics, with one study of 84 overdoses of 1g or more showing no convulsions. Seizures have been reported at therapeutic doses of **amoxapine**.

3.4.3 Anxiolytics and hypnotics

17. **Benzodiazepines** have an intrinsic anticonvulsant activity (see *1.15*).

18. **Buspirone** is contraindicated in epilepsy but there is no evidence that it is actually epileptogenic.

19. A weak anticonvulsant activity for **zopiclone** has been shown. **Zolpidem** is not reported to have any anticonvulsant activity. There is no data on **zaleplon**.

20. There are no apparent problems with the **beta-blockers**.

21. For **chloral** and **clomethiazole**, see *1.15.1* and *1.15.2*.

3.4.4 Others

22. Cholinomimetics (eg. anticholinesterases) may have some potential for

causing seizures so care is needed with **donepezil** and **rivastigmine** in pre-existing seizure activity (MI), although there are no reported problems with **galantamine** (UK SPC). **Memantine** should be used with care.

23. There are no problems reported with the **anticholinergics**.

24. The UK SPC for **disulfiram** recommends caution in epilepsy. There are no known problems with **acamprosate**.

25. **Lithium** has a marked epileptogenic activity in overdose, but probably has no effect at standard dose. **Carbamazepine** and **valproate** are obvious alternatives.

26. **Methylphenidate** is not associated with significant risk at therapeutic dose, but the UK SPC suggests caution. There are no apparent problems with **modafinil**.

27. **Bupropion** has some epileptogenic activity. Doses should not exceed 450mg/d, no single dose should be above 200mg and doses should not be increased at more than 150mg/d (SPC). The risk of seizures is about 4 in 1000 and there appears to be correlation between plasma concentration and the risk for seizures.

3.5 Glaucoma

	Lower risk	Moderate risk	High risk
Antipsychotics	Butyrophenones[2] Risperidone[3] Sulpiride[3] Thioxanthenes[2]	Clozapine[2] Loxapine[2] Phenothiazines[1] Zotepine[3]	Olanzapine[3]
Antidepressants	Flupentixol[5] MAOIs[5] Mirtazapine[5] Moclobemide[5] Trazodone[5] Tryptophan[5] Venlafaxine[5]	SSRIs[5]	Tricyclics[4]
Others	Acamprosate[6] Benzodiazepines[6] Caffeine[8] Clomethiazole[6] Disulfiram[6] Gabapentin[6] Lithium[6] Lofexidine[6] Naltrexone[6] Phenobarbital[6] Phenytoin[6] Tiagabine[6] Topiramate[6] Valproate[6] Vigabatrin[6]	Carbamazepine[6]	Anticholinergics[10] Dexamfetamine[7] Methylphenidate[9]

Angle-closure glaucoma occurs in eyes with a narrow anterior chamber angle, where drainage of the aqueous fluid through the anterior chamber angle is reduced or blocked. Drugs with anticholinergic properties have the potential to either induce angle-closure glaucoma or to worsen it. Although the degree of anticholinergic effect of a drug is of relevance, the individual's susceptibility to those effects is of greater importance.

General advice: Patients with glaucoma may be treated with drugs with anticholinergic properties provided intraocular pressure is monitored, an ophthalmologist is involved and information given on the symptoms of acute-angle closure, with advice to stop the drug and seek medical attention immediately should those symptoms occur eg. blurred vision, 'coloured haloes' around bright lights, intense pain, lacrimation, lid oedema, red eye, nausea and vomiting.

3.5.1 Antipsychotics

1. **Phenothiazines** are weak anticholinergics so some potential for problems exists. Some academics have recommended screening for glaucoma before initiating therapy (see introduction).

2. Other antipsychotics with similar anticholinergic effects would include **clozapine, loxapine, flupentixol** and **zuclopenthixol**. **Zotepine** has anticholinergic effects and should be used with caution in narrow-angle glaucoma.

3. **Antipsychotics** with little or no anticholinergic effect must still be considered to have a potential for problems, albeit probably at a low level, eg. **sulpiride, amisulpride, haloperidol** and **risperidone**. **Olanzapine**, is, however, contraindicated in angle-closure glaucoma in the UK.

3.5.2 Antidepressants

4. **Tricyclics** have a greater anticholinergic effect than phenothiazines. If patients are at risk of angle-closure glaucoma, pre-treatment examination by an ophthalmologist is recommended. See introduction.

5. Antidepressants which can cause dilation of the pupil, include the **SSRIs, mirtazapine, moclobemide, trazodone** and **MAOIs**. Acute angle-closure glaucoma associated with **paroxetine** has been reported. There is limited experience with **reboxetine** but the SPC recommends close supervision. Raised intraocular pressure or narrow-angle glaucoma is now a **venlafaxine** UK SPC warning.

3.5.3 Others

6. There are no reported problems with any of the **anticonvulsants, mood stabilisers, anxiolytics** nor **hypnotics**.

7. **Amfetamine** causes a transient rise in intraocular pressure but which is not associated with closure of the angle.

8. **Caffeine** has been reported to cause a transient rise in intraocular pressure.

9. **Methylphenidate** causes a transient rise in intraocular pressure but which is not associated with closure of the angle.

10. **Anticholinergics** are contraindicated in angle-closure glaucoma. There is no mention in the SPC of problems with **memantine**.

3.6   Liver disease

	Lower risk	Moderate risk	High risk
Antipsychotics	Amisulpride[5] Aripiprazole[2] Flupentixol[4] Haloperidol[6] Pimozide[8] Sulpiride[5] Zuclopenthixol[4]	Clozapine[3] Loxapine[8] Olanzapine[2] Phenothiazines[7] Quetiapine[2] Risperidone[1] Sertindole[2]	Zotepine[2]
Antidepressants	Mianserin[16] Paroxetine[9] Tryptophan[16]	Mirtazapine[11] Moclobemide[16] Reboxetine[14] SSRIs[9] St. John's wort[16] Trazodone[13] Tricyclics[12] Venlafaxine[10]	Lofepramine[12] MAOIs[15]

Anxiolytics and hypnotics	Lorazepam LD[17]
	Oxazepam LD[17]
	Temazepam LD[17]
		Buspirone[18]
		Benzodiazepines
		  (short-acting)[17]
		Clomethiazole[21]
		Propranolol LD[20]
		Zaleplon[19]
		Zolpidem[19]
		Zopiclone[19]
			Benzodiazepines
			  (long-acting)[17]
			Chloral[21]
			Propranolol HD[20]

Anticonvulsants	Carbamazepine[22]
	Ethosuximide[28]
	Gabapentin[26]
	Topiramate?[27]
	Vigabatrin[27]
		Acetazolamide[28]
		Benzodiazepines
		  (short-acting)[17]
		Lamotrigine[27]
		Levetiracetam[27]
		Oxcarbazepine[22]
		Tiagabine[27]
			Barbiturates[25]
			Benzodiazepines
			  (long-acting)[17]
			Phenytoin[24]
			Valproate[23]

Others	Donepezil[29] Lithium[32] Memantine[29]	Acamprosate[31] Anticholinergics[30] Bupropion[35] Disulfiram[31] Galantamine[29] Methylphenidate[34] Modafinil[33] Rivastigmine[29]	

LD = Low dose; HD = High dose

General Principals (*adapted from Maudsley Guidelines, 2003*)

1. The greater the degree of hepatic impairment, the greater the degree of impaired drug metabolism, the greater the risk of drug toxicity, the lower should be the starting and final dose. People may be more sensitive to common or predictable side-effects.

2. Start low, go slow and monitor LFTs regularly (eg. weekly).
3. LFTs do not necessarily correlate well with metabolic impairment, although give a reasonable indication.
4. Care is needed with drugs with a high first-pass clearance effect, as the half-life may be longer.
5. In severe liver disease, avoid drugs with marked side-effects of sedation and constipation.

3.6.1 Antipsychotics

1. Unbound **risperidone** increases in liver disease and so initial doses and dose increments should be halved, and a dose of 4mg/d not exceeded in patients with liver impairment (UK SPC).
2. A lower **olanzapine** starting dose of 5mg/d may be appropriate in patients with risk factors (eg. hepatic impairment, concomitant hepatotoxic drugs). Asymptomatic changes in some liver enzymes may occur with **quetiapine**, so the starting dose should be 25mg/d, with dose increments of 25–50mg/d. **Zotepine** levels may be 2–3 times higher in patients with liver impairment. Start at 25mg bd up to maximum of 75mg bd and measure LFTs weekly for the first three months of therapy for patients with hepatic impairment (MI). Dose changes are unnecessary for **aripiprazole**. Use slower dose titrations and lower maintenance doses with **sertindole** and contraindicate in severe hepatic failure.
3. Severe hepatic disease is a contraindication for **clozapine**, and so lower doses and regular plasma level monitoring would be necessary if used.
4. No dosage adjustments are necessary for **flupentixol** nor **zuclopenthixol**, perhaps except in significant hepatic impairment.
5. **Sulpiride** and **amisulpride** are virtually unmetabolised, with little or no biliary excretion, and so dosage adjustments are unnecessary (UK SPCs).
6. There are no apparent problems with **haloperidol**, although the UK SPC states liver disease to be a caution.

7. **Phenothiazines** may cause hepatocanalicular cholestasis and there have been suggestions of possible immunological liver damage. Onset is usually during the first month of therapy. Phenothiazines may precipitate coma due to increased cerebral neurone sensitivity. **Chlorpromazine** is particularly hepatotoxic and should be avoided.
8. No specific problems are known in liver damage with **loxapine** but extensive hepatic metabolism indicates a higher risk.

3.6.2 Antidepressants

9. With hepatic impairment, alternate day dosing of **fluoxetine** is recommended due to prolonged half-lives and higher plasma levels. **Citalopram** and **escitalopram** are metabolised extensively by the liver, and so doses at the lower end of the therapeutic range should be used. **Sertraline** is extensively metabolised by the liver and so is contraindicated (due to lack of safety evidence). **Fluvoxamine** should be started at 50mg/d and monitored carefully, as raised hepatic enzymes have been reported. **Paroxetine** is probably the drug of choice, although there are isolated cases of hepatotoxicity.
10. **Venlafaxine** is contraindicated in severe hepatic impairment and doses should be reduced by about 25–50% in mild to moderate impairment, although there is much inter-patient variability.
11. **Mirtazapine** clearance can be decreased by 33% in hepatic impairment and so dosage reduction may be necessary.
12. Most **tricyclics** have a high first-pass clearance by the liver, and so lower starting doses are necessary. Increased sedation with **tricyclics** is likely in liver damage due to decreased metabolism and increased blood levels due to reduced plasma protein binding, eg. **amitriptyline** has been reported to have doubled or tripled plasma levels in patients with cirrhosis. Cholestatic jaundice has been noted with **imipramine**, **amitriptyline** and **nortriptyline**. **Lofepramine** is contraindicated. SSRIs such as **paroxetine**

would appear to be easier to use than tricyclics in liver disease.

13. **Trazodone** should be used with care in severe hepatic impairment.

14. **Reboxetine** half-life and plasma levels appear to rise in severe hepatic insufficiency and dose adjustment may be necessary. A starting dose of 2mg BD is recommended.

15. **MAOIs** are hepatotoxic and may precipitate coma. Patients may also be more sensitive to side-effects. If essential, start with a low dose, increase gradually and observe carefully. **Isocarboxazid** is contraindicated with any degree of impaired hepatic function.

16. **Moclobemide** clearance can be reduced and half-life increased in cirrhosis, so doses should be reduced by a half or third to avoid accumulation. There are no apparent problems with **mianserin** and **tryptophan**. **St. John's wort** levels may rise in moderate cirrhosis and absorption decreased.

3.6.3 Anxiolytics and hypnotics

17. The metabolism of **diazepam** and **chlordiazepoxide** is impaired in liver disease. The half-lives of their metabolites are reported to be substantially prolonged and such metabolite accumulation in liver damage has been reported to induce coma. Impaired metabolism has been reported with **alprazolam, clobazam** and **midazolam**. The metabolism of **lorazepam, temazepam** and **oxazepam** are unchanged and these are the benzodiazepines of choice in low dose.

18. The **buspirone** UK SPC recommends caution with a history of hepatic impairment and contraindicates in severe hepatic disease.

19. Elimination of **zopiclone** can be reduced with hepatic dysfunction but a lower dose of 3.75mg to 7.5mg (but no higher) can be used with caution. **Zolpidem** is contraindicated in severe hepatic insufficiency and reduced doses are recommended in cirrhosis and other hepatic impairment due to increases in half-life and peak plasma concentrations.

Zaleplon is contraindicated in severe hepatic insufficiency and the dose should be reduced to 5mg in patients with mild to moderate hepatic impairment.

20. **Propranolol** metabolism is impaired in liver disease and may increase the risk of developing hepatic encephalopathy. Reduced oral doses are needed.

21. A ten-fold increase in blood levels of **clomethiazole** can occur in severe liver disease, so reduced doses are needed. Care is needed as sedation can mask the onset of coma. **Chloral** is contraindicated in marked hepatic impairment.

3.6.4 Anticonvulsants

22. Serious hepatic disorders from **carbamazepine** are rare, although jaundice, hepatitis and liver function disorders have been reported, and so use should be with caution. Although **oxcarbazepine** is rapidly and extensively metabolised, no dose adjustments are generally needed in mild to moderate hepatic impairment. **Oxcarbazepine** has not been studied in severe hepatic impairment (SPC).

23. **Valproate** is contraindicated in active liver disease (SPC), as it can be hepatotoxic and liver failure can occur in about 1 in 10,000 cases. The risk is higher early on in therapy and lessens after a couple of months. Hepatotoxicity occurs mostly in children and presents as worsening epilepsy, drowsiness and with biochemical and/or clinical evidence of liver failure. Some fatal cases have been reported. Care needs to be taken if valproate is used in children, especially if used with other anticonvulsants.

24. **Phenytoin** can accumulate and toxicity may occur in severe liver disease, so use minimal doses and monitor carefully for toxicity. In uraemia, protein binding may be reduced but active/free levels remain unchanged and so therapeutic control may then be possible at plasma levels below the normal range. Severe cardiovascular ADRs have been reported with **fosphenytoin IV**.

25. Increased cerebral sensitivity and impaired metabolism of **barbiturates** may precipitate coma.

26. **Gabapentin** is virtually unmetabolised and so dose adjustments are unnecessary. Initial and maintenance doses of **lamotrigine** should be reduced by 50% in moderate (Child-Pugh grade B) hepatic impairment, and by 75% in severe (Child-Pugh grade C) impairment.

27. **Vigabatrin** can cause decreased SGOT and SGPT levels but there is no evidence of hepatic toxicity. **Topiramate** is not extensively metabolised and dose reductions are not normally necessary. **Tiagabine** is metabolised by the liver. Initial doses in mild to moderate hepatic impairment should be lower and use in severe hepatic impairment is not recommended. No dose adjustment is needed with **levetiracetam** in mild to moderate hepatic impairment, but a 50% dose reduction is recommended in severe impairment due to concomitant renal impairment (UK SPC).

28. There are no apparent problems with **ethosuximide**. **Acetazolamide** should be used with caution.

3.6.5 Others

29. No change in dose is necessary with **donepezil** in mild to moderate hepatic impairment (MI). **Rivastigmine** is contraindicated in severe liver impairment (MI). In moderate to severe impaired hepatic function, start **galantamine** at 4mg/d, increasing slowly to a maximum of 8mg BD, as the half-life may be increased by about 30%. In severe (Child-Pugh > 9) impairment, galantamine is contraindicated (due to current lack of safety data). No dosage reduction is necessary for mild impairment (SPC). **Memantine** is metabolised by the liver only to inactive metabolites and so hepatic impairment is unlikely to have any adverse effect.

30. The UK SPCs for the **anticholinergics** all urge some caution in hepatic disease.

31. The UK SPC for **disulfiram** recommends caution in liver disease. There is little problem with **acamprosate** in mild to moderate hepatic impairment, but it is contraindicated in severe hepatic failure.

32. There are no problems with **lithium** in liver disease.

33. The maximum **modafinil** dose of 400mg/d should only be used in the absence of hepatic impairment (UK SPC).

34. There is no data on **methylphenidate**.

35. **Bupropion** is extensively metabolised and there are rare reports of abnormalities as a prolonged half-life has been reported in hepatic failure. Reduced initial doses and close monitoring is required.

3.7 Old age

	Lower risk	Moderate risk	High risk
Antipsychotics	Amisulpride[5] Aripiprazole[2] Risperidone?[1] Sulpiride[5]	Butyrophenones[6] Olanzapine?[2] Phenothiazines[7] Quetiapine[2] Sertindole[2] Thioxanthenes[4]	Clozapine[4] Thioridazine[7] Zotepine[2]
Antidepressants	Lofepramine[12] Mirtazapine[11] Moclobemide[16] SSRIs[9] Tryptophan[16] Venlafaxine[10]	Flupentixol[4] MAOIs[15] Mianserin[16] Nortriptyline[12] Reboxetine[14] Trazodone	Tricyclics (most)[12]
Anxiolytics and hypnotics	Alprazolam[17] Buspirone[18] Clobazam[17] Lorazepam[17] Oxazepam[17] Oxprenolol[20] Zaleplon[19] Zopiclone[19]	Clomethiazole[21] Flunitrazepam[17] Flurazepam[17] Propranolol[20] Temazepam[17] Zolpidem[19]	Benzodiazepines (long-acting)[21]
Anticonvulsants[7]	Carbamazepine[22] Clobazam[17] Oxcarbazepine[22] Tiagabine[27] Topiramate?[27]	Barbiturates[25] Clonazepam[17] Gabapentin[26] Lamotrigine[26] Levetiracetam[27] Piracetam?[27] Valproate[23]	Acetazolamide[28] Benzodiazepine (most)[17] Fosphenytoin[24] Phenytoin[24] Vigabatrin[27]
Others	Anticholinesterases[29] Bupropion[35] Memantine[29] Modafinil[33]	Anticholinergics[29] Lithium[32]	Acamprosate?[31] Methylphenidate[34]

General Principals (*adapted from Maudsley Guidelines, 2003*)

In the elderly, drug absorption, metabolism and distribution are altered, metabolism, cardiac output and renal perfusion are reduced and tissue sensitivity is usually increased. The over 70s have about twice as many adverse drug reactions as the under 50s, eg. postural hypotension with antipsychotics, prolonged sedation with hypnotics, increased sensitivity to anticholinergic side-effects of drugs etc. All these can lead additionally to falls. Thus, with the elderly, the main principles are to *start with the lowest dose* that can be thought to be beneficial, lower than the adult dose. Only use drugs when necessary, decide a treatment aim, keep therapy simple, use the smallest effective doses and *discontinue gradually if no apparent benefit* can be seen. Monitor effects (both positive and negative) regularly and frequently. 'Start low and go slow' is a useful motto. Avoid drugs with sedative and hypotensive effects, which can increase the under-rated risks of falls.

3.7.1 Antipsychotics

Antipsychotics can relieve psychotic symptoms in older adults but frequent assessments for potential side-effects are very useful before treatment, and then every 3–6 months. Side-effects such as postural hypotension, anticholinergic effects and Parkinsonism are common. Single daily doses are usually appropriate once the person is stable (as indeed they are in younger adults). Doses should be reviewed regularly, and periodic reduction in dose (eg. by 10–25% every four weeks) for some patients may be indicated.

1. Lower doses of **risperidone** may be needed only if hepatic impairment is also present (see *3.6.1*). There is good evidence for risperidone being useful for treating behavioural and other symptoms of dementia and the UK SPC now states that risperidone is well tolerated in the elderly when used with a starting dose of 0.5mg BD (or even lower) and adjusted up to 2mg BD.

2. A lower **olanzapine** starting dose of 5mg/d is recommended in some patients as half-life and plasma levels are higher in the elderly and transient sedation and somnolence are more marked in the elderly. Blood pressure monitoring is recommended periodically and there may be a slightly higher risk of seizures in people over 65. The starting dose for **quetiapine** should be 25mg/d, with dose increments of 25–50mg/d and the final dose is likely to be less than in younger patients, although it appears well tolerated in the elderly. **Zotepine** levels are higher in the elderly so start at 25mg bd up to a maximum of 75mg bd for elderly patients. No **aripiprazole** dose changes are necessary in the elderly. A slower dose titration and perhaps lower final doses may be needed with **sertindole**.

3. **Clozapine** may be safe, tolerated and effective in the elderly at doses as low as 50–100mg/d, but as there may be an increased incidence of agranulocytosis, great care should be taken.

4. **Zuclopenthixol** and **flupentixol** should be used with caution in renal disease.

5. Single doses of **amisulpride** are well tolerated and show a similar pharmacokinetic profile in healthy elderly and young subjects.

6. An increased severity of side-effects, including oversedation, hypotension and respiratory depression, may occur with **haloperidol** and so lower starting doses are indicated.

7. No more than one half to one third the normal adult dose of **phenothiazines** should be used for elderly patients, who are more susceptible to Parkinsonian side-effects. **Chlorpromazine**, except in very low dose, should be **avoided** as Parkinsonian side-effects, hypotension and sedation are much more likely to occur. **Levomepromazine** is not recommended for use in people over 50 unless the risk of hypotensive reaction has been assessed (SPC).

8. **Loxapine** should generally be avoided.

3.7.2 Antidepressants

Depression increases mortality in the elderly with cardiac disease, especially if long-standing and severe. Drugs with anticholinergic side-effects may further harm an already compromised cholinergic system.

9. **SSRIs** have obvious benefits in the elderly (fewer anticholinergic effects, a benign cardiovascular profile, ease of use and safety in overdose) but some unappreciated risks, including hyponatraemia, weight loss, sexual dysfunction and drug interactions (especially fluoxetine and paroxetine). The half-life of **fluoxetine** appears not significantly different in the elderly. No dosage changes are necessary for **fluoxetine, fluvoxamine** and **sertraline**. Initially lower doses of 10mg/d are recommended for **paroxetine** as blood levels with 20mg/d in the elderly can be similar to those of 30mg/d in younger

people. A prolonged **citalopram** and **escitalopram** half-life may occur and maximum doses of 40mg/d and 10mg/d respectively are recommended.

10. Care is needed with **venlafaxine** as cardiac side-effects and postural hypotension may be more common in the elderly.

11. **Mirtazapine** dosage is the same in the elderly as younger adults, although the SPC recommends care with dosage increments and a quicker onset of action has been reported compared with paroxetine.

12. Reduced initial doses of **tricyclics** are recommended, with perhaps slightly lower final doses, depending upon tolerance, as cognitive and central effects are enhanced in the elderly, eg. with **amitriptyline, dothiepin/dosulepin, imipramine** and **doxepin. Nortriptyline** appears much less affected by age and dose changes may not be needed. Elderly patients may respond to lower doses of **lofepramine** but low dose lofepramine (70mg/d) is no better than placebo, so that full, or at least higher, doses are necessary. Anticholinergic side-effects are more common but a proper therapeutic dose is still needed as doses such as 75mg/d are generally subtherapeutic. It has been noted that when tricyclic non-response has occurred in an elderly person, response to an alternative antidepressant may take up to 5–6 weeks, rather than the 3–4 weeks normally expected, so do not give up too soon.

13. Single daily dosing of **trazodone** may not be appropriate in the elderly, and reduced doses may be required, eg. 150mg/d may be the optimum in the elderly. Half-life is increased in elderly men, but not women.

14. For **reboxetine**, start at 2mg BD as peak plasma levels are higher in the elderly. Frail elderly may need dose reduction. The UK SPC does not recommend use in the elderly, for lack of positive information rather than the presence of negative information. Lowered potassium levels and tachycardia have also been reported.

15. **MAOIs** are often considered as more toxic to the elderly, mainly due to postural hypotension and dizziness although MAOIs have been used by specialists to great effect in resistant depression in the elderly.

16. There are no problems with **moclobemide**. Reduced doses of **mianserin** may be needed although reduced receptor sensitivity may not lead to increased side-effects. There are no apparent problems with **tryptophan**.

3.7.3 Anxiolytics and hypnotics

17. All benzodiazepines should be used with care in the elderly, as side-effects are likely to be enhanced. Reduced doses are generally recommended for **flunitrazepam** and other longer-acting benzodiazepines, eg. **clobazam** and **chlordiazepoxide**. The half-life of nitrazepam is extended and steady state can be reached in 4–5 days in the elderly (with increased daytime cognitive impairment and CNS side-effects) and so reduced doses are necessary if it cannot be avoided. Reduced doses of **diazepam** should also be used in the elderly, eg. diazepam 2.5mg produced significant memory impairment, reduced psychomotor performance and sedation in the elderly in one study. Reduced doses of **temazepam** are usually recommended as the half-life can reach 24 hours in elderly people, not to mention its well-publicised use as a pension supplement by being sold to relatives etc. Slightly reduced doses of **lorazepam** are suggested, particularly if used as a hypnotic. Normal adult doses of **oxazepam** and **loprazolam** can be used and may be the benzodiazepines of choice in the elderly.

18. Dose adjustments are not considered necessary for **buspirone.**

19. There appears to be no problem with **zaleplon** in the elderly. Normal adult doses of **zopiclone** can be used if moderate-to-severe hepatic impairment is present. A 5mg dose of **zolpidem** (half the healthy adult dose) is recommended, with studies

showing good efficacy and lack of adverse effects in an elderly population.

20. Increased **propranolol** side-effects have been reported in the elderly and so reduced initial doses are generally recommended, but **oxprenolol** can be used normally.

21. **Clomethiazole** doses should be reduced, as plasma levels can be up to five times higher than in young adults.

3.7.4 Anticonvulsants

For **anticonvulsants**, it is best to avoid renally excreted drugs (eg. **vigabatrin** and **gabapentin**) as the renal excretion may be reduced in the elderly, sometimes to one sixth compared with younger people. Hepatically metabolised drugs, such as **valproate, carbamazepine** and **lamotrigine**, are not influenced by age (review of epilepsy in old age by Bene, *Prescriber* 1997, **8**, 31–36).

22. **Carbamazepine** levels in the elderly are likely to be the same as in younger adults although they may be more susceptible to cardiac arrhythmias with the drug. Although **oxcarbazepine** levels may be higher in the elderly, no dose recommendations exist, other than gradual dose titration, particularly in patients with compromised renal function (UK SPC).

23. The half-life of **valproate** may be doubled in old age, possibly via reduced metabolism but total blood levels are similar to younger adults, so no dose changes are recommended.

24. Reduced doses of **phenytoin** are needed in the elderly. Great care in monitoring is necessary, especially in those with hypoalbuminaemia or renal disease as this may induce an increased level of side-effects and toxicity eg. cardiac arrhythmias. In people aged from 60 to 80, doses 20% lower will maintain blood levels, compared to younger adults. Severe cardiovascular ADRs have been reported with **fosphenytoin IV** (see *3.2*), so reduced doses are recommended.

25. Reduced doses of **phenobarbital/ primidone** should be used.

26. **Lamotrigine** is hepatically metabolised and so reduced doses may be needed as the half-life may be extended in the elderly. **Gabapentin** clearance is reduced in old age, probably via reduced renal clearance.

27. **Vigabatrin** is renally excreted and excretion may be reduced in the elderly to one sixth compared to younger people. Reduced doses have been recommended in people with a creatinine clearance of less than 60ml/min and some have recommended that it should be avoided entirely in the elderly. No age-related changes in pharmacokinetics have been detected with **topiramate**. The half-live of **piracetam** and **tiagabine** are extended in the elderly, but no dose changes are recommended. Since renal impairment may occur, reduced doses of **levetiracetam** are recommended (see *3.9.4*), as the half-life may increase by about 40%.

28. Lower **acetazolamide** doses are indicated.

3.7.5 Others

29. There are no specific problems with **donepezil, galantamine, rivastigmine** and **memantine**, provided the dose titration guidelines are followed.

30. For the anticholinergics, an initial low dose is usually recommended for **benzhexol/trihexyphenidyl**. **Procyclidine** should be used as a BD rather than TDS dosing. No dose changes are necessary with **orphenadrine**. Confusion can be induced in the elderly by all these drugs by further reducing an already potentially compromised cholinergic system.

31. The UK SPC for **acamprosate** states that it should not be used in the elderly, due more to lack of data rather than specific reported problems.

32. Reduced **lithium** clearance and lengthened half-life in the elderly mean that doses reduced by as much as 50% may be necessary. The elderly may also develop symptoms of lithium toxicity at standard therapeutic blood levels. However, lithium can be safely used in the

elderly if monitored *carefully* (ie. it actually gets done!) and *frequently* (eg. every 1–2 months), along with renal and thyroid function. Hypothyroidism can also occur.

33. In the elderly, a **modafinil** starting dose of 100mg/d is recommended (MI).

34. There is no data for **methylphenidate**, although it has been used successfully to treat resistant depression in the elderly.

35. **Bupropion** appears well tolerated in the elderly, although some accumulation may occur and greater side-effects might occur.

3.8 Pregnancy

	Lower risk (FDA = A)	Moderate risk (FDA = B or C)	High risk (FDA = D or X)
Antipsychotics		Aripiprazole[2] Butyrophenones[6] Clozapine[3] Olanzapine?[2] Phenothiazines[7] Quetiapine[2] Risperidone[1] Sulpiride[5] Thioxanthenes[4]	Zotepine[2]
Antidepressants	Flupentixol?[4] Tryptophan?[16]	MAOIs[15] Mianserin[16] Mirtazapine[11] Moclobemide[16] SSRIs[9] St. John's wort[16] Trazodone[13] Tricyclics[12] Venlafaxine[10]	
Anxiolytics and hypnotics		Beta-blockers[20] Buspirone[18] Chloral[21] Clomethiazole[21] Clonazepam[17] Promethazine[21] Zaleplon[19] Zopiclone[19]	Alprazolam[17] Chlordiazepoxide[17] Lorazepam[17] Oxazepam[17] Temazepam[17] Zolpidem[19]
Anticonvulsants[9]		Acetazolamide[28] Carbamazepine[22] Clonazepam?[17] Ethosuximide[28] Gabapentin[25] Lamotrigine[25] Oxcarbazepine[22] Tiagabine[27]	Benzodiazepines[17] Phenobarbital[25] Phenytoin[24] Topiramate[27] Valproate[23] Vigabatrin[27]
Others		Anticholinergics[31] Anticholinesterases[29] Bupropion[35] Dexamfetamine[42] Disulfiram[38] Lithium[36] Memantine[2] Methadone LD[35] Methylphenidate[36]	Acamprosate[31] Lithium[32] Methadone HD[34] Modafinil?[33]

All drugs should be avoided in the first three months of pregnancy if at all possible. With most drugs, however, the lack of quality data means only an approximate assessment of the relative risks can be made. The **FDA in the USA** has established five really useful categories to indicate a drugs potential for teratogenicity:

A — controlled studies in women have *failed to show a risk* in the first trimester and the risk of foetal harm seems remote.

B — *Either* animal tests do not show a risk but there are no human studies *or* animal studies show a risk but human studies have failed to show a risk to the foetus.

C — *Either* animal studies show teratogenic or embryocidal effects but there are no controlled studies in women *or* there are no studies in either animals or humans (the default classification).

D — Definite evidence of a risk to the foetus exists but the benefits in certain circumstances (eg. life threatening situations) may make use acceptable.

X — Foetal abnormalities have been shown in animals or humans or both and the *risk outweighs any possible benefits*.

Where known or available, these classifications are noted in the text.

Spontaneous major or gross malformations (usually defined as incompatible with life or requiring surgical correction) occur in 2–4% of pregnancies and spontaneous abortions in about 10–20% of clinically recognised pregnancies. In the first trimester, teratogenicity is the main drug risk, in the 2–3rd, growth retardation and neurological damage may occur. After birth, drug withdrawal effects may occur and there may be evidence of delayed development.

General Principals (*adapted from Maudsley Guidelines, 2003*)

Pre-conception:

1. For planned conception, discuss the risks and benefits of discontinuing or continuing medication, eg. relapse, teratogenicity etc, the unpredictability of the pre-conceptual duration, and that no decision is risk-free. Avoiding all drugs during the first trimester is the ideal. Other options include continuing at the lowest possible dose or switching to a drug with a shorter half-life.

2. Consider the risk of pregnancy even if not currently planned, eg. carry out a pregnancy test before starting teratogenic drugs in a woman of child-bearing age. Up to 50% of pregnancies are unplanned, so document the patient's birth control method and document potential risks for pregnancy exposure to drug(s). Encourage proper nutrition, exercise and vitamin supplementation, any other substances taken, eg. excess caffeine, alcohol, natural products etc and educate about the potential risks. Enquire about any pregnancy plans and emphasise the need for pre-pregnancy consultation.

3. Consider switching to lowest-risk drugs before conception.

During pregnancy:

1. Avoid all drugs during the first trimester if possible. The maximum teratogenic potential is from days 17-60 after conception, and decisions must balance the relative *vs* absolute risk.

2. Subtle functional disturbances (eg. learning difficulties, neurological deficits, developmental delay etc), and an effect on labour and delivery may occur with drugs in the second and third trimesters.

3. Use the lowest possible (maintenance) dose and monitor effects (adverse and desired) carefully.

4. In many cases, the risk of relapse (and subsequent higher dose drug use) will be higher than the risk of foetal damage.

5. Avoid polypharmacy, as synergistic teratogenicity can occur.

6. The pharmacokinetics of drugs may change during pregnancy and so doses may need to be adjusted (see lithium, tricyclics), especially close to delivery date.

7. Discontinuation effects have been reported in the newborn (see benzodiazepines, tricyclics, SSRIs etc) and these psychotropics should, if possible, be gradually reduced or withdrawn over the weeks before delivery is due.

Unexpected pregnancy

If a woman discovers or reports that she is pregnant while taking a drug:

- Don't panic
- If before day 17, consider immediate stopping or temporary discontinuation
- If after day 60, the major risk has passed and so decisions are less urgent
- Institute immediate nutritional supplements (eg. folic acid)
- Reduce the dose if possible, at least during the high risk period
- Discontinue any non-essential treatments, particularly any that might be at sub-therapeutic doses
- Do not stop lithium abruptly (see point 32) and beware of stopping some SSRIs and anticonvulsants
- Seek specific specialist advice, and discuss the risk of the possible consequences of relapse versus the published risk to the foetus.

Further information should be sought on individual drugs to balance the risk-benefit ratio, eg. from a National Teratology Information Service in Newcastle on 0191-232-1525 (reminder from Bateman and McElhatton, *Br Med J* 1997, **314**, 1414–15) and would be delighted to answer all your questions. NTIS carries out individual risk assessments for pregnant women exposed to drugs or chemicals and offers pre-conceptual advice, research and follow-up information.

3.8.1 Antipsychotics

Low folate intake and serum levels have been reported in women taking atypical antipsychotics and so dietary advice and/or folate supplements pre-conception would be essential.

1. **Risperidone** (FDA = C) has no reported teratogenicity in animal tests but little human data is available as yet.

2. From 23 documented pregnancies to 2002 with **olanzapine** (FDA = C), 5% were premature, spontaneous abortion occurred in 13% and stillbirth in 5%, but with no major malformations; all these are within normal ranges. It should only be used when the potential benefit outweighs the potential risk (SPC). No information is available for **quetiapine** (FDA = C) and the SPC recommends using only if the benefits justify the risk. **Zotepine** crosses the placenta and although there are no indications of teratogenicity, the drug is contraindicated in pregnancy. No human data is available for **aripiprazole** (FDA = C) although the animal data is unremarkable. **Sertindole** is contraindicated.

3. Women are more likely to conceive on **clozapine** (FDA = B) than other antipsychotics due to the relative lack of effect of clozapine on prolactin. Novartis have had 84 reports of pregnancy with known outcomes to date, and although no firm conclusions can be drawn, it appears that clozapine is not a major teratogen. Naturally the manufacturers do not recommend it, and the *BNF* notes that the manufacturers advise avoiding.

4. **Thioxanthenes**
(FDA classifications not available)
Flupentixol passes across the placenta and foetal levels are about a quarter of the mother's but there is no positive evidence of teratogenicity (although Lundbeck obviously do not recommend it's use).

Studies in 3 species have not shown malformations. A total of fifteen cases of variable birth defects have been reported. With **zuclopenthixol**, few birth defects have been recorded, at a rate consistent with the spontaneous levels of malformations.

5. **Sulpiride** (FDA N/A) has been used as an antinauseant in pregnancy. There are no published reports of abnormalities in animals or humans.

6. **Butyrophenones** (FDA = C)
The safety of **haloperidol** in pregnancy has not been established although it was once used in hyperemesis gravidarum with no reports of teratogenicity. Although there are isolated cases of alleged teratogenicity with haloperidol (eg. unproven limb malformations), no cause-effect relationship has been established and there are no reports of haloperidol alone causing abnormalities (MI).

7. **Phenothiazines**
(FDA: chlorpromazine = C, levomepromazine = C, trifluoperazine = C, promazine = C, thioridazine = C, trifluoperazine = C, fluphenazine = C, others not available)
The phenothiazines have been studied in detail, although most of the data is based on low dose use and thus not necessarily applicable to higher dose use. The phenothiazines are considered by some as of lowest risk, although the potential for hypotension, sedation and anticholinergic effects means that any use must be with extreme care. Severe congenital abnormalities were not significantly different in the studies of 543 women taking low-dose phenothiazines other than prochlorperazine for nausea and in 1309 mothers, mostly taking prochlorperazine. The largest study, of 315 pregnancies, where phenothiazines were taken in the first trimester, showed a statistically significant difference in malformation rate of 3.5% in the aliphatic (**chlorpromazine** and **promazine**) phenothiazine-treated group (11 malformed infants) compared with 1.6% in the control group. There was no apparent trend in the type of abnormality and the risk is still considered low. There

was no difference with the other phenothiazines, which appear to have an incidence of malformations similar to the background incidence. In the neonate, lethargy, jaundice and extrapyramidal symptoms have been reported, as has respiratory depression when given in high dose (above 500mg chlorpromazine equivalents) close to term. There is a case of apparent withdrawal symptoms (jitteriness, abnormal movements and irritability) in an infant, reversed by diphenhydramine, in a mother taking chlorpromazine (up to 1200mg/d) and fluphenazine decanoate (100mg a week). Symptoms resolved by about 9 months. In the longer term, a lack of impaired mental or physical development has been shown at 2 and 7 years in a 16-child follow-up study.

8. **Loxapine** (FDA = C) data is lacking.

3.8.2 Antidepressants

9. **SSRIs**
(FDA: citalopram = C, escitalopram = C, fluoxetine = B, fluvoxamine = C, paroxetine = B, sertraline = B; but the *BNF* notes adverse effects in animals for all SSRIs and manufacturers advise to avoid).
No embryotoxic or teratogenic effects have been seen in animals with **paroxetine** and in the limited human data available no abnormalities have been seen yet. However, a withdrawal syndrome in the new-born child seems likely and so gradual dose reduction before delivery should be considered. Information is available on over 2000 **fluoxetine**-exposed pregnancies, reported in 3 prospective cohort-controlled studies and 4 prospective surveys. Based on published studies, there is no increased risk of malformations occurring in women exposed to fluoxetine and no evidence of teratogenicity (eg. study and review, Nulman and Koren, *Teratology* 1996, **53**, 304-8). There is an absence of perinatal sequleae and no evidence of an increase in major malformations, spontaneous abortion, poor perinatal state or neurodevelopmental delay. No long-term effect on IQ

nor language and behaviour development have been shown, whereas untreated depression is associated with poorer cognitive and language development. The UK SPC naturally states caution and use should only be if clearly needed. There is no human information available for **sertraline** at present nor **citalopram** or **escitalopram**.

In a prospective, multicentre cohort study of 267 women exposed to an SSRI antidepressant (fluvoxamine, sertraline and paroxetine) during pregnancy and 267 controls, exposure to SSRIs at recommended doses did not appear to be associated with increased teratogenicity (relative risk 1.06, 95% CI, 0.43–2.62) or higher rates of miscarriage, stillbirth or prematurity. Gestational ages and birth weights were similar amongst offspring of both groups of women (Kulin *et al, JAMA* 1998, **279**, 609–10).

10. Data on 150 **venlafaxine** (FDA = C) pregnancies indicates a slightly higher spontaneous abortion rate but no increase in malformations.

11. Animal tests do not show **mirtazapine** (FDA = C) to be teratogenic nor cause foetal harm. There are 7 reported human cases with no adverse consequences.

12. **Tricyclic antidepressants** (FDA: amitriptyline = C, amoxapine = C, clomipramine = C, doxepin = C, maprotiline = B, nortriptyline = D, trimipramine = C) There is no convincing evidence that the **tricyclics** are teratogenic in the first trimester, with early retrospective studies showing no connection with limb deformities. Evidence from studies shows no increase in spontaneous abortions, malformations nor pattern of defects from tricyclics and a meta-analysis of the use of tricyclics in pregnancy, reviewing over 300,000 live births including 414 first trimester exposures, failed to show a significant association between tricyclics and congenital malformations. **Amitriptyline** and **imipramine** are considered the tricyclics of choice, based on cumulative data on their relative safety. Discontinuation effects have been noted,

sometimes requiring active treatment, eg. withdrawal symptoms from clomipramine in the neonate have been reported widely, eg. jittery/twitchy, lethargic infants. One study has shown that tricyclic levels decrease during the third trimester and then rise rapidly immediately after birth (probably due to decreased metabolism) and so one needs to observe for toxic effects and adjust doses rapidly if needed.

Postnatal development:
A careful study of children (assessed between 18 and 86 months) whose mothers had taken either a tricyclic (n = 84) or no drug (n = 80) showed tricyclics to have no effect on global IQ, language development or behavioural development compared to no drug (Nulman *et al, NEJM* 1997, **336**, 258–62), whereas untreated depression is associated with poorer cognitive and language development.

13. For **trazodone** (FDA = C) at very high doses (15+ times the maximum human dose), there appears to be some foetal resorption and congenital abnormalities but little human data exists to support this.

14. No teratogenic effects have been noted with **reboxetine** in animal studies but little human data exists so the drug should be avoided in pregnancy (SPC).

15. **MAOIs:**
(FDA: isocarboxazid = C, phenelzine = C, tranylcypromine = C). The *BNF* notes no evidence of harm but the manufacturers recommend avoiding unless compelling reasons. There are no reports of human teratogenicity with **phenelzine** nor **tranylcypromine**, although it has been suggested that the risk of teratogenic problems may be roughly doubled if tranylcypromine is taken in the first trimester. **MAOIs** should be avoided if at all possible due to maternal toxicity and lack of published safety data. MAOIs may interact with drugs used in labour (see pethidine under MAOIs in *4.3.4)*

16. There is no evidence of teratogenicity with **mianserin** in animals except at toxic doses but no human data is available (FDA = N/A). No human data is available

for **tryptophan** which is, after all, an amino-acid. No data is available yet on the use of **moclobemide** in pregnancy. The *BNF* notes no evidence of harm but that the manufacturers recommend avoiding unless compelling reasons exist. Slight *in vitro* uterotonic activity has been reported and the lack of safety and toxicity data suggests that **St. John's wort** is currently best avoided in pregnancy.

3.8.3 Anxiolytics and hypnotics

17. Benzodiazepines:
(FDA: alprazolam = D, chlordiazepoxide = D, clonazepam = C, diazepam = D, lorazepam = D, oxazepam = D, temazepam = X, others not available). The *BNF* notes neonatal respiratory depression, hypotonia and withdrawal symptoms, and to avoid regular use of longer-acting benzodiazepines, preferring short-acting benzodiazepines.

Assessment of 104,000 births in the USA has shown a higher incidence of teratogenicity in women taking benzodiazepines but multiple alcohol and illicit substance exposure could account for this. With **alprazolam** there are no reports of teratogenicity. With **chlordiazepoxide**, an increased risk of teratogenicity has been suggested if chlordiazepoxide is taken during the first 42 days of pregnancy (11.4 per 100 live births) compared to after 42 days (3.6 per 100 live births, 175 studied), although others have failed to repeat this link. **Clobazam** is known to pass the placenta and benzodiazepine withdrawal symptoms in the neonate have been suggested. For **diazepam**, studies show a varying risk of oral clefts, with the worst case scenario bringing the risk to 7 in 1000. In late pregnancy, doses of 30mg or more of diazepam IM or IV during the last 15 hours of labour can induce neonatal respiratory depression and feeding problems. 10mg given IV within 10 minutes of birth has been shown not to affect Apgar scores. As with other benzodiazepines, withdrawal symptoms in the neonate have been seen. As **lorazepam** crosses the placenta, the floppy baby syndrome and respiratory depression can occur, especially if IV doses are used close to birth. Oral use during later pregnancy may show delayed feeding in full-term infants but premature infants may have lower Apgar scores and respiratory depression. In 1997, the UK CSM restated the danger of high doses and use during pregnancy or labour due to the effects on the neonate such as hypothermia, hypotonia, respiratory depression and withdrawal symptoms (*Curr Prob* 1997, **23**, 10).

After birth, benzodiazepine withdrawal symptoms have been noticed in the neonate with many benzodiazepines. The 'floppy baby' syndrome, as it is often termed, includes facial features and CNS dysfunction and can occur particularly with higher doses (eg. > 30mg diazepam equivalent per day) of longer-acting benzodiazepines, eg. **nitrazepam.**

Thus, shorter acting benzodiazepines on a 'when required' basis may be acceptable later in pregnancy, but the first trimester should be avoided if at all possible.
18. There is no evidence of a teratogenic effect from **buspirone** (FDA = B) but some effects on survival and weight has been noted in animal tests. This is a UK SPC contraindication.
19. **Zopiclone** has not been contraindicated in pregnancy, animal tests have shown no abnormalities and the limited human data is unremarkable. Little information is currently available on **zolpidem** (FDA = B) and **zaleplon** (FDA = C). Until more is known, they should be avoided in pregnancy, especially during the first trimester.
20. **Beta-blockers**
(FDA: propranolol = C, oxprenolol = C). The *BNF* notes they may cause intrauterine growth retardation, neonatal hypoglycaemia and bradycardia. **Beta-blockers** are not generally considered major teratogens but there may be a connection between **propranolol** use in pregnancy and tracheosophageal fistulas and intrauterine growth retardation. Direct

effects on the foetus would also occur, eg. bradycardia etc. Use in the second and third trimesters may aggravate or produce neonatal hypoglycaemia. Foetal and neonatal bradycardia may occur especially in pregnancies already complicated by placental insufficiency (eg. severe maternal hypertension). Due to direct cardiac effects, hypoglycaemia and apnoea, it may be prudent to discontinue treatment 1–2 weeks before delivery.

21. Maternally administered **chloral** lowers bilirubin concentrations in the infant (FDA = C), but no increase in congenital anomalies was seen in a large comparative study in women who took chloral at some time in pregnancy. The manufacturers state that **clomethiazole** should not be used, particularly in the first and third trimesters, although it has been used widely for pre-eclampsia. Adverse effects of platelet aggregation in the neonate have been reported with **promethazine** (FDA = C), although overall promethazine may be safe and appropriate as a hypnotic.

3.8.4 Anticonvulsants

Children of women who have seizures during pregnancy are at a 2.5 times higher risk of seizures later in life. Increased seizures occur in about 25–30% of pregnant women with epilepsy, partly because of marked alterations in plasma protein binding of drugs as pregnancy progresses, resulting in declining plasma levels. A prospective study of 211 women with epilepsy treated with anticonvulsants showed that the risk of abnormal outcomes (10.7%) was three times that for controls (3.4%), with phenobarbital showing the highest risk, although most have an uncomplicated pregnancy and normal healthy offspring. A retrospective cohort study of children born to epileptic mothers showed that most antiepileptic drugs were associated with an increased risk of major congenital abnormalities, in particular valproate, carbamazepine, benzodiazepines and phenobarbital. A review of anticonvulsants in pregnancy concluded that the lowest dose of one of the major drugs probably has less risk than that of recurrent seizures. Smoking increases the risk of pre-term delivery, lower birthweight, length and head circumference. A recent survey has suggested that children exposed to anticonvulsants during pregnancy have a higher frequency of educational needs statements (10.3% drug exposed cf 5.7% non-drug-exposed). The figure for valproate (30%), and possibly also polypharmacy, were much higher, again suggesting a drug effect (Adab *et al, J Neurol Neurosurg Psychiatry* 2001, **70**, 15–21).

Summary of the risks of pregnancy in women with epilepsy:
- 25–33% increase in maternal seizure frequency
- 10% risk of vaginal bleeding
- 7% risk of neonatal hemorrhage if no vitamin K is given
- 10% risk of infant facial dysmorphism
- 4–6% risk of major malformations (30% of which are oral facial defects)
- 1–2% risk of spina bifida with valproate
- 0.5–1% risk of spina bifida with carbamazepine.

Summary of risk minimisation strategies:
1. Pre-conception:
- education of the patient to risks/benefits
- adequate oral contraceptive dosage (see *4.5*) until conception planned
- **regular multivitamins with folate** before oral contraceptives stopped to reduce the chance of spina bifida
- diagnosis verified and the need for anticonvulsants confirmed
- seizure control with lowest dose monotherapy targeted.

2. After conception:
- education of the patient to risks/benefits.

3. Seizure control without toxicity:
- do not change drugs if the patient is stabilised
- multivitamins with folate continued

- frequent monitoring of free anticonvulsant concentrations and dose adjustment if necessary
- monotherapy if possible
- vitamin K given during last week of pregnancy
- ultrasound and AFPs carried out.

22. **Carbamazepine** (FDA = C) was considered by many to be the anticonvulsant of choice in epilepsy, but there is now evidence of an association with neural tube defects, particularly spina bifida (1% incidence), and a pattern of minor problems such as craniofacial defects (11%), fingernail hypoplasia (27%) and developmental delay (20%) has been noted although all these cases were in women on polytherapy and so an interaction effect is possible, and the effect of the epilepsy itself is not definitely known. Polytherapy has been separately reported to increase the risk of malformations. The **BNF/CSM** recommends the need for counselling, adequate folate supplements (eg. 5mg/d) and screening for neural tube defects (*Curr Problems* 1993, **19**, 8), which can detect 90–95% of neural tube defects if carried out with AFP levels at 16–18 weeks. Two studies have shown no adverse long-term effects from carbamazepine on the children eg. similar IQs and language abilities to controls, suggesting the lack of a clinically important adverse effect in cognitive development. In late pregnancy, routine vitamin K to mothers is usually recommended because of a neonatal bleeding tendency. **Oxcarbazepine** (FDA = C) is closely related to carbamazepine. The placenta may contribute to the metabolism of oxcarbazepine and the UK SPC suggests that oxcarbazepine may cause serious birth defects.

23. **Valproate** (FDA = D; the *BNF* notes increased neural tube defects plus neonatal bleeding and hepatotoxicity). Valproate crosses the placenta easily and teratogenicity, specifically neural tube defects such as spina bifida, has been strongly suggested. A 'foetal valproate syndrome' has been shown, presenting as congenital heart defects and a withdrawal syndrome of irritability, jitteriness, hypotonia and feeding problems. UK rates with valproate are stated to be about 1%, which is 50 times the prevalent untreated rate. Incidence rates are reported to be 1–2% in the USA. The **BNF/CSM** recommends the need for counselling and screening for neural tube defects (*Curr Problems* 1993, **19**, 8), which should take place in a specialist centre with high resolution ultrasound and experienced technicians. The UK SPC now states that there have been rare reports of a haemorrhagic syndrome in neonates whose mothers took valproate in pregnancy. *In utero* exposure to valproate may lead to a higher than expected incidence of education needs statements, although a prospective study would be needed to confirm this. Dividing daily doses and using SR preparations to reduce the peak levels may be wise. Folic acid supplementation at 4mg/d before and during pregnancy has also been recommended. A recent study has suggested that the valproate syndrome only occurs at valproate doses above 1000mg/d, a useful and important finding (Mawer *et al, Seizure* 2002, **11**, 512–18).

24. **Phenytoin** (FDA = D; the *BNF* notes screening required, folate supplements, K_1 pre-delivery and caution with plasma level interpreting). Phenytoin crosses the placenta freely and teratogenicity is well established, including the 'foetal hydantoin syndrome'. This syndrome includes retarded intrauterine growth, microcephaly, mental retardation, facial defects including cleft lip and/or palate, digit hypoplasia and inguinal hernia, plus cardiovascular gastrointestinal or genitourinary anomalies. The full syndrome occurs in about 8–10% of children born to mothers who take phenytoin in the first trimester and a part syndrome in a further 30% of children. It appears not to be dose-related. A withdrawal syndrome, including irritability and haemorrhage has also been reported. It has also been noted that epileptic fathers taking phenytoin have increased rates of malformed children.

In the 3rd trimester phenytoin also inhibits the synthesis of Vitamin K-dependent clotting factors and neonatal haemorrhage may occur. Vitamin K for the mother during the last 2 weeks of pregnancy and to the neonate after birth are recommended.

The kinetics of phenytoin change in pregnancy, with up to 45% of women having an increased seizure frequency and total blood levels may be low but still be active. As with other anticonvulsants, foetal hypoxia presents a significant risk.

Risk reduction of phenytoin in pregnancy:

Where seizures are proven to be controlled only by phenytoin, then the risks of withdrawal are probably greater than the continued use of phenytoin and the risk can be reduced by:

1. Use of minimal effective doses. Monitor monthly both during pregnancy and for up to six months to avoid toxicity and increased teratogenic risk.
2. Use of folic acid 5mg/d from before conception. One study resulted in **no** birth defects in the 33 mothers who took folic acid from before conception or immediately upon becoming pregnant, but there were 10 children with malformations from the 66 born to mothers who did not take folic acid, a *clinically significant and important* difference. The neural tube closes around the time of the first missed period and so folic acid supplements need to be started **before** pregnancy is detected.
3. Vitamin K supplementation (see above). Developmental impairment and reduced growth and head circumference have been reported at 7 years, a clinically important adverse effect.

25. Phenobarbital

(FDA = D; the *BNF* notes congenital malformations, neonatal bleeding tendency, and suggests prophylactic vitamin K before delivery)

Phenobarbital has been implicated as a teratogen, although in many cases that have occurred it has been as part of combination therapy. Minor digital deformities,

hip and facial abnormalities, smaller head size at birth and persistent learning problems are higher compared to controls. There may be a direct neurotoxic effect by phenobarbital on developing foetal neurones. Withdrawal symptoms such as seizures and irritability have occurred in the neonate, some delayed by up to two weeks after birth. There is also some evidence of longer-term learning difficulties, based on psychological tests on 7-year-old children. However, antenatal exposure has not been shown to affect neurodevelopment at 2 years.

26. The incidence of major malformations with **lamotrigine** (FDA = C) is about 1.8% (in line with other monotherapy studies), but may be as high as 10% if taken with valproate. Increased doses may be necessary as pregnancy progresses as clearance may increase by 50%. Human data (n = 11) indicates no major problem with **gabapentin** (FDA = C)

27. **Vigabatrin** is contraindicated due to a slight increase in the incidence of cleft palate at high doses in one animal test. No human data is available on **tiagabine** (FDA = C) in pregnancy and so use should only be where clearly indicated. **Topiramate** (FDA = C) has shown some teratogenicity in animals at high dose, similar to **acetazolamide** (MI) and so should not be used in pregnancy unless the benefit clearly outweighs the risk. Some animal studies show animal reproductive toxicity, and so **levetiracetam** (FDA = C) should not be used unless clearly necessary (MI).

28. **Acetazolamide** (FDA = C) may be teratogenic and so if use is essential, maternal electrolyte balance should be monitored. There are reported cases of malformations with **ethosuximide** (FDA = C, BNF = may possibly be teratogenic) alone and when combined with other drugs but no cause-effect relationship has been proven.

4.8.5 Others

29. Very high doses of **donepezil** (FDA = C) may have some minor effects in pregnancy but no teratogenicity has been

detected (MI). The safety of **rivastigmine** (FDA = C) in pregnancy has not been established (MI). There is no data on **galantamine** nor **memantine** in pregnancy (SPC).

30. **Anticholinergics:**
(FDA: benzhexol = C, procyclidine = C)
There is little data available on these drugs.

31. For **disulfiram** (FDA = C) there have been isolated reports of congenital abnormalities, although other drugs were often taken and the symptoms were similar to the foetal alcohol syndrome. The risk:benefit ratio for the foetus for the risks of high alcohol consumption against disulfiram must be assessed carefully. The UK SPC for **acamprosate** states that use in pregnancy is a contraindication. Animal studies have not shown any evidence of teratogenicity.

32. **Lithium** (FDA = D)
Lithium readily crosses the placenta and cases of cardiac arrhythmia, hypotonia and hypothyroidism have been reported. The most well-known risk is of Ebstein's anomaly of the heart (a rare congenital downward displacement of the tricuspid valve into the right ventricle) which can occur if the drug is taken during weeks 2 to 6 post-conception. Ebstein's anomaly is 20 times more common with lithium, but the risk rises from 1 in 20,000 to 1 in 1,000, and must be weighed against the 50% chance of relapsing if lithium is stopped. Several decades ago a raised incidence of foetal malformations in the first trimester was reported but a more recent 148-patient study showed that congenital malformation rates with lithium (2.8%) were similar to control rates (2.4%), suggesting that lithium is not an important human teratogen if used with *adequate screening* (including level II ultrasound and foetal echocardiography) to detect Ebstein's anomaly. During pregnancy, thyroid suppression may also produce neonatal goitre and cardiac arrhythmias may occur. Renal clearance is increased early in pregnancy and so higher doses are needed but clearance reduces

markedly near end of term and the dose may need to be reduced by up to 30–50% in the last few weeks, so measure plasma levels carefully and frequently.

A recent study (n = 101, retrospective, Viguera *et al, Am J Psych* 2000, **157,** 179–84) has noted that:

- the heart is formed very early, so stopping lithium when pregnancy is confirmed is too late
- relapse rates of 50% within 35 weeks of stopping lithium are high, and the risk from consequentially needed drugs is also high
- the known relapse rates after lithium discontinuation are similar for pregnant (52%) and non-pregnant (58%) women, but much higher than the year before discontinuation (21%), so pregnancy is relatively 'risk neutral'
- women who remain stable for 10 months after lithium discontinuation are 3 times more likely to relapse than non-pregnant women during the next 5 months (70% vs 24%)
- the rates are much higher in rapid (less than 2 weeks) rather than gradual (4 weeks or longer) discontinuation
- there were no major malformations in the children born to the women (n = 9) who continued lithium throughout pregnancy in this study.

A study of 60 healthy children born to mothers who took lithium during the first trimester did not reveal any increased frequency of physical or mental anomalies among the lithium children compared to their non-lithium exposed siblings over 5–10 years.

33. **Modafinil** (FDA = C) is contraindicated in pregnancy (SPC). Pre-clinical studies have shown no teratogenicity but more information is required.

34. **Methadone** (FDA = B, or D if used in high dose or for prolonged periods) at maintenance doses has been used successfully, does not appear to be overtly teratogenic and reduces the risk of poor quality street drugs being used. With potential illicit drug using mothers, teratogenicity with methadone will obviously be

very difficult to ascertain but there does not appear to be a clear association with malformations. Predictably, a foetal withdrawal syndrome, occurring within the first 24 hours has been seen. Symptoms include tremor, irritability, hyperactivity, jitteriness, shrill cry, vomiting, diarrhoea and convulsions. Long-term developmental outcome seems unaffected. There have been numerous reports of withdrawal reactions, sudden death, reduced body weight and head circumference etc. but these are virtually all in uncontrolled situations and so other effects can not be excluded. In a study of methadone maintenance in pregnancy, head circumference and birth weight were slightly lower with methadone compared to controls (n = 32, Brown *et al, Am J Obs Gynecol* 1998, **179**, 459–63). Stopping opiates abruptly is dangerous as withdrawal reactions can damage the foetus more than the methadone.

35. No teratogenic effects have been reported in patients who took **dexamfetamine** (FDA = C) before knowing they were pregnant.

36. There is little information available for **methylphenidate** (FDA = C), and the few reported cases are unremarkable, but the UK SPC advises caution.

37. For **bupropion** (FDA = B), animal studies have shown no definitive evidence of teratogenicity nor impaired fertility.

3.9   Renal impairment

	Lower risk	Moderate risk	High risk
Antipsychotics	Aripiprazole[2] Loxapine[8] Sertindole[2]	Butyrophenones[6] Clozapine[3] Olanzapine[2] Phenothiazines[7] Quetiapine[2] Thioxanthenes[4]	Amisulpride[5] Risperidone[1] Sulpiride[5] Zotepine[2]
Antidepressants	Mianserin[16] Moclobemide[16] Trazodone[13] Tricyclics[12] Tryptophan[16]	MAOIs[15] Mirtazapine[11] Reboxetine[14] SSRIs[9]	Fluoxetine[9] Venlafaxine[10]
Anxiolytics and hypnotics	Zaleplon[19] Zopiclone[19]	Benzodiazepines[17] Beta-blockers[20] Clomethiazole[21] Zolpidem[19]	Buspirone[18] Chloral[21]
Anticonvulsants	Phenytoin[24] Tiagabine[27]	Barbiturates[25] Benzodiazepines[17] Carbamazepine[22] Ethosuximide[28] Fosphenytoin[24] Lamotrigine[26] Piracetam[27] Topiramate[27]	Gabapentin[26] Levetiracetam[27] Midazolam[17] Oxcarbazepine[22] Valproate[23] Vigabatrin[27]
Others	Anticholinesterases[29]	Anticholinergics[30] Bupropion[34] Disulfiram[31] Memantine[29] Modafinil[33]	Acamprosate[31] Lithium[32]

Grade of renal impairment	GFR ml/min	Serum creatinine micromol/L
Mild	20–50	150–300
Moderate	10–20	300–700
Severe	<10	>700

General Principals (*adapted from Maudsley Guidelines, 2003*)

1. Renal impairment will lead to accumulation of drugs — the greater the impairment, the greater the potential for accumulation.

2. Serum creatinine may not be raised in the elderly, although renal impairment may be present.

3. Care is needed with drugs or active metabolites predominantly cleared by the kidney, eg. antidepressants and

antipsychotics (except sulpiride and amisulpride).

4. Start low and go slow, adjusting doses to tolerance.

5. Adverse effects such as postural hypotension, sedation and confusion may be more common.

6. Care is needed with drugs with marked anticholinergic activity, which may cause urinary retention and interfere with U&E measurements.

3.9.1 Antipsychotics

Lower doses of all antipsychotics should be used as increased cerebral sensitivity and EPSEs may occur.

1. **Risperidone** elimination is reduced in renal disease and so initial doses and dose increments should be halved, up to about 4mg/d.

2. **Olanzapine** is excreted primarily via the renal pathway and so a lower starting dose of 5mg/d may be appropriate in renal impairment (UK SPC). **Quetiapine** should be started at 25mg/d, with dose increments of 25–50mg/d, as clearance is reduced by 25% in severe renal impairment. Some **zotepine** is excreted through the kidneys and levels may be 2–3 times higher in patients with renal impairment. Start at 25mg BD up to a maximum of 75mg BD. Dose adjustments of **aripiprazole** and **sertindole** are not necessary even in severe renal impairment.

3. **Clozapine** is contraindicated in severe renal disease.

4. **Zuclopenthixol** and **flupentixol** should be used with caution in renal impairment (UK SPC), as some accumulation of metabolites has been reported.

5. **Sulpiride** is mainly cleared by the kidneys. Reduce the dose by 35–70% or extend the dosage interval by a factor of 1.5 to 3 if necessary. **Amisulpride** is principally cleared unchanged through the kidneys, so care is needed in moderate to severe renal insufficiency (GFR 10–30ml/min). It is not appreciably removed during haemodialysis.

6. There are no apparent problems with **haloperidol**, and is less sedative and

causes little postural hypotension. The UK SPC recommends caution as some accumulation might occur.

7. There is little information on **phenothiazines**, but excretion may be slower and accumulation may occur, causing sedation, postural hypotension etc. **Levomepromazine** (methotrimeprazine) should be used with care in renal disease, and **chlorpromazine** and **thioridazine** avoided.

8. **Loxapine** is 70% excreted via the kidneys and 30% via faeces. No specific problems in renal damage are known.

3.9.2 Antidepressants

9. If the GFR is less than 10ml/min do **not** use **fluoxetine**, unless the patient is on dialysis. If the GFR is 10–50ml/min, alternate day dosing is suggested, with care. In moderate renal impairment, reduce the initial dose of **paroxetine**. **Citalopram** and **escitalopram** doses do not need to be reduced in mild to moderate renal impairment. In severe renal failure, a lower dosage of citalopram may be appropriate. The use of **sertraline** in renal disease is not recommended by the manufacturers, although they have 'data on file' that there are no such problems. **Fluvoxamine** should be used with care, starting at 50mg/d and increasing only slowly. An unpublished report indicated that fluvoxamine does not accumulate at 100mg/d in renal impairment, although this is probably a sub-therapeutic dose.

10. About 1–10% of a dose of **venlafaxine** is cleared unchanged by the kidney and 30% renally excreted as the major metabolite. Total clearance is reduced by about 35% in mild to moderate renal impairment (GFR 10–30ml/min) and so doses should be reduced by about 25–50%. Daily doses should also be reduced by 50% in dialysis and doses separated from dialysis itself. It is not recommended in severe renal failure.

11. **Mirtazapine** clearance was reduced by 33% in moderate and by 50% in severe renal failure in a single dose study, and so care with higher doses is recommended,

but standard doses can be used in mild renal failure.

12. **Tricyclics** should be started at low dose and increased slowly, with divided doses. Avoid **lofepramine** in severe renal impairment, as 50% is renally excreted.

13. No dosage adjustment is necessary for **trazodone**.

14. **Reboxetine's** half-life and plasma levels appear to rise (up to two fold), particularly in severe renal impairment, so a starting dose of 2mg BD in patients with moderate to severe renal dysfunction has been suggested.

15. No dosage adjustments are usually necessary for the **MAOIs**, although isocarboxazid should be used with caution with impaired renal function to prevent accumulation (UK SPC).

16. Dosage adjustments in renal disease are not necessary for **moclobemide, mianserin** nor **tryptophan**.

3.9.3 Anxiolytics and hypnotics

17. Low dose anticonvulsant use of **benzodiazepines** may be acceptable as higher doses produce an increase in CNS side-effects. **Chlordiazepoxide** can be given in normal doses. In severe renal failure doses of **oxazepam** should be reduced to 75%. No dose changes are necessary for **clobazam**.

18. **Buspirone** is contraindicated in moderate or severe renal impairment, as plasma levels have been shown to be higher in patients with renal failure.

19. The pharmacokinetics of **zaleplon** and **zopiclone** are not significantly different in renal insufficiency, and so dose alteration is not required. Plasma protein binding of **zolpidem** is reduced in renal failure and half-life doubled. No dosage adjustments are recommended by the manufacturers in mild renal dysfunction but care would seem prudent.

20. In severe renal disease plasma levels of **beta-blockers** may be higher and so starting doses should be lower. Beta-blockers may also reduce renal blood flow and adversely affect existing renal function.

21. Caution is needed with **clomethiazole** in chronic renal disease. **Chloral** is contraindicated in moderate to marked renal impairment.

3.9.4 Anticonvulsants

22. **Carbamazepine** rarely causes renal disturbances although it has been suggested that doses should be reduced by 25% in severe renal failure. For **oxcarbazepine** in renal impairment (creatinine clearance less than 30ml/min), start at half the usual dose (300mg/day), increasing at no more frequently than weekly intervals. In patients with pre-existing renal conditions associated with low sodium or in patients treated concomitantly with sodium-lowering drugs (eg. diuretics, desmopressin) as well as NSAIDs, serum sodium levels should be monitored (see UK SPC).

23. **Valproate** is eliminated mainly through the kidneys and the UK SPC now states that it may be necessary to decrease the dosage in renal insufficiency.

24. No specific dose adjustments are required for **phenytoin**, but it's protein binding is altered in uraemia which can be problematic in accurately assessing serum levels. Severe cardiovascular ADRs have been reported with **fosphenytoin** IV (see *3.2*).

25. High-dose **phenobarbital** in particular causes increased sedation and the dosage interval should be increased to at least 12 to 16 hours in severe renal failure and large doses avoided. Active metabolites of **amylobarbital** accumulate in severe renal disease.

26. Most of a dose of **gabapentin** is excreted unchanged in the urine and the manufacturers recommend dose reductions as follows:

Creatinine clearance	Dose
60–90ml/min	400mg tds
30–60ml/min	300mg bd
15–30ml/min	300mg/d
<15ml/min	300mg alternate days

Patients undergoing haemodialysis should receive a loading dose of 400mg and 200–300mg of gabapentin for every four hours of dialysis. A reduced maintenance dose of **lamotrigine** is usually recommended in severe renal impairment, but the dose probably needs little adjustment in mild to moderate impairment and even in end stage renal failure (SPC).

27. **Vigabatrin** is excreted by the kidneys and so reduced doses are recommended with a creatinine clearance of < 60mL/min. The time to steady state may be increased with **topiramate**, and there is an increased risk of renal stone formation. Supplemental doses of 50% of the daily dose should be given on haemodialysis days. There are no apparent problems with **tiagabine**. Some dose reduction may be necessary with **piracetam** in renal impairment. Since 66% of a dose of **levetiracetam** is excreted unchanged in the urine, dose reductions are necessary in impaired renal function, and a supplemental dose of 250–500mg given after dialysis.

28. **Ethosuximide** doses should be reduced by 25% in severe renal failure.

3.9.5 Others

29. No change in dose is necessary with **donepezil** or **rivastigmine** in mild to moderate renal impairment (MI). No dosage reduction of **galantamine** is necessary for creatinine clearance greater than 9ml/min. In severe impairment (< 9ml/min) galantamine is contra-indicated (due to lack of safety data, UK SPC). **Memantine** dose adjustment is not necessary except in moderate renal impairment (when the maximum dose should be 10mg/d) and should not be used in severe renal impairment.

30. The UK SPCs recommend some caution in renal disease with the **anticholinergics**.

31. The UK SPC for **disulfiram** recommends caution in renal disease. The UK SPC for **acamprosate** states that use in renal insufficiency (serum creatinine > 120 micromol/L) is a contraindication.

32. **Lithium** is contraindicated in severe renal impairment. If lithium use is, however, unavoidable, alternate day dosing, use of very low doses (25–75% normal) and frequent (ie. at least monthly) plasma level estimating is *essential.*

33. The maximum **modafinil** dose of 400mg/d should only be used in the absence of renal impairment (MI).

34. **Bupropion** and metabolites are almost exclusively (85%) excreted through the kidneys and so, in renal failure, the initial dose should be reduced and close monitoring for toxicity carried out.

4.
Drug interactions

Full reviews, assessments and references for most of these interactions can be found in standard reference books and one can do no better than refer to *Drug Interactions in Psychiatry*, edited by Ciraulo, Shader, Greenblatt and Creelman (Williams & Wilkins, Maryland) for accurate and unbiased reviews of many of these interactions.

Absolute classification of interactions is virtually impossible. In order to give some guidance, interactions with the drugs in **CAPITAL LETTERS** are those which could be:

- potentially hazardous
- where a dosage adjustment is likely to have to be made
- well established and documented
- of clinical significance
- rare but important.

How to use this section
1. Look up the psychiatric drug or group.
2. Look up the drug group of the potentially interacting drug.
3. If nothing there, look up the actual drug.
4. If still nothing, no interaction has been reported.

4.1   Hypnotics & Anxiolytics

4.1.1 Benzodiazepines

Acamprosate + benzodiazepines
See acamprosate (*4.6.1*).

ALCOHOL + BENZODIAZEPINES
See alcohol (*4.7.1*).

Aminophylline + benzodiazepines
See xanthines + benzodiazepines.

Amiodarone + clonazepam
A single case exists of clonazepam toxicity at low dose with amiodarone.

Antacids + benzodiazepines
Benzodiazepine absorption is slightly delayed (but not reduced) by antacids.

Anticholinergics + benzodiazepines
Benzodiazepine absorption may be delayed by anticholinergics.

Anticoagulants + benzodiazepines
Lack of interaction has been shown but there are isolated cases of adverse reactions reported.

Antidepressants + benzodiazepines
Enhanced sedation is possible.

Antihistamines + benzodiazepines
Enhanced sedation is possible.

Antihypertensives + benzodiazepines
Enhanced hypotension could occur.

Antipsychotics + benzodiazepines
See antipsychotics (*4.2.1*).

Baclofen + benzodiazepines
Enhanced sedation can occur.

Beta-blockers + benzodiazepines
Some beta-blockers may produce a small but significant reduction in diazepam clearance and patients may become more 'accident-prone' on the combination.

Buprenorphine + benzodiazepines
Lack of interaction has been reported.

Buspirone + benzodiazepines
See buspirone (*4.1.2*).

CALCIUM-CHANNEL BLOCKERS + BENZODIAZEPINES
Diltiazem and verapamil can significantly raise diazepam levels but nimodipine doesn't appear to interact.

Cannabis + benzodiazepines
See cannabis (*4.7.2*).

Carbamazepine + benzodiazepines
See carbamazepine (*4.5.1*).

Charcoal (activated) + benzodiazepines
25g activated charcoal given 30 minutes after diazepam reduces the total absorbed, but not the peak levels, although gastric lavage doesn't help much.

Citalopram/escitalopram + benzodiazepines
See (es)citalopram (*4.3.2.1*).

Clarithromycin + benzodiazepines
Clarithromycin may increase benzodiazepine levels.

CLOZAPINE + BENZODIAZEPINES
See clozapine (*4.2.3*).

Cyclophosphamide + benzodiazepines
Increased cyclophosphamide toxicity is possible.

Dextropropoxyphene + benzodiazepines
Increased sedation can occur.

Diflunisal + benzodiazepines
Diflunisal may reduce the effect of some benzodiazepines by increasing their metabolism.

Disulfiram + benzodiazepines
See disulfiram (*4.6.6*).

Escitalopram + benzodiazepines
See (es)citalopram (*4.3.2.1*).

Fluoxetine + benzodiazepines
See fluoxetine (*4.3.2.2*).

Fluvoxamine + benzodiazepines
See fluvoxamine (*4.3.2.3*).

Food + benzodiazepines
Food delays the absorption of benzodiazepines, only clinically significant if a rapid action is needed.

Gabapentin + benzodiazepines
See gabapentin (*4.5.3*).

Grapefruit juice + benzodiazepines
Lots of concentrated grapefruit juice could increase benzodiazepine levels.

H2-blockers + benzodiazepines
Cimetidine inhibits the metabolism of long-acting benzodiazepines (eg. chlordiazepoxide, diazepam etc) but not oxazepam and temazepam. Only a few patients experience increased side-effects and the clinical effect is probably negligible. The other H2-blockers, eg. ranitidine do not interact this way.

Indometacin + diazepam
Increased dizziness may occur.

Isoniazid + benzodiazepines
Isoniazid reduces the clearance of diazepam, but not of oxazepam.

Itraconazole + benzodiazepines
Itraconazole and ketoconazole significantly increase midazolam levels, and perhaps other benzodiazepines.

Ketoconazole + benzodiazepines
See itraconazole above.

Lamotrigine + benzodiazepines
See lamotrigine (*4.5.4*).

LEVODOPA + BENZODIAZEPINE
Levodopa can be antagonised by diazepam, chlordiazepoxide and nitrazepam,

much reducing its effect. It is thus best to observe the patient for worsening parkinsonian symptoms.

Lithium + benzodiazepines

See lithium (4.4).

MAOIs + benzodiazepines

See MAOIs (4.3.4).

Methadone + diazepam

See methadone (4.6.8).

Metronidazole + benzodiazepines

No interaction occurs.

Mianserin + benzodiazepines

See mianserin (4.3.3.1).

Mirtazapine + benzodiazepines

See mirtazapine (4.3.3.2)

Moclobemide + benzodiazepines

See moclobemide (4.3.3.3).

Modafinil + benzodiazepines

See modafinil (4.6.10).

Nimodipine + benzodiazepines

No clinically significant interaction.

Olanzapine + benzodiazepines

See olanzapine (4.2.4).

Ondansetron + benzodiazepines

Lack of interaction has been shown.

Opioids + benzodiazepines

Enhanced sedation can occur.

Oral contraceptives + benzodiazepines

OCs may slightly *increase* the effects of chlordiazepoxide, diazepam and nitrazepam but *reduce* those of oxazepam, lorazepam and temazepam.

Paroxetine + benzodiazepines

See paroxetine (4.3.2.4).

Phenobarbital + benzodiazepines

Enhanced sedation can occur.

Phenytoin + benzodiazepines

See phenytoin (4.5.8).

PROTON-PUMP INHIBITORS + DIAZEPAM

Omeprazole, but not pantoprazole, may raise diazepam levels by up to 50%.

Quetiapine + benzodiazepines

See quetiapine (4.2.5).

Reboxetine + benzodiazepines

See reboxetine (4.3.3.5).

Rifampicin + diazepam

The effect of diazepam can be reduced.

Ritonavir + benzodiazepines

Raised benzodiazepine levels may occur.

Rivastigmine + benzodiazepines

See rivastigmine (4.6.3.3).

Sertindole + benzodiazepines

See sertindole (4.2.7).

Sertraline + benzodiazepines

See sertraline (4.3.2.5).

Smoking + benzodiazepines

See smoking (4.7.4).

Tiagabine + benzodiazepines

See tiagabine (4.5.10).

Tricyclics + benzodiazepines

Enhanced sedation has predictably been reported. Monitor carefully and reduce benzodiazepine dose if necessary.

Valproate + benzodiazepines

Valproate may enhance the effectiveness of both lorazepam and diazepam and doses of both may need to be reduced.

Venlafaxine + diazepam

See venlafaxine (4.3.3.7).

Warfarin + benzodiazepines

Theoretical only.

Xanthines + benzodiazepines

Xanthines eg. theophylline, aminophylline and caffeine antagonise the sedative (and possibly anxiolytic) effects of benzodiazepines.

Zotepine + benzodiazepines
See zotepine (*4.2.8*).

4.1.2 Buspirone (Buspar®)

Alcohol + buspirone
See alcohol (*4.7.1*).

Benzodiazepines + buspirone
Minimal enhanced sedation may occur.

Calcium-channel blockers + buspirone
Verapamil and diltiazem may increase buspirone plasma levels 3–5 fold, enhancing the therapeutic and adverse effects.

Cimetidine + buspirone
Lack of interaction has been shown.

Citalopram + buspirone
See (es)citalopram (*4.3.2.1*).

Clozapine + buspirone
An isolated but near fatal interaction has been reported.

Erythromycin + buspirone
Erythromycin and itraconazole can both increase buspirone levels dramatically.

Escitalopram + buspirone.
See (es)citalopram (*4.3.2.1*).

Fluoxetine + buspirone
A case of reduced anxiolytic effect when fluoxetine was started has been reported, as has dystonia and akathisia.

Fluvoxamine + buspirone
Fluvoxamine increases buspirone levels slightly.

Grapefruit juice + buspirone
200mls double-strength grapefruit juice may raise buspirone levels significantly.

Itraconazole + buspirone
See erythromycin + buspirone above.

MAOIs + BUSPIRONE
See MAOIs (*4.3.4*).

NSAIDs + buspirone
GI and CNS side-effects may be more common.

Phenytoin + buspirone
No interaction occurs.

Propranolol + buspirone
No interaction occurs.

Rifampicin + buspirone
Buspirone levels may be significantly lower with rifampicin.

St. John's wort + buspirone
There is an isolated case of a serotonin syndrome.

Trazodone + buspirone
Serotonin syndrome and raised LFTs have been reported.

Warfarin + buspirone
No interaction occurs.

Zudovudine + buspirone
No interaction occurs.

4.1.3 Chloral (Welldorm®)

ALCOHOL + CHLORAL
See alcohol (*4.7.1*).

Fluvoxamine + chloral
See fluvoxamine (*4.3.2.3*).

Furosemide + chloral
Diaphoresis, facial flushing and agitation have been reported.

MAOIs + chloral
See MAOIs (*4.3.4*).

Methadone + chloral
See methadone (*4.6.8*).

Nicoumalone + chloral
An enhanced anticoagulant effect can occur. See also warfarin.

Phenytoin + chloral
See phenytoin (*4.5.8*).

Warfarin + chloral
The anticoagulant effects of warfarin are increased slightly by chloral, probably by

plasma protein displacement. This can be particularly important if chloral is taken as a 'PRN' hypnotic.

4.1.4 Zaleplon (Sonata®)

As with similar drugs, use with other CNS-depressants needs care.

Alcohol + zaleplon

See alcohol (4.7.1).

Antipsychotics + zaleplon

Additive psychomotor effects may occur with thioridazine.

CARBAMAZEPINE + ZALEPLON

A four-fold reduction in zaleplon levels can occur, minimising its effect.

Cimetidine + zaleplon

Raised zaleplon levels can occur with cimetidine.

Digoxin + zaleplon

Lack of interaction has been shown.

Erythromycin + zaleplon

Raised zaleplon levels can occur.

Ibuprofen + zaleplon

Lack of significant interaction has been shown.

Ketoconazole + zaleplon

Raised zaleplon levels can occur.

Narcotics + zaleplon

Enhanced euphoria is possible.

Rifampicin + zaleplon

A four-fold reduction in zaleplon levels can occur.

Phenobarbital + zaleplon

Reduced zaleplon levels can occur.

Warfarin + zaleplon

No interaction occurs (SPC).

4.1.5 Zolpidem (Stilnoct®)

As with similar drugs, use of zolpidem with other CNS-depressants needs care.

Alcohol + zolpidem

See alcohol (4.7.1).

Antipsychotics + zolpidem

Excessive sedation has been reported.

BUPROPION + ZOLPIDEM

See bupropion (4.6.4).

Caffeine + zolpidem

Caffeine does not appear to antagonise the sedative effects of zolpidem.

Fluconazole + zolpidem

See itraconazole + zolpidem.

Food + zolpidem

The rate of absorption of zolpidem is slowed significantly by food.

H2-blockers + zolpidem

Lack of interaction has been shown with cimetidine and ranitidine.

Ketoconazole + zolpidem

Ketoconazole lengthens the half-life of zolpidem by about 25%.

Itraconazole + zolpidem

Itraconazole and fluconazole may lengthen the half-life of zolpidem, but probably not significantly.

Rifampicin + zolpidem

Rifampicin may significantly reduce zolpidem plasma levels and therapeutic effect.

Smoking + zolpidem

Zolpidem half-life may be 30% shorter in smokers.

SSRIs + zolpidem

SSRIs may enhance zolpidem-associated hallucinations and there may be a quicker zolpidem onset with sertraline but lack of significant interaction with fluoxetine has been shown.

4.1.6 Zopiclone (Zimovane®)

Alcohol + zopiclone

See alcohol (4.7.1).

Aspirin + zopiclone

Lack of interaction reported (MI).

Caffeine + zopiclone

Caffeine has been reported to moderately antagonise the psychomotor effects of zopiclone.

Erythromycin + zopiclone

The absorption and onset of action of zopiclone may be more rapid, of significance perhaps in the elderly.

Itraconazole + zopiclone

Itraconazole significantly increased zopiclone's plasma levels and half-life, of significance perhaps in the elderly.

Metoclopramide + zopiclone

Zopiclone levels are significantly increased by metoclopramide.

Ranitidine + zopiclone

Lack of interaction reported (MI).

Rifampicin + zopiclone

Rifampicin significantly reduces zopiclone plasma levels and therapeutic effect.

Tricyclics + zopiclone

One study showed slightly decreased levels of both drugs.

4.2 Antipsychotics

See also aripiprazole (*4.2.2*), clozapine (*4.2.3*), olanzapine (*4.2.4*), risperidone (*4.2.5*), quetiapine (*4.2.6*), sertindole (*4.2.7*) and zotepine (*4.2.8*).

4.2.1 Antipsychotics (general, typical)

ACE inhibitors + phenothiazines

Enhanced hypotension can occur, with severe postural hypotension reported with chlorpromazine and possibly other phenothiazines.

ALCOHOL + ANTIPSYCHOTICS

See alcohol (*4.7.1*).

Amfetamines + neuroleptics

The antipsychotic effects of phenothiazines can be antagonised by amfetamines.

Amiodarone + phenothiazines

The *BNF* notes an increased risk of ventricular arrhythmias with phenothiazines.

Antacids + antipsychotics

Antacids reduce chlorpromazine and haloperidol serum levels. Sulpiride absorption may be reduced by antacids containing sucralfate or aluminium. The problem can be avoided by separating doses by a couple of hours.

Anticholinergics + antipsychotics

Anticholinergics, eg. procyclidine may antagonise the effect of neuroleptics in acute treatment, partly by lowering their serum levels. Other complications include neuroleptic malignant syndrome and severe constipation. Routine use of anticholinergics thus seems unwarranted. It is more appropriate to use them if Parkinsonian side-effects occur and then taper them off over about three months.

Anticonvulsants + antipsychotics

Antipsychotics lower the seizure threshold and may antagonise anticonvulsant actions.

ANTIHISTAMINES + ANTIPSYCHOTICS

QT prolongation can occur with some antihistamines and so loratadine and chlorphenamine are the preferred alternative.

Antihypertensives + phenothiazines

Enhanced hypotension can occur.

Antimalarials + chlorpromazine

Markedly increased chlorpromazine levels can occur with antimalarials, eg. chloroquine and Fansidar®.

Benzodiazepines + antipsychotics

Enhanced sedation and impaired psychomotor function can occur.

Beta-blockers + antipsychotics

Blood levels of both can rise, leading to hypotension, eg. chlorpromazine levels may rise by 100–500% with propranolol so use with care. Thioridazine is now contraindicated with propranolol due to QTc prolongation.

Betel nut + antipsychotics

Betel nut (Areca catechu), which contains a cholinergic alkaloid arecoline, may cause rigidity, bradykinesia, tremor, stiffness and akathisia with flupenthixol and fluphenazine.

Bromocriptine + antipsychotics

Mutual antagonism can occur, eg. reversal of the antipsychotic effect and antagonism of the hypo-prolactinaemic and antiparkinsonian effects of bromocriptine.

Calcium-channel blockers + antipsychotics

Enhanced hypotension can occur.

Cannabis + chlorpromazine

See cannabis (4.7.2).

CARBAMAZEPINE + ANTIPSYCHOTICS

See carbamazepine (4.5.1).

Citalopram + methotrimeprazine/levomepromazine

See citalopram (4.3.2.1).

CLARITHROMYCIN + ANTIPSYCHOTICS

The BNF notes an increased risk of arrhythmias with phenothiazines and recommends avoiding the combination. Deaths have been reported with pimozide.

CLOZAPINE + ANTIPSYCHOTICS

See clozapine (4.2.3).

Cocaine + antipsychotics

See cocaine (4.7.3).

Desferrioxamine + prochlorperazine

Avoid the combination as prolonged unconsciousness may occur (SPC).

Diazoxide + chlorpromazine

A single case indicates possible enhanced hypoglycaemia from both drugs.

Disopyramine + antipsychotics

Increased anticholinergic effects may occur.

Disulfiram + antipsychotics

See disulfiram (4.6.6).

Domperidone + antipsychotics

Enhanced risk of parkinsonian effects.

Donepezil + antipsychotics

See donepezil (4.6.3.1).

Erythromycin + antipsychotics

See clarithromycin + antipsychotics.

Escitalopram + methotrimeprazine/levomepromazine

See citalopram (4.3.2.1).

FLUOXETINE + ANTIPSYCHOTICS

Cases have been reported of severe EPSEs (haloperidol), dystonia (fluphenazine) and myoclonic jerks (clozapine). Two cases exist of enhanced pimozide side-effects (eg. stupor, confusion, severe bradycardia and drowsiness) after fluoxetine was added and this combination should be avoided. Citalopram and sertraline would be suitable alternatives. Fluoxetine may significantly increase clozapine and norclozapine levels, with several case reports (including fatalities), so be wary for clozapine toxicity.

Fluvoxamine + antipsychotics

See fluvoxamine (4.3.2.3).

Ginseng + haloperidol

Ginseng may potentiate the general effects of haloperidol.

H2-blockers + antipsychotics

Chlorpromazine levels may be reduced by 30% by cimetidine. Ranitidine is a suitable alternative.

Haloperidol + phenothiazines

Haloperidol levels may be raised.

Hydroxyzine + phenothiazines

The antipsychotic effect of phenothiazines may be decreased.

Hypoglycaemics + chlorpromazine

Chlorpromazine in doses of 100mg or more can occasionally induce hyperglycaemia and upset the control of diabetes with oral hypoglycaemics.

Indometacin + haloperidol

One study showed profound drowsiness and confusion on the combination.

Itraconazole + haloperidol

Itraconazole 200mg/d significantly increases haloperidol levels, enhancing side effects.

LEVODOPA + ANTIPSYCHOTICS

Mutual therapeutic antagonism can occur via the dopamine system. Levodopa may worsen antipsychotic-induced EPSEs.

LITHIUM + ANTIPSYCHOTICS

See lithium (*4.4*).

MAOIs + antipsychotics

See MAOIs (*4.3.4*).

Methyldopa + haloperidol

Three cases of pseudo-dementia have been reported. There is an enhanced risk of EPSEs and postural hypotension.

Metoclopramide + antipsychotics

An enhanced risk of EPSEs exists.

Minocycline + phenothiazines

A case report of discoloured galactorrhoea exists.

Naltrexone + phenothiazines

Severe drowsiness with naltrexone and either thioridazine or chlorpromazine have been reported.

Olanzapine + antipsychotics

See olanzapine (*4.2.4*).

Oral contraceptives + chlorpromazine

Significantly raised chlorpromazine levels have been reported.

Orlistat + haloperidol

No interaction reported.

Oxcarbazepine + antipsychotics

See oxcarbazepine (*4.5.6*).

Paroxetine + antipsychotics

See paroxetine (*4.3.2.4*).

Pethidine + phenothiazines

Increased CNS toxicity and hypotension can occur.

PHENOBARBITAL + ANTIPSYCHOTICS

Additive sedative effects can occur, as well as 25–75% lower plasma levels of some antipsychotics, eg. haloperidol and thioridazine. Antagonism of the barbiturate anticonvulsant effects may also occur.

Phenylpropanolamine + thioridazine

A single fatal case of arrhythmia exists.

PHENYTOIN + ANTIPSYCHOTICS

See phenytoin (*4.5.8*).

Procarbazine + antipsychotics

Enhanced sedation is possible.

Quetiapine + antipsychotics

See quetiapine (*4.2.5*).

Reboxetine + antipsychotics

See reboxetine (*4.3.3.5*).

RIFAMPICIN + HALOPERIDOL

Rifampicin may reduce the serum levels of haloperidol by a third.

Sertindole + antipsychotics

See sertindole (*4.2.7*).

Smoking + antipsychotics

See smoking (*4.7.4*).

Tea or coffee + antipsychotics

Studies show that many antipsychotics precipitate out of solution to form a tannin complex with tea and coffee but the clinical significance is thought to be minimal.

Tetrabenazine + chlorpromazine

Enhanced EPSEs have (predictably) been reported in a Huntington's patient.

Thiazide diuretics + antipsychotics

Although no case reports exist, enhanced thioridazine cardiotoxicity has been suggested.

Trazodone + antipsychotics

See trazodone (*4.3.3.6*).

TRICYCLICS + ANTIPSYCHOTICS

See tricyclics (*4.3.1*).

Valproate + antipsychotics

See antipsychotics + valproate (*4.5.12*).

Venlafaxine + antipsychotics

See venlafaxine (*4.3.3.7*).

Warfarin + antipsychotics

An interaction is theoretically possible.

Zaleplon + antipsychotics

See zaleplon (*4.1.4*).

Zolpidem + antipsychotics

See zolpidem (*4.1.5*).

Zotepine + antipsychotics

See zotepine (*4.2.8*).

4.2.2 Aripiprazole (Abilify®)

Aripiprazole is metabolised by many enzyme systems but has no effect on them so drug interactions are uncommon.

Alcohol + aripiprazole

See alcohol (see *4.7.1*).

Carbamazepine + aripiprazole

See antipsychotics + carbamazepine (*4.5.1*).

Dextromethorphan + aripiprazole

Lack of interaction has been shown (MI).

H2-blockers + aripiprazole

Lack of significant interaction has been shown with famotidine.

Ketoconazole + aripiprazole

Ketoconazole increases aripiprazole metabolism and so an aripiprazole dose should be decreased by a half during co-administration.

Lithium + aripiprazole

See antipsychotics + lithium (*4.4*).

Omeprazole + aripiprazole

Lack of interaction has been shown.

Quinidine + aripiprazole

Quinidine increases aripiprazole metabolism and so aripiprazole doses should be halved.

Smoking + aripiprazole

See smoking (*4.7.4*).

Valproate + aripiprazole

See valproate + antipsychotics (*4.2.1*).

Warfarin + aripiprazole

No known interaction.

4.2.3 Clozapine (Clozaril® etc, see also *4.2.1* for more general interactions)

Whilst most clozapine will be prescribed and dispensed by secondary care, clozapine has a number of important and potentially dangerous or fatal interactions of which GPs should be aware.

ACE inhibitors + clozapine

Clozapine may enhance the hypotension caused by diltiazem or enalapril and lisinopril has caused clozapine toxicity.

Alcohol + clozapine

See antipsychotics + alcohol (*4.7.1*).

ANTIBIOTICS + CLOZAPINE

Some antibiotics are reported to cause leucopenia/neutropenia with clozapine and might enhance the likelihood of clozapine-induced (potentially fatal) neutropenia and hence **should be avoided** if possible. Those **less likely** to cause neutropenia and hence which are safer to use include the penicillins (except benzylpenicillin G), all tetracyclines, amino-glycosides, clarithromycin, some anti-TBs, sodium fusidate, spectinomycin and polymixin B.

Those which can cause leucopenia/neutropenia and are **more likely** to adversely interact include the cephalosporins, cephamycins, clindamycin, lincomycin, trimethoprim, some anti-TBs, metronidazole, tinidazole, 4-Quinolones (ciprofloxacin, nalidixic acid etc.), nitrofurantoin, chloramphenicol and vancomycin. There is a single reported case of a seizure occurring 7 days after erythromycin 250mg/d was added to clozapine 800mg/d.

Choose antibiotics from the top list as first choice and seek specialist advice if other drugs are needed.

ANTIPSYCHOTICS (other) + CLOZAPINE

There is an enhanced risk of agranulocytosis (UK SPC) which would be complicated by the long-term nature of a depot. There have been some cases of raised clozapine levels with risperidone, including sudden agranulocytosis so care with this combination is essential. There are also reports of problems with haloperidol and fluphenazine.

BENZODIAZEPINES + CLOZAPINE

There are cases of severe hypotension, sedation and respiratory depression. Monitor for enhanced sedation and take particular care with lorazepam and when a clozapine dose is being increased.

Buspirone + clozapine

See buspirone (*4.1.2*).

CAFFEINE + CLOZAPINE

Caffeine and clozapine are both metabolised by the same enzyme (CYP1A2) and caffeine in doses of 400–1000mg may inhibit the metabolism of clozapine to an extent that might be significant in some people.

CARBAMAZEPINE + CLOZAPINE

See antipsychotics + carbamazepine (*4.5.1*).

Chloramphenicol + clozapine

Enhanced risk of clozapine agranulocytosis (mandatory precaution in the UK SPC).

Cocaine + clozapine

See cocaine (*4.7.3*).

Co-trimoxazole + clozapine

There is an enhanced risk of agranulocytosis (mandatory precaution in the UK SPC).

Cytotoxic agents + clozapine

There is an enhanced risk of agranulocytosis (mandatory precaution in the UK SPC).

Digoxin + clozapine

The UK SPC for clozapine advises caution with highly bound drugs, which would include digoxin. Monitor for adverse effects and adjust doses as necessary.

ERYTHROMYCIN + CLOZAPINE

See antibiotics + clozapine. Raised clozapine levels and toxicity have been reported.

FLUOXETINE + CLOZAPINE

See fluoxetine + antipsychotics (*4.2.1*).

FLUVOXAMINE + CLOZAPINE

Clozapine plasma levels may rise up to 9-fold with fluvoxamine (even at very low doses), via enzyme inhibition. This combination should be avoided unless really close monitoring is occurring.

Grapefruit juice + clozapine

No interaction occurs.

H2-blockers + clozapine

Clozapine levels may rise by up to 50%, with ranitidine a safer alternative.

Influenza vaccine + clozapine

No interaction occurs.

Itraconazole/ketoconazole + clozapine

No interaction noted.

LAMOTRIGINE + CLOZAPINE

There is one reported case of toxic clozapine levels occurring two weeks after 100mg/d lamotrigine was added to a stable clozapine regimen, so be careful.

Lithium + clozapine

See lithium (*4.4*).

MAOIs + clozapine

Enhanced sedation may occur with all CNS depressants (MI).

Oral contraceptives + clozapine

Raised clozapine levels have been reported.

Orlistat + clozapine

No interaction occurs.

PAROXETINE + CLOZAPINE

Paroxetine may significantly increase plasma clozapine levels so be aware of possible toxicity.

Penicillamine + clozapine

There is an enhanced risk of agranulocytosis (mandatory precaution in the UK SPC).

Phenobarbital + clozapine

Raised clozapine levels (requiring dose reduction) have been reported after discontinuation of phenobarbital.

Phenylbutazone + clozapine

There is an enhanced risk of agranulocytosis (mandatory precaution in the UK SPC).

PHENYTOIN + CLOZAPINE

Phenytoin may markedly reduce clozapine levels.

PPIs + clozapine

Only minor changes in clozapine levels have been reported.

Rifampicin + clozapine

Dramatic reductions in clozapine levels over 2–3 weeks with rifampicin have been reported.

RISPERIDONE + CLOZAPINE

See antipsychotics + clozapine (*4.2.3*).

Sertraline + clozapine

Sertraline may significantly raise clozapine levels, so the risk of clozapine toxicity must be considered carefully.

Smoking + clozapine

See antipsychotics + smoking (*4.7.4*).

Sulphonamides + clozapine

There is an enhanced risk of agranulocytosis (SPC).

Tricyclics + clozapine

See antipsychotics + tricyclics (*4.3.1*).

Valproate + clozapine

See antipsychotics + valproate (*4.5.12*).

Venlafaxine + clozapine

See venlafaxine (*4.3.3.8*).

Warfarin + clozapine

The clozapine UK SPC advises caution with highly bound drugs, which would include warfarin.

4.2.4 Olanzapine (Zyprexa®, see also *4.2.1* for more general interactions)

Olanzapine is metabolised mainly by glucuronidation, and the main metabolites have little or no clinical activity.

Alcohol + olanzapine

See alcohol (*4.7.1*).

Antacids + olanzapine

There is no effect on olanzapine bioavailability.

Antipsychotics (other) + olanzapine

NMS and seizures have been reported rarely.

Benzodiazepines + olanzapine

Lack of significant interaction has been shown. Mild increases in heart rate, sedation and dry mouth were noted with the combination, but no dose adjustment deemed necessary.

Biperiden + olanzapine

No interaction has been detected.

Carbamazepine + olanzapine

See carbamazepine + antipsychotics (*4.5.1*).

Charcoal (activated) + olanzapine

Activated charcoal reduces olanzapine bioavailability by 50–60%.

Cimetidine + olanzapine

There is no effect on olanzapine bioavailability.

Ciprofloxacin + olanzapine

Raised olanzapine levels have been reported, possibly caused by ciprofloxacin.

Lithium + olanzapine

See antipsychotics + lithium (*4.4*).

Probenecid + olanzapine

Olanzapine levels may be slightly raised.

Smoking + olanzapine

See antipsychotics + smoking (*4.7.4*).

SSRIs + olanzapine

Fluvoxamine and high-dose fluoxetine (but not sertraline) may raise olanzapine levels. Melancholic depression has been reported with fluoxetine, but the combination is marketed in USA for psychotic depression.

Tricyclics + olanzapine

Single dose studies show no effect of olanzapine on the metabolism of imipramine. Seizures have been reported with clomipramine and olanzapine.

Warfarin + olanzapine

Single dose studies show no effect of olanzapine on the metabolism of warfarin.

Xanthines + olanzapine

Lack of interaction with aminophylline and theophylline has been shown.

4.2.5 Quetiapine (Seroquel®, see also *4.2.1* for more general interactions)

Quetiapine is metabolised primarily by the CYP3A4 enzyme.

Alcohol + quetiapine

See alcohol (*4.7.1*).

Antipsychotics (other) + quetiapine

Haloperidol and risperidone have no effect on quetiapine but thioridazine reduces quetiapine levels, probably by enzyme induction.

Benzodiazepines + quetiapine

Single doses of lorazepam and diazepam are unaffected by quetiapine.

Carbamazepine + quetiapine

See antipsychotics + carbamazepine (*4.5.1*).

Cimetidine + quetiapine

No interaction occurs.

Erythromycin + quetiapine

Raised quetiapine levels are likely via enzyme inhibition.

Ketoconazole + quetiapine

Raised quetiapine levels are likely via enzyme inhibition.

Lithium + quetiapine

See antipsychotics + lithium (*4.4*).

Lovastatin + quetiapine

A prolonged QT interval has been reported.

Phenobarbital + quetiapine

Lower levels of quetiapine would be expected, due to enzyme induction by barbiturates.

Phenytoin + quetiapine

Lower levels of quetiapine would be expected, due to enzyme induction by phenytoin.

Rifampicin + quetiapine

Lower levels of quetiapine would be expected, due to enzyme induction by rifampicin.

SSRIs + quetiapine

No interaction with fluoxetine has been shown.

Tricyclics + quetiapine

No interaction with imipramine has been shown.

Warfarin + quetiapine

Lack of interaction has been proposed, but there is an isolated case report.

4.2.6 Risperidone (Risperdal®, see also 4.2.1 for more general interactions)

CARBAMAZEPINE + RISPERIDONE

See antipsychotics + carbamazepine (4.5.1).

CLOZAPINE + RISPERIDONE

See antipsychotics + clozapine (4.2.3).

Donepezil + risperidone

See antipsychotics + donepezil (4.6.3.1).

FLUOXETINE + RISPERIDONE

A 75% increase in risperidone levels and increased side effects has been reported in one study.

FLUVOXAMINE + RISPERIDONE

A case of neurotoxicity has been reported.

Galantamine + risperidone

See galantamine (4.6.3.2).

Lithium + risperidone

See antipsychotics + lithium (4.4).

Methadone + risperidone

See methadone (4.6.8).

Mirtazapine + risperidone

See mirtazapine (4.3.3.2).

Paroxetine + risperidone

A 60% increase in risperidone levels and increased side effects has been reported in one study.

Phenytoin + risperidone

See antipsychotics + phenytoin (4.5.8).

Quetiapine + risperidone

See quetiapine (4.2.5).

Ritonavir/indinavir + risperidone

Cases of EPSE and coma have been reported with the combination.

Tricyclics + risperidone

See antipsychotics + tricyclics (4.3.1).

Valproate + risperidone

See antipsychotics + valproate (4.5.12).

Venlafaxine + risperidone

Slightly raised risperidone levels have been reported.

4.2.7 Sertindole (Serdolect®, see also 4.2.1 for more general interactions)

Sertindole is metabolised by CYP2D6 and 3A4 and is contraindicated in patients also receiving drugs known to prolong the QT interval. Whilst any sertindole use is likely to be via clinical trials until 2005, co-prescribing of other drugs could cause significant problems.

Aluminium-magnesium antacids + sertindole

No interaction occurs.

ANTIPSYCHOTICS (other) + SERTINDOLE

The UK SPC for sertindole states that it is contraindicated with drugs known to prolong the QT interval eg. thioridazine.

ANTIARRHYTHMICS + SERTINDOLE

The UK SPC for sertindole states that it is contraindicated with drugs known to prolong the QT interval eg. class Ia and III antiarrhythmics eg. quinidine, amiodarone, sotalol, dofetilide etc.

Benzodiazepines + sertindole

Lack of interaction has been reported.

Calcium-channel blockers + sertindole

Non-significant increases in sertindole levels have been detected with calcium-channel antagonists via CYP3A4 inhibition.

CARBAMAZEPINE + SERTINDOLE

Carbamazepine can reduce sertindole levels 2–3-fold by CYP3A4 induction, so higher maintenance sertindole doses might be needed.

CIMETIDINE + SERTINDOLE

Cimetidine is contraindicated, but ranitidine would be a suitable alternative.

Citalopram + sertindole

No interaction appears to occur.

Escitalopram + sertindole

See citalopram above.

MACROLIDES + SERTINDOLE

The QT prolongation potential makes this combination a contraindication.

FLUOXETINE + SERTINDOLE

Plasma levels of sertindole are increased 2–3-fold via CYP2D6 inhibition, so lower maintenance doses might be needed or use of a non-2D6 inhibiting antidepressant (eg. citalopram, escitalopram or sertraline).

HIV PROTEASE INHIBITORS + SERTINDOLE

The UK SPC for sertindole states that it is contraindicated with drugs such as indinavir due to 3A4 inhibition.

ITRACONAZOLE/KETOCONA-ZOLE + SERTINDOLE

The UK SPC for sertindole states that it is contraindicated for use with systemic itraconazole and ketoconazole due to CYP3A4 inhibition.

LITHIUM + SERTINDOLE

See antipsychotics + lithium (*4.2.1*).

PAROXETINE + SERTINDOLE

As for fluoxetine, plasma levels of sertindole are increased 2–3-fold via CYP2D6 inhibition, so lower maintenance doses might be needed or use a non-2D6 inhibiting antidepressant (eg. citalopram, escitalopram or sertraline).

PHENYTOIN + SERTINDOLE

Phenytoin can reduce sertindole levels 2–3-fold by 3A4 induction, so higher maintenance doses might be needed.

Propranolol + sertindole

No interaction occurs.

QUINIDINE + SERTINDOLE

Sertindole levels are increased 2–3-fold via 2D6 inhibition, so this combination is contraindicated.

QUINOLONE ANTIBIOTICS + SERTINDOLE

QT prolongation potential makes the combination with eg. gatifloxacin a contraindication.

Sertraline + sertindole

No interaction via CYP2D6 appears occur.

TRICYCLICS + SERTINDOLE

The UK SPC for sertindole states that it is contraindicated with drugs known to prolong the QT interval eg. some tricyclics.

4.2.8 Zotepine (Zoleptil®, see also 4.2.1 for more general interactions)

Alcohol + zotepine

See antipsychotics + alcohol (*4.7.1*).

Anticonvulsants + zotepine

Zotepine lowers the seizure threshold, especially at doses of 300mg/d or above.

Anticholinergics + zotepine

Lack of interaction has been shown.

Anticoagulants + zotepine

The Japanese SPC notes that zotepine has been reported to enhance the risk of bleeding when given with anticoagulants, eg. with nicoumalone, dicoumarol and warfarin, possibly via a change in protein binding.

Antipsychotics (other) + zotepine

The incidence of seizures may rise.

Benzodiazepines + zotepine

Diazepam may increase zotepine levels by 10%.

Carbamazepine + zotepine

See antipsychotics + carbamazepine (*4.5.1*).

Clonidine + zotepine

Zotepine may decrease the hypotensive actions of clonidine.

Hypotensive drugs + zotepine

Zotepine has alpha-1 blocking activity and care is needed with other hypotensive agents.

Phenytoin + zotepine

See antipsychotics + phenytoin (*4.5.8*).

Smoking + zotepine

See antipsychotics + smoking (*4.7.4*).

SSRIs + zotepine

Fluoxetine increases zotepine levels by 10% (UK SPC). Deep vein thrombosis possibly linked to concurrent paroxetine and zotepine has been reported.

Tricyclics + zotepine

Desipramine does not seem to affect zotepine levels (UK SPC).

Valproate + zotepine

See antipsychotics + valproate (*4.5.12*).

4.3 Antidepressants

4.3.1 Tricyclic antidepressants

Tricyclics are metabolised by the CYP2D6, of interest only to pharmacists and anyone co-prescribing an SSRI such as fluoxetine or paroxetine, which both inhibit this enzyme and double or triple tricyclic levels.

Acamprosate + tricyclics

See acamprosate (*4.6.1*).

ALCOHOL + TRICYCLICS

See alcohol (*4.7.1*).

Amiodarone + tricyclics

The *BNF* notes an increased risk of ventricular arrhythmias with tricyclics.

ANTICHOLINERGICS + TRICYCLICS

Enhanced anticholinergic effects may occur, especially in the elderly.

Antihistamines + tricyclics

Enhanced sedation can occur.

ANTIPSYCHOTICS + TRICYCLICS

Serum levels of both may rise when used together giving enhanced anticholinergic side-effects. Antidepressants may even be counter-productive in psychosis. Tricyclic levels may be up to twice as high if haloperidol is taken concurrently so care with side-effects is needed. No interaction has been reported with the thioxanthenes (eg. flupentixol and zuclopenthixol) nor risperidone.

Aspirin + tricyclics

Imipramine levels may rise with aspirin.

Baclofen + tricyclics

A patient with MS lost muscle tone when a tricyclic was added to baclofen.

Benzodiazepines + tricyclics

See benzodiazepines (*4.1.1*).

Beta-blockers + tricyclics

Enhanced tricyclic toxicity has been reported, eg. labetolol may increase tricyclic plasma levels by up to 28%. Use care at higher tricyclic doses.

Buprenorphine + amitriptyline

No enhanced CNS depressant or respiratory effects have been seen.

Bupropion + tricyclics

See bupropion (*4.6.4*).

Calcium-channel blockers + tricyclics

Amitriptyline clearance was reduced by diltiazem and verapamil in one study, with adverse effects increased. Enhanced cardiac side-effects are also possible.

Cannabis + tricyclics

See antidepressants + cannabis (*4.7.2*).

CARBAMAZEPINE + TRICYCLICS

See carbamazepine (*4.5.1*).

Charcoal, activated + tricyclics

5–10g may reduce absorption of tricyclics by up to 75% if given within 30 minutes of ingestion and may be an effective treatment for overdose even up to two hours after the overdose was taken.

Cholestyramine + doxepin

A single case doxepin levels reduced to a third has been reported.

CLONIDINE + TRICYCLICS

Tricyclics can be expected to antagonise the hypotensive effects of clonidine.

Cocaine + tricyclics

See antidepressants + cocaine (*4.7.3*).

Co-trimoxazole + tricyclics

Five cases exist of relapse when cotrimoxazole was added to a tricyclic.

Dextropropoxyphene + doxepin

One case exists of raised doxepin plasma levels with co-proxamol.

Dicoumarol + tricyclics

An enhanced dicoumarol half-life is possible with some tricyclics.

Disopyramine + tricyclics

Increased anticholinergic effects may occur.

Disulfiram + tricyclics

Amitriptyline may enhance the effects of disulfiram but tricyclic levels may also be increased by about 30%.

Fibre + tricyclics

Several cases of a high fibre diet reducing tricyclic levels by up to a third (and hence to inactive levels) have been reported and may explain non-response in some patients.

Fluconazole + nortriptyline

Inhibition of tricyclic metabolism has resulted in toxic nortriptyline levels.

Glyceryl trinitrate + tricyclics

See nitrates below.

H2-blockers + tricyclics

Cimetidine may increase tricyclic half-lives and raise blood levels by 30–100%. Dose reductions may be necessary if side-effects develop or use ranitidine instead.

Hypoglycaemics + tricyclics

Enhanced hypoglycaemia may occur so monitor blood glucose regularly.

Levodopa + tricyclics

A small reduction in the effect of levodopa may be seen but this is unlikely to be of clinical significance.

Levothyroxine/thyroxine + tricyclics

This is usually a synergistic interaction but a few isolated cases of tachycardia and hypothyroidism have been reported.

Lithium + tricyclics

The combination is obviously widely used but some adverse reactions have been reported, eg. myoclonus, neurotoxicity, NMS and seizures.

MAOIs + TRICYCLICS

See MAOIs (*4.3.4*).

Methadone + tricyclics

See methadone (*4.6.8*).

Methylphenidate + tricyclics

See methylphenidate (*4.6.9*).

Mirtazapine + tricyclics

See mirtazapine (*4.3.3.2*)

Moclobemide + tricyclics

See moclobemide (*4.3.3.3*).

Modafinil + tricyclics

See modafinil (*4.6.10*).

Morphine + tricyclics

Tricyclics increase the bioavailability and potentiate the analgesia of morphine, a usually beneficial effect.

Nitrates (sublingual) + tricyclics

Dry mouth as a side-effect may reduce the dissolution of sublingual nitrates.

Olanzapine + tricyclics

See olanzapine (*4.2.4*).

Oral Contraceptives/estrogens+ tricyclics

Restlessness, reduced tricyclic effectiveness and enhanced tricyclic toxicity have all been reported so monitor closely.

Orlistat + tricyclics

No interaction has been reported.

Phenindione + tricyclics

An enhanced risk of bleeding may occur with this combination.

PHENOBARBITAL + TRICYCLICS

Barbiturates can reduce the serum levels of many tricyclics by up to 60% via enzyme induction. Use an alternative to barbiturates or monitor the tricyclic carefully. Tricyclics may also lower the seizure threshold and thus antagonise the anticonvulsant effects.

Phenylbutazone + tricyclics

Tricyclic absorption may be delayed or reduced by phenylbutazone.

PHENYTOIN + TRICYCLICS

See phenytoin (*4.5.8*).

Quetiapine + tricyclics

See quetiapine (*4.2.5*).

Quinine and quinidine + nortriptyline

One study showed a much reduced clearance of nortriptyline with quinidine and quinine so monitor tricyclic carefully.

Reboxetine + tricyclics

See reboxetine (*4.3.3.5*).

SERTINDOLE + TRICYCLICS

See sertindole (*4.2.7*).

Smoking + tricyclics

See smoking (*4.7.4*).

SSRIs + TRICYCLICS

Fluoxetine, paroxetine and, to a lesser extent fluvoxamine, inhibit the metabolism of tricyclics, doubling or **tripling tricyclic plasma levels** and are thus contraindicated together to avoid toxic reactions. Citalopram and sertraline may also have some effect but this is really only clinically relevant at high SSRI doses. Use the combination only with **great** care, eg. tricyclic dosage should be reduced by about 75% when fluoxetine or paroxetine is added. Standard dose citalopram, escitalopram and sertraline are safer alternatives.

St. John's wort + tricyclics

See St. John's wort (*4.3.3.8*).

Sucralfate + amitriptyline

Reduced tricyclic absorption may occur.

Tea or coffee + tricyclics

Some tricyclics may precipitate out of solution to form an insoluble complex with tea and coffee but the clinical significance is thought to be minimal.

Terbinafine + tricyclics

Tricyclic levels may double or triple with terbinafine.

Valproate + tricyclics

See antidepressants + valproate (*4.5.12*).

VASOCONSTRICTOR SYMPATHOMIMETICS + TRICYCLICS

Although a greatly enhanced response, eg. hypertension and arrhythmias, to phenylephrine has been shown in patients taking tricyclics, in practice moderate doses of cold cures containing sympathomimetics should present little risk in healthy patients. Local anaesthetics with adrenaline appear safe.

Venlafaxine + tricyclics

Tricyclic levels may rise slightly and fits and serotonin syndrome have been reported.

Warfarin + tricyclics

Occasional control problems have been reported with lofepramine.

YOHIMBINE + TRICYCLICS

Tricyclics can potentiate the blood pressure changes caused by yohimbine, especially if blood pressure is already raised.

Zopiclone + tricyclics

See zopiclone (*4.1.6*).

Zotepine + tricyclics

See zotepine (*4.2.8*).

4.3.2 SSRIs (selective serotonin reuptake inhibitors)

Drug-drug interactions involving the cytochrome P450 system, the enzymes which metabolise many drugs, have been noted for all SSRIs but there are significant differences in the isoenzymes inhibited and the potency of inhibition. Fluoxetine and paroxetine are most likely to interact this way and citalopram (20mg/d), escitalopram (10mg/d) and sertraline (at 50mg/d) least likely. This is of particular importance when switching antidepressants (see *Chapter 2.2.2*), in overdose and when co-administering drugs also metabolised by the same P450 enzymes.

4.3.2.1 Citalopram (Cipramil®) + escitalopram (Cipralex®)

Citalopram and escitalopram are less potent enzyme inhibitors than the other SSRIs and appear to have a lower incidence of interactions. Lack of interaction has so far been shown with benzodiazepines, antipsychotics, analgesics, antihistamines, antihypertensives, beta-blockers and other cardiovascular drugs. As far as is known, all interactions apply to both escitalopram and citalopram.

Alcohol + (es)citalopram

See alcohol (*4.7.1*).

Alimemazine/trimeprazine + (es)citalopram

See antipsychotics + (es)citalopram.

Antipsychotics + (es)citalopram

Levomepromazine may increase plasma levels of citalopram by about a third, of limited clinical significance. There has been no detectable effect from (es)citalopram on clozapine and risperidone.

Benzodiazepines + (es)citalopram

Lack of interaction has been shown.

Buspirone + (es)citalopram

Hyponatraemia and serotonin syndrome has been reported with the combination.

Carbamazepine + (es)citalopram

Carbamazepine may reduce the effect of citalopram.

Charcoal, activated + (es)citalopram

25g activated charcoal given 30 minutes after citalopram reduces citalopram peak and total levels by about 50%. Concurrent gastric lavage does not provide any additional reductions.

Ciclosporin + (es)citalopram

No interaction has been reported.

Digoxin + (es)citalopram

No interaction has been reported.

Donepezil + (es)citalopram

See SSRIs + donepezil (*4.6.3.1*).

Fluvoxamine + citalopram

Fluvoxamine may slightly enhance the effect of citalopram.

Ketoconazole + (es)citalopram

No interaction has been reported.

Lithium + (es)citalopram

See SSRIs + lithium (*4.4*).

MAOIs + (ES)CITALOPRAM

See citalopram + MAOIs (*4.3.4*).

Moclobemide + (es)citalopram

See SSRIs + moclobemide (*4.3.3.3*).

OXCARBAZEPINE + (ES)CITALOPRAM

See oxcarbazepine (*4.5.6*).

Selegiline + (es)citalopram

Lack of interaction has been shown.

Sertindole + (es)citalopram

No interaction has been reported.

St. John's wort + (es)citalopram

See SSRIs + St. John's wort (*4.3.3.8*).

Sympathomimetics + (es)citalopram

Augmentation of amfetamines is theoretically possible.

Tricyclics + (es)citalopram

See SSRIs + tricyclics (*4.3.1*).

Triptans + (es)citalopram

The *BNF* notes an increased risk of CNS toxicity and recommends avoiding the combination. See also triptans + fluoxetine (*4.3.2.2*).

Warfarin + (es)citalopram

Citalopram 40mg/d may produce a small increase in prothrombin time, probably clinically insignificant.

Zolpidem + (es)citalopram

See SSRIs + zolpidem (*4.1.5*).

4.3.2.2 Fluoxetine (Prozac®)

Fluoxetine and its metabolite norfluoxetine potently inhibit CYP2D6 and thus have a high incidence of interactions with drugs metabolised by this and other enzymes.

Alcohol + fluoxetine

See alcohol (*4.7.1*).

Alosetron + fluoxetine

No interaction has been reported.

Amfetamines + fluoxetine

See sympathomimetics + fluoxetine.

ANTIPSYCHOTICS + FLUOXETINE

See fluoxetine + antipsychotics (*4.2.1*), clozapine (*4.2.3*), olanzapine (*4.2.4*),

risperidone (*4.2.6*), sertindole (*4.2.7*) and zotepine (*4.2.8*).

Beta-blockers + fluoxetine

Bradycardia with fluoxetine and metoprolol has been reported. Atenolol or sotalol may be suitable alternatives.

Benzodiazepines + fluoxetine

Fluoxetine may slightly increase levels of benzodiazepines and hence their effects. No special precautions seem necessary.

Bupropion + fluoxetine

See bupropion (*4.6.4*).

Buspirone + fluoxetine

See buspirone (*4.1.2*).

Calcium-channel blockers + fluoxetine

Oedema, weight gain and headache have occurred with verapamil and fluoxetine so use lower doses if an interaction is suspected.

Cannabis + fluoxetine

See antidepressants + cannabis (*4.7.2*).

Carbamazepine + fluoxetine

Fluoxetine may inhibit carbamazepine metabolism, increasing levels by up to 25%. Best to monitor carbamazepine levels regularly.

Ciclosporin + fluoxetine

Ciclosporin levels may be doubled by fluoxetine.

Clarithromycin + fluoxetine

There is a single case of delirium with the combination.

Cocaine + fluoxetine

See antidepressants + cocaine (*4.7.3*).

Cyproheptadine + fluoxetine

There are case reports of relapse of depression.

Dextromethorphan + fluoxetine

Visual hallucinations lasting 6–8 hrs occurred in one patient on fluoxetine who took a cough mixture containing dextromethorphan.

Donepezil + fluoxetine
See SSRIs + donepezil (*4.6.3.1*).

Lithium + fluoxetine
See lithium (*4.4*).

LSD + fluoxetine
Grand mal convulsions occurred in one patient who took LSD while on fluoxetine.

MAOIs + FLUOXETINE
See MAOIs (*4.3.4.1*).

Methadone + fluoxetine
See methadone (*4.6.8*).

Mirtazapine + fluoxetine
See fluoxetine (*4.3.3.2*).

Moclobemide + fluoxetine
See SSRIs + moclobemide (*4.3.3.3*).

Morphine + fluoxetine
Fluoxetine may enhance the analgesic effect of morphine.

Olanzapine + fluoxetine
See fluoxetine (*4.2.4*).

Oral contraceptives + fluoxetine
No interaction has been shown.

Pentazocine + fluoxetine
An unproven case of rapid toxicity with the combination exists.

PHENYTOIN + FLUOXETINE
See phenytoin (*4.5.8*).

Quetiapine + fluoxetine
See SSRIs + quetiapine (*4.2.5*).

Reboxetine + fluoxetine
See reboxetine (*4.3.3.4*).

RISPERIDONE + FLUOXETINE
See risperidone (*4.2.6*).

Rivastigmine + fluoxetine
See rivastigmine (*4.6.3.3*).

Selegiline + fluoxetine
Three cases exist of toxic reactions, eg. hypomania, shivering, ataxia and hypertension. Discontinue one or both drugs if an adverse reaction occurs.

SERTINDOLE + FLUOXETINE
See sertindole (*4.2.7*).

Sertraline + fluoxetine
See sertraline (*4.3.2.5*).

St. John's wort + fluoxetine
See SSRIs + St. John's wort (*4.3.3.8*).

Sympathomimetics + fluoxetine
A possible toxic interaction has been suggested by several case reports of extreme agitation.

Tolterodine + fluoxetine
Fluoxetine has been shown to inhibit the metabolism of tolterodine.

Tramadol + fluoxetine
Serotonin syndrome and mania have been reported with the combination.

Trazodone + fluoxetine
Trazodone toxicity eg. myoclonus may occur.

TRICYCLICS + FLUOXETINE
See SSRIs + tricyclics (*4.3.1*).

Triptans + fluoxetine
Lack of significant interaction has been reported with sumatriptan although post-marketing surveillance in Canada indicated that a serotonin-like syndrome may occur rarely with the combination. The *BNF* notes an increased risk of CNS toxicity and recommends avoiding the combination.

Tryptophan + fluoxetine
Cases of central toxicity with the combination of an SSRI and tryptophan have been reported.

Valproate + fluoxetine
In one case valproate levels rose by nearly 50% when fluoxetine was added, although no adverse reactions were seen. Perversely, reduced valproate levels have also been reported.

Venlafaxine + fluoxetine

Serotonin syndrome has been reported when venlafaxine was started immediately after fluoxetine was discontinued and severe anticholinergic side-effects may occur with the combination.

WARFARIN + FLUOXETINE

There is published evidence that no change in bleeding occurs although four cases of raised INR within ten days of starting fluoxetine have been reported.

Zolpidem + fluoxetine

See SSRIs + zolpidem (*4.1.5*).

Zotepine + fluoxetine

See SSRIs + zotepine (*4.2.8*).

4.3.2.3 Fluvoxamine *(Faverin®)*

Fluvoxamine strongly inhibits CYP1A2, CYP2D6, CYP3A and CYP2C19 activity and may have a high incidence of significant interactions with drugs metabolised by these enzymes.

Alcohol + fluvoxamine

See alcohol (*4.7.1*).

Antipsychotics + fluvoxamine

Seizures have been reported with levomepromazine (methotrimeprazine) and fluvoxamine. Thioridazine is now contraindicated with fluvoxamine due to QTc prolongation.

Benzodiazepines + fluvoxamine

Plasma concentrations of some benzodiazepines may be increased but lorazepam is unaffected. Reduce doses if necessary.

Beta-blockers + fluvoxamine

Propranolol, but not atenolol, plasma levels can be raised by fluvoxamine.

Buspirone + fluvoxamine

See buspirone (*4.1.2*).

Caffeine + fluvoxamine

Even low-dose fluvoxamine may enhance caffeine's effects via enzyme inhibition, possibly resulting in toxicity.

Carbamazepine + fluvoxamine

Carbamazepine levels may be increased by fluvoxamine, possibly resulting in toxicity.

Ciclosporin + fluvoxamine

There is a case report of ciclosporin levels elevated by the introduction of fluvoxamine to a ciclosporin-treated allograft recipient. Intensive monitoring of the serum creatinine and ciclosporin level was indicated, along with appropriate dose reduction.

Chloral + fluvoxamine

Lack of interaction has been reported.

CLOZAPINE + FLUVOXAMINE

See clozapine (*4.2.3*).

Citalopram + fluvoxamine

See citalopram (*4.3.2.1*).

Digoxin + fluvoxamine

Lack of interaction has been reported.

Donepezil + fluvoxamine

See SSRIs + donepezil (*4.6.3.1*).

Escitalopram + fluvoxamine

See citalopram (*4.3.2.1*).

Glimepiride + fluvoxamine

Fluvoxamine may increase glimepiride levels slightly.

Lithium + fluvoxamine

Lack of interaction has been shown, but cases of serotonin syndrome and somnolence exist.

MAOIs + FLUVOXAMINE

See MAOIs (*4.3.4*).

Melatonin + fluvoxamine

Fluvoxamine 50mg inhibits the metabolism of oral melatonin 5mg, and combining the treatments may improve sleep.

Methadone + fluvoxamine

See methadone (*4.6.8*).

Metoclopramide + fluvoxamine

Acute dystonia has been associated with the combination.

Mirtazapine + fluvoxamine

See mirtazapine (*4.3.3.2*).

Moclobemide + fluvoxamine

See moclobemide (*4.3.3.3*).

NICOUMALONE + FLUVOXAMINE

The anticoagulant effects may be enhanced by fluvoxamine.

Olanzapine + fluvoxamine

See SSRIs + olanzapine (*4.2.4*).

PHENYTOIN + FLUVOXAMINE

See phenytoin (*4.5.8*).

Quinidine + fluvoxamine

Fluvoxamine significantly inhibits the clearance of quinidine.

Reboxetine + fluvoxamine

See reboxetine (*4.3.3.5*).

Risperidone + fluvoxamine

See risperidone (*4.2.6*).

Smoking + fluvoxamine

See smoking (*4.7.4*).

St. John's wort + fluvoxamine

See SSRIs + St. John's wort (*4.3.3.8*).

Sympathomimetics + fluvoxamine

Augmentation of amfetamines is theoretically possible (see also fluoxetine, *4.3.2.2*).

THEOPHYLLINE + FLUVOXAMINE

Two cases of theophylline toxicity induced by fluvoxamine have been reported and the CSM recommends avoiding the combination.

Tolbutamide + fluvoxamine

Tolbutamide levels may rise by 20% with fluvoxamine.

TRICYCLICS + FLUVOXAMINE

See SSRIs + tricyclics (*4.3.1*).

Triptans + fluvoxamine

The *BNF* notes an increased risk of CNS toxicity with sumatriptan and recommends avoiding the combination. See also fluoxetine (*4.3.2.2*).

Tryptophan + fluvoxamine

See fluoxetine + tryptophan (*4.3.2.2*).

Valproate + fluvoxamine

Augmentation of fluvoxamine has been seen with valproate.

WARFARIN + FLUVOXAMINE

Fluvoxamine can increase warfarin levels by up to 65% and elevated INR has been reported.

Zolpidem + fluvoxamine

See SSRIs + zolpidem (*4.1.5*).

Zotepine + fluvoxamine

See zotepine (*4.2.8*).

4.3.2.4 Paroxetine (Seroxat®)

Paroxetine is probably the most potent SSRI inhibitor of CYP2D6 and may thus have a higher incidence of interactions with drugs metabolised by this enzyme.

Alcohol + paroxetine

See alcohol (*4.7.1*).

Anticholinergics + paroxetine

See SSRIs + anticholinergics (*4.6.2*).

Antipsychotics + paroxetine

No interaction occurs with haloperidol, flupentixol nor zuclopenthixol.

Benzodiazepines + paroxetine

Lack of interaction has been shown.

Beta-blockers + paroxetine

Paroxetine 20 mg/d increases the effects of metoprolol and so reduced metoprolol doses might be needed. Raised paroxetine levels after the addition of pindolol has been reported, probably via 2D6 inhibition.

Bupropion + paroxetine

See bupropion (*4.6.4*).

Cannabis + paroxetine

See antidepressants + cannabis (*4.7.2*).

Carbamazepine + paroxetine

No significant interaction occurs.

CLOZAPINE + PAROXETINE

See clozapine (*4.2.3*).

Dextromethorphan + paroxetine

Paroxetine may increase dextromethorphan levels by CYP2D6 inhibition (see fluoxetine, *4.3.2.2*).

Digoxin + paroxetine

Lack of interaction has been shown.

Donepezil + paroxetine

See SSRIs + donepezil (*4.6.3.1*).

Galantamine + paroxetine

See galantamine (*4.6.3.2*).

H2-blockers + paroxetine

Cimetidine may inhibit the metabolism of paroxetine, increasing bioavailability by up to 50%, so use ranitidine.

Interferon alpha + paroxetine

Previous good response to paroxetine and trazodone was reversed in one woman by interferon alpha.

Lithium + paroxetine

See SSRIs + lithium (*4.4*).

MAOIs + PAROXETINE

See MAOIs (*4.3.4*).

Methadone + paroxetine

Steady-state methadone levels may rise with paroxetine, but only in slow CYP2D6 metabolisers.

Mirtazapine + paroxetine

See mirtazapine (*4.3.3.2*).

Moclobemide + paroxetine

See SSRIs + moclobemide (*4.3.3.3*).

Olanzapine + paroxetine

See SSRIs + olanzapine (*4.2.4*).

Oral contraceptives + paroxetine

Lack of interaction has been shown.

Phenytoin + paroxetine

Paroxetine levels may be decreased slightly.

Phenobarbital + paroxetine

Paroxetine levels may be decreased by about 25%.

Risperidone + paroxetine

See risperidone (*4.2.5*).

SERTINDOLE + PAROXETINE

See sertindole (*4.2.7*).

St. John's wort + paroxetine

See SSRIs + St. John's wort (*4.3.3.8*).

Sympathomimetics + paroxetine

Augmentation of amfetamines is theoretically possible (see sympathomimetics + fluoxetine *4.3.2.2*).

TRICYCLICS + PAROXETINE

See SSRIs + tricyclics (*4.3.1*).

Triptans + paroxetine

The *BNF* notes an increased risk of CNS toxicity with sumatriptan and recommends avoiding the combination, although lack of interaction has been shown with rizatriptan. See also fluoxetine (*4.3.2.2*).

Valproate + paroxetine

No interaction has been noted.

Warfarin + paroxetine

The possibility of an interaction has been suggested but not shown yet.

Zolpidem + paroxetine

See SSRIs + zolpidem (*4.1.5*).

Zotepine + paroxetine

See SSRIs + zotepine (*4.2.8*).

4.3.2.5 Sertraline *(Lustral®)*

Sertraline appears a less potent inhibitor of CYP2D6 than most other SSRIs and has, at 50–100 mg/d, a low incidence of interactions with drugs metabolised by CYP2D6.

Alcohol + sertraline

See alcohol (*4.7.1*).

Anticholinergics + sertraline

See SSRIs + anticholinergics (*4.6.2*).

Atenolol + sertraline

Lack of interaction has been shown.

Benzodiazepines + sertraline

Lack of clinically significant interaction has been shown.

Beta-blockers + sertraline

Lack of clinically significant interaction has been shown.

Carbamazepine + sertraline

One study showed no significant interaction but there are reported cases of increased carbamazepine plasma levels and lack of sertraline efficacy via reduced levels.

Clozapine + sertraline

See clozapine (*4.2.3*).

Digoxin + sertraline

Lack of interaction has been noted.

Donepezil + sertraline

See donepezil (*4.6.3.1*).

Erythromycin + sertraline

Serotonin syndrome has been reported in a child on erythromycin and sertraline.

Fluoxetine + sertraline

In a report of a 'therapeutic substitution', out-patients were abruptly swapped from fluoxetine to sertraline. 20 failed, including 10 with intolerable adverse effects (nervousness, jitters, nausea and headache). The authors correctly suggest that a serotonin-like syndrome just might be responsible for this.

Lamotrigine + sertraline

See lamotrigine (*4.5.4*).

Lithium + sertraline

See SSRIs + lithium (*4.4*).

MAOIs + SERTRALINE

See MAOIs (*4.3.4*).

Mirtazapine + sertraline

See SSRIs + mirtazapine (*4.3.3.2*).

Moclobemide + sertraline

See SSRIs + moclobemide (*4.3.3.3*).

Olanzapine + sertraline

See SSRIs + olanzapine (*4.2.4*).

Phenytoin + sertraline

Lack of significant interaction has been shown, but there are case reports of significantly raised phenytoin levels and reduced sertraline levels.

Quetiapine + sertraline

See SSRIs + quetiapine (*4.2.5*).

Sertindole + sertraline

See sertindole (*4.2.7*).

St. John's wort + sertraline

See SSRIs + St. John's wort (*4.3.3.8*).

Sympathomimetics + sertraline

Augmentation of amfetamines is theoretically possible (see sympathomimetics + fluoxetine, *4.3.2.2*).

Tolbutamide + sertraline

200 mg/d sertraline has been shown to produce a 16% decrease in tolbutamide clearance.

Tramadol + sertraline

Serotonin syndrome has been reported with the combination.

Tricyclics + sertraline

See SSRIs + tricyclics (*4.3.1*).

Triptans + sertraline

The *BNF* notes an increased risk of CNS toxicity with sumatriptan and recommends avoiding the combination. See also fluoxetine (*4.3.2.2*).

Venlafaxine + sertraline

Acute liver damage possibly related to sertraline and venlafaxine ingestion has been reported.

Warfarin + sertraline

Although sertraline is probably the SSRI of choice with warfarin, prothrombin time can be increased slightly, probably of minimal clinical importance.

Zolpidem + sertraline

See SSRIs + zolpidem (*4.1.5*).

Zotepine + sertraline

See SSRIs + zotepine (*4.2.8*).

4.3.3 Related antidepressants

4.3.3.1 Mianserin

Alcohol + mianserin

See alcohol (*4.7.1*).

Benzodiazepines + mianserin

Enhanced sedation may occur.

Carbamazepine + mianserin

Mianserin levels may be halved by carbamazepine.

Warfarin + mianserin

There is normally no problem but occasional control problems have been experienced with mianserin.

4.3.3.2 Mirtazapine (Zispin®)

Mirtazapine has multiple metabolic routes and does not inhibit major liver enzymes and so interactions via these enzymes are unlikely. It has linear kinetics from 15–75mg/d, with 100% excreted via the urine and faeces

ALCOHOL + MIRTAZAPINE

Mirtazapine causes drowsiness, enhanced considerably by alcohol.

Benzodiazepines + mirtazapine

The combination of diazepam and mirtazapine, not surprisingly, produces an additive sedative effect and so anyone on the combination should be warned about driving etc.

Carbamazepine + mirtazapine

Carbamazepine may produce a 60% decrease in mirtazapine levels, and so raised mirtazapine doses might be needed.

Cimetidine + mirtazapine

Lack of significant interaction has been shown.

Fluoxetine + mirtazapine

Lack of clinically significant interaction has been shown, although mania has been reported with the combination.

Fluvoxamine + mirtazapine

Mirtazapine levels may be increased 3–4 fold, a significant effect.

Lithium + mirtazapine

Lack of interaction has been shown.

MAOIs + mirtazapine

The manufacturers cautiously recommend a two-week gap between stopping an MAOI and starting mirtazapine.

Paroxetine + mirtazapine

Lack of interaction has been shown.

Phenytoin + mirtazapine

Lack of significant interaction has been shown.

Risperidone + mirtazapine

Lack of interaction has been shown.

Sertraline + mirtazapine

There is an isolated case of hypomania with the combination.

Tricyclics + mirtazapine

Lack of significant interaction has been shown.

Venlafaxine + mirtazapine

Serotonin syndrome has been reported with the combination.

Warfarin + mirtazapine

No interaction is known or suspected, but there is insufficient information to confirm this at present.

4.3.3.3 Moclobemide (Manerix® — Reversible Inhibitor of Monoamine Oxidase-A or a RIMA)

Alcohol + moclobemide

See alcohol (*4.7.1*).

Benzodiazepines + moclobemide

No significant interaction occurs.

Bupropion + moclobemide

See MAOIs + bupropion (*4.6.4*).

CIMETIDINE + MOCLOBEMIDE

Cimetidine reduces the clearance and prolongs the half-life of moclobemide so start with a low dose of moclobemide and monitor closely.

Digoxin + moclobemide

Lack of interaction has been reported.

Ibuprofen + moclobemide

Moclobemide is alleged to potentiate the effect of ibuprofen (manufacturers' information, pre-clinical studies only).

Metoprolol + moclobemide

Concurrent metoprolol and moclobemide results in further lowering of blood pressure so monitor carefully.

Nifedipine + moclobemide

Lack of significant interaction has been reported.

Opiates + moclobemide

Moclobemide is alleged to potentiate the effect of opiates (UK SPC) and opiate dose reductions may be necessary.

Oral contraceptives + moclobemide

Lack of interaction has been reported.

SELEGILINE + MOCLOBEMIDE

Selegiline (an MAO-**B** inhibitor) combined with moclobemide (an MAO-**A** inhibitor) could produce full MAO inhibition. The combination is not recommended but if the two need to be used together then full MAOI dietary precautions would be required.

SSRIs + moclobemide

The UK SPCs contraindicate the combination as cases of fatal serotonin syndrome have been reported after moclobemide and citalopram overdose. Insomnia and dysphoria has been reported with fluvoxamine and moclobemide. However, a study of fluoxetine and moclobemide was unable to show any such problems. SSRIs should be avoided with moclobemide unless carefully supervised.

Sympathomimetics + moclobemide

The UK SPC recommends avoiding the combination and the pressor effect has been slightly enhanced.

Tricyclics + moclobemide

The moclobemide UK SPC contraindicates this combination if the tricyclic (or metabolite) is a 5-HT reuptake inhibitor, eg. clomipramine, amitriptyline or imipramine. There are several cases of serotonin syndrome with moclobemide and clomipramine, imipramine or an SSRI.

Triptans + moclobemide

Moclobemide may significantly potentiate the effects of zolmitriptan, rizatriptan or sumatriptan and the combination is not recommended, although a small study with sumatriptan suggested combined use was safe with care (Blier and Bergeron, *J Clin Psychopharmacol* 1995, **15**, 106–9).

Tyramine + moclobemide

Moclobemide does not appear to significantly potentiate the pressor effects of tyramine. Dietary restrictions are generally **not** required, but it is recommended that patients should avoid eating excessive amounts of tyramine containing foods, especially if they have pre-existing hypertension. Minor pressor effects are not usually seen until an intake of about 100mg tyramine, quite difficult to eat with a normal life-style. The author was sadly not involved with the naturalistic study staged in a variety of high class restaurants to prove this point.

Venlafaxine + moclobemide

See venlafaxine (*4.3.3.7*).

Warfarin + moclobemide

No interaction is reported, although the potential exists.

4.3.3.4 Reboxetine (Edronax®)

Reboxetine is extensively protein bound (97%) and so may interact with drugs such as dipyridamole, propranolol, methadone, imipramine, chlorpromazine and local anaesthetics. It appears not to be affected by changes in liver metabolism.

Alcohol + reboxetine

See alcohol (*4.7.1*).

Antipsychotics + reboxetine

An interaction is possible eg. with chlorpromazine (see p.149).

Benzodiazepines + reboxetine

Lack of interaction has been reported (SPC), although some mild to moderate drowsiness and transient increases in heart rate were noted.

Chlorpromazine + reboxetine

An interaction is possible (see p. 149).

Dipyridamole + reboxetine

An interaction is possible (see p. 149).

Disopyramide + reboxetine

The manufacturers of reboxetine advise caution with the combination (*BNF*).

Diuretics + reboxetine

There may be an increased risk of hypokalaemia with loop diuretics or thiazides (*BNF*).

Erythromycin + reboxetine

The manufacturers of reboxetine advise avoiding the combination (*BNF*).

Flecainide + reboxetine

The manufacturers of reboxetine advise avoiding the combination (*BNF*).

Fluoxetine + reboxetine

Lack of significant interaction has been shown.

Fluvoxamine + reboxetine

The manufacturers of reboxetine advise avoiding the combination (*BNF*).

Ketoconazole + reboxetine

Reboxetine clearance may be reduced slightly, and so some caution may be advisable.

Lidocaine + reboxetine

An interaction is possible (see above) with lidocaine and other local anaesthetics.

MAOIs + reboxetine

No information so avoid until further notice.

Methadone + reboxetine

An interaction is possible (see p. 149).

Potassium-losing diuretics + reboxetine

Hypokalaemia is possible (SPC).

Propranolol + reboxetine

An interaction is possible (see p. 149).

Tricyclics + reboxetine

An interaction is possible (see p. 149).

Warfarin + reboxetine

No interaction is known or suspected, but there is insufficient information to confirm this at present.

4.3.3.5 Trazodone *(Molipaxin*®*)*

Trazodone is metabolised by CYP2D6 and inhibits CYP3A4.

ALCOHOL + TRAZODONE

See alcohol (*4.7.1*).

Antipsychotics + trazodone

Two cases of enhanced hypotension with chlorpromazine and trifluoperazine have been reported.

Buspirone + trazodone

See buspirone (*4.1.2*).

Carbamazepine + trazodone

See carbamazepine (*4.5.1*).

Cocaine + trazodone

See antidepressants + cocaine (*4.7.3*).

Digoxin + trazodone

Isolated cases of digoxin toxicity exist.

Fluoxetine + trazodone

See fluoxetine (*4.3.2.2*).

Gingko biloba + trazodone

Coma has been reported with the combination.

Interferon alpha + trazodone

See paroxetine + interferon alpha (*4.3.2.4*).

MAOIs + trazodone

See MAOIs (*4.3.4*).

Phenytoin + trazodone

See phenytoin (*4.5.8*).

Venlafaxine + trazodone

See venlafaxine (*4.3.3.7*).

Warfarin + trazodone

There are reported cases of 30% reduction in prothrombin time.

4.3.3.6 Tryptophan (Optimax®)

Fluoxetine + tryptophan

See fluoxetine (*4.3.2.2*).

Fluvoxamine + tryptophan

See tryptophan + fluoxetine (*4.3.2.3*).

MAOIs + tryptophan

See MAOIs (*4.3.4*).

4.3.3.7 Venlafaxine (Efexor®)

Venlafaxine does not appear to have a significant effect on the P450 enzyme system, although it is metabolised by P450 isoenzymes and its levels can be affected by other drugs inhibiting or competing for these enzymes.

Alcohol + venlafaxine

See alcohol (*4.7.1*).

Antipsychotics + venlafaxine

Urinary retention has been reported with haloperidol, probably by raised haloperidol levels. Increased clozapine levels and adverse effects have also been reported.

Benzodiazepines + venlafaxine

No significant interaction has been shown.

Bupropion + venlafaxine

See bupropion (*4.6.4*).

Carbamazepine + venlafaxine

Lack of interaction has been shown in a manufacturers study.

Cimetidine + venlafaxine

Cimetidine can reduce venlafaxine clearance by up to 43% and result in increased venlafaxine levels. Patients should be monitored for dose-related side-effects, eg. nausea, drowsiness.

Fluoxetine + venlafaxine

See fluoxetine (*4.3.2.2*).

Indinavir + venlafaxine

Peak indinavir levels may be reduced by 35% by venlafaxine, potentially significant.

Lithium + venlafaxine

Venlafaxine has been shown to have no effect on lithium (SPC). Lithium reduces the renal clearance of venlafaxine but without apparent clinical significance.

MAOIs + VENLAFAXINE

See MAOIs (*4.3.4*).

Mirtazapine + venlafaxine

See mirtazapine (*4.3.3.2*).

Moclobemide + venlafaxine

Do not use together and leave a 7–14-day gap if switching (see *Chapter 2.2.2*).

Risperidone + venlafaxine

See risperidone (*4.1.6*).

Selegiline + venlafaxine

Do not use together and leave a 7–14-day gap between the drugs.

Sertraline + venlafaxine

See sertraline (*4.2.5*).

Trazodone + venlafaxine

A serotonin syndrome has been reported.

Tricyclics + venlafaxine

See tricyclics (*4.3.1*).

Verapamil + venlafaxine

An isolated case of a fatality has been reported.

Warfarin + venlafaxine

No problems reported, although the UK SPC notes that warfarin potentiation can occur.

4.3.3.8 St. John's wort

Although not licensed for depression in the UK, this section has been included because queries about it's interactions are frequently raised. Minor serotonin, noradrenaline and dopamine reuptake inhibition activity has been detected from St. John's wort (SJW) and might thus potentiate any antidepressants, and so should in theory best be avoided, particularly at high dose. The UK CSM issued advice about potential interactions in February 2000 (*Curr Prob Pharmacovig* 2000, **26**, 6–7).

Anticonvulsants + St. John's wort

SJW may induce the metabolism of carbamazepine, phenobarbital and phenytoin, increasing the risk of seizures, and so should not be taken together (CSM warning, 2000), although suddenly stopping SJW may require dose adjustment of any anticonvulsant. Check anticonvulsant levels before and after stopping SJW.

Anti-HIV drugs + St. John's wort

SJW may induce the metabolism of anti-HIV drugs, reducing efficacy, and so should not be taken together (CSM warning, 2000), although suddenly stopping SJW may require dose adjustment of any anti-HIV drug.

Buspirone + St. John's wort

See buspirone (*4.1.2*).

Carbamazepine + St. John's wort

See anticonvulsants + SJW (above).

Ciclosporin + St. John's wort

SJW may induce the metabolism of ciclosporin, reducing plasma levels significantly, and so should not be taken together (CSM warning, 2000). Heart transplant rejection due to SJW has been reported.

Digoxin + St. John's wort

SJW may induce the metabolism of digoxin, reducing AUC by up to 25%, and so should not be taken together. Suddenly stopping SJW may also require dose adjustment of digoxin.

Fexofenadine + St. John's wort

Lack of interaction has been shown.

Indinavir + St. John's wort

SJW may reduce the levels of indinavir by 57%, and so SJW should be avoided in patients receiving indinavir as their sole protease inhibitor. The same would probably be true for other protease inhibitors eg. ritonavir and saquinavir.

MAOIs + St. John's wort

Minor MAOI activity has been detected from SJW and might thus potentiate existing MAOI therapy, and should be avoided, particularly at high dose.

Oral contraceptives + St. John's wort

The UK CSM has recommended that, since SJW reduces the effectiveness of oral contraceptives, the two should not be taken together. Contraceptive failure has been reported.

SSRIs + St. John's wort

Minor serotonin reuptake inhibition activity has been detected from SJW and might thus potentiate existing SSRI therapy and so should, in theory, be avoided, particularly at high dose.

Statins + St. John's wort

SJW may reduce the levels of simvastatin, but not pravastatin.

Theophylline + St. John's wort

SJW may induce the metabolism of theophylline, reducing efficacy, and so should not be taken together (CSM warning, 2000), although suddenly stopping SJW may require dose adjustment of theophylline. Check theophylline levels before and after stopping SJW.

Tricyclics + St. John's wort

Minor serotonin and noradrenaline reuptake inhibition activity has been detected from SJW and might thus potentiate existing tricyclic therapy, and so should, in theory, be avoided, particularly at high dose.

Triptans + St. John's wort

The CSM has warned that SJW may increase the serotonergic effects of sumatriptan, naratriptan, rizatriptan and zolmitriptan, with increased adverse effects and so the two should not be used together.

Tyramine + St. John's wort

There is not thought to be an interaction.

Warfarin + St. John's wort

SJW may induce the metabolism of warfarin, reducing efficacy, and so should not be taken together (CSM warning, 2000). Suddenly stopping SJW may require dose adjustment of warfarin so check INR before and after stopping SJW and adjust doses as necessary.

4.3.4 Mono-amine oxidase inhibitors (isocarboxazid, phenelzine and tranylcypromine)

4.3.4.1 Drug-drug interactions

Adrenaline + MAOIs

See noradrenaline + MAOIs.

ALCOHOL + MAOIs

See alcohol (*4.7.1*).

Amantadine + MAOIs

Isolated cases of hypertension have been reported.

AMFETAMINES + MAOIs

See dexamfetamine + MAOIs.

Anaesthetics + MAOIs

With proper monitoring, general and local anaesthesia can be given safely with MAOIs, although occasional problems have been reported.

Anticholinergics + MAOIs

Enhanced anticholinergic effects have been postulated.

Antipsychotics + MAOIs

This combination is a risk factor for neuroleptic malignant syndrome and may enhance anticholinergic and extrapyramidal side-effects.

Aspartame + MAOIs

A single case exists of recurrent headaches following aspartame ingestion.

Benzodiazepines + MAOIs

There are isolated cases of toxicity, eg. oedema and hepatotoxicity but this is normally considered a safe combination.

Beta-blockers + MAOIs

Propranolol used with MAOIs has caused severe hypertension and slight bradycardia so monitor bp carefully, especially in the elderly.

Bupropion + MAOIs

See bupropion (*4.6.4*).

BUSPIRONE + MAOIs

There are four reports of increased bp and possible CVA so care is needed.

Caffeine + MAOIs

Case reports exist of increased jitteriness with caffeine taken while on MAOIs.

Carbamazepine + MAOIs

A few cases of raised carbamazepine levels have been reported so monitor regularly.

Chloral + MAOIs

There are two poorly documented case reports of fatal interaction but this is not thought to be an important interaction.

CITALOPRAM + MAOIs

There are many reported cases of serotonin syndrome with other SSRIs and MAOIs and so care is needed if this combination is used. The manufacturers state this to be a contraindication.

Clozapine + MAOIs

See clozapine (*4.2.3*).

Cyproheptadine + MAOIs

An isolated case of hallucinations exist.

DEXAMFETAMINE + MAOIs

There are case reports of death with phenelzine plus dexamfetamine or amfetamine so avoid the combination.

Dextromethorphan + MAOIs

Although mainly extrapolation from pethidine, two fatal cases of alleged interaction have been reported so it is probably best to avoid this combination. See also dextropropoxyphene.

Dextropropoxyphene + MAOIs

Dextropropoxyphene sedation was enhanced by phenelzine in one case and severe hypotension, ataxia and impaired coordination occurred in another patient when propoxyphene was added to phenelzine.

Disulfiram + MAOIs

See disulfiram (*4.6.6*).

Ecstasy/MDMA + MAOIs

There are cases of hypertensive crisis, muscle tension, coma and delirium with MDMA (Ecstasy) and phenelzine.

EPHEDRINE + MAOIs

See sympathomimetics + MAOIs.

ESCITALOPRAM + MAOIs

See citalopram above.

FLUOXETINE + MAOIs

There are several reported interactions, including 4 deaths, so do not use together and allow **at least** five weeks after stopping fluoxetine before starting an MAOI. Allow two weeks vice versa, starting with a low dose of fluoxetine, eg. 20mg on alternate days.

FLUVOXAMINE + MAOIs

There is a UK SPC recommendation to allow a two-week gap between therapies.

Ginseng + MAOIs

There are two cases of headache, tremor and mania with Ginseng and phenelzine.

Hypoglycaemics + MAOIs

An enhanced hypoglycaemic effect with insulin and sulphonylureas has been noted, so care is needed.

Indoramin + MAOIs

The manufacturers of indoramin state this to be a contraindication.

LEVODOPA + MAOIs

Low dose Sinemet® and Madopar® seem safe but avoid higher doses and levodopa on its own.

Lithium + MAOIs

Lack of an interaction has been shown.

MAOIs + MAOIs

There is some evidence that different MAOIs may interact with each other, eg. if abruptly changed, mostly where the MAOI is changed to tranylcypromine.

Methadone + MAOIs

Lack of an interaction has been reported.

Methylphenidate + MAOIs

A minor interaction has been reported, eg. headache and hyperventilation.

Mirtazapine + MAOIs

See mirtazapine (*4.3.3.2*).

Morphine + MAOIs

This is mainly extrapolation from pethidine, but cases exist of hypotension and loss of consciousness with IV morphine, responsive to naloxone. Low dose morphine and other narcotics, eg. codeine, methadone and fentanyl are probably safe, as other studies show little interaction. If narcotics are used, it is best to start at a third or half the normal dose of opiate and titrate carefully, noting blood pressure and levels of consciousness.

NEFOPAM + MAOIs

The manufacturers recommend avoiding this combination.

Oxcarbazepine + MAOIs

See oxcarbazepine (*4.5.6*).

PAROXETINE + MAOIs

Nothing has been reported with paroxetine although there has been interactions reported with fluoxetine and fluvoxamine.

PETHIDINE + MAOIs

A well documented, rapid, severe and **potentially fatal** interaction which may not be well known among junior medical staff.

Phenobarbital + MAOIs

Barbiturate sedation may be prolonged so be aware, as one fatality has been reported.

Reboxetine + MAOIs

See reboxetine (*4.3.3.4*).

Salbutamol + MAOIs

No interaction occurs.

SERTRALINE + MAOIs

The manufacturers suggest a one week wash-out period after sertraline before an MAOI is used, so care is advised.

St. John's wort + MAOIs

See St. John's wort (*4.3.3.8*).

Sulphonamides + MAOIs

An isolated case of adverse effects with sulphafurazole and phenelzine exists.

SYMPATHOMIMETICS + MAOIs

Hypertension has been reported with many indirectly-acting sympathomimetic amines, eg. ephedrine, metaraminol, pseudoephedrine, phenylephrine and phenylpropanolamine. Phenylephrine is found in many over-the-counter cough and cold remedies and can cause a massive rise in blood pressure with MAOIs. Use in nasal sprays and drops is not recommended although there are no case reports.

Trazodone + MAOIs

There are many reported cases of serotonin syndrome (see p. 56) with SSRIs and MAOIs and so care is needed if this combination is used.

TRICYCLICS + MAOIs

The combination of tranylcypromine and clomipramine has caused death in four cases. Other MAOI/TCA combinations have been used with extreme care and with strict supervision by hospital specialists but should be avoided by others. Excitation, seizures, hyperpyrexia and serotonin syndrome have also been reported.

TRIPTANS + MAOIs

The UK SPC recommends triptans are not used with MAOIs.

Tryptophan + MAOIs

There are cases of behavioural and neurological toxicity with high doses of tryptophan. Potentiation of the therapeutic effect is well known. If used together it is best to monitor **very** carefully.

TYRAMINE + MAOIs

For advice on dietary tyramine see the next section.

VENLAFAXINE + MAOIs

The manufacturers state that venlafaxine and MAOIs should not be used together. They recommend a 14-day gap after stopping an MAOI before starting venlafaxine, and a 7-day gap after venlafaxine before an MAOI is used.

Warfarin + MAOIs

No interaction is known, although tranylcypromine is known to inhibit CYP2C19 and so some potential exists.

Xanthines + MAOIs

There is a single case report of possible hypertension with phenelzine and oxtriphylline, a theophylline derivative.

4.3.4.2 Treatments for MAOI hypertensive crisis

1. Phentolamine (Rogitine®) 2–10mg by slow IV infusion (adults), repeated if necessary.
2. If no phentolamine, chlorpromazine 50–100mg IM can be used, as can diazoxide (50–100mg by IV injection). Repeat after 10 minutes if necessary.
3. Alternately, bite open a 10mg capsule of nifedipine, swallow the contents with water and immediately go to a hospital casualty department. Nifedipine produces a consistent and prompt fall in arterial blood pressure but should be used with great care due to possible adverse effects.
4. Cool any fever with external cooling. Blood pressure should be monitored frequently and refer to A&E department.

4.3.4.3. Patient information

Warning signs of a reaction to an MAOI

If a patient experiences any of the following symptoms, especially if after eating, taking drugs of any type or if unexpected or severe, a reaction should be suspected and appropriate medical attention sought immediately:

- headache (especially at the back of the head)
- lightheadedness or dizziness
- flushing of the face
- pounding of the heart
- numbness or tingling of the hands or feet
- pain or stiffness in the neck
- photophobia
- chest pain
- nausea and vomiting.

Such symptoms usually occur about two hours after ingestion of the compound.

Foods to avoid with an MAOI
General principles:

Avoid foods which are matured, might be 'going off' or contain tyramine. Generally, the more 'convenience' the food, the safer it is, eg. packet soups are generally safe. Although many foods have only small amounts of tyramine, it is possible to have local concentrations which might give a reaction.

Tyramine-containing foods:

The dietary information on the RPSGB/BMA card is very brief and the following may be of use as general guidelines:

● **Dairy products:**
Avoid hard cheeses, soft cheeses and cheese spreads (eg. Philadelphia®) and foods containing cheese (eg. pizzas, pies, etc), which are a known cause of inadvertent ingestion and death. Cottage cheese and 'Dairylea®' cream cheese contain only minute amounts of tyramine and large quantities would be needed to produce a reaction.

● **Game, meat and fish:**
Pickled or salted dried herrings and any hung or badly stored game, poultry or other meat which might be 'going off' or spoiling must be avoided.

● **Meat products/Offal:**
Avoid chicken liver pâté, liver pâté and any other liver which is not fresh. Fresh chicken liver, fresh beef liver and fresh pâté, however, should be safe.

● **Fruit and vegetables:**
Broad bean pods (but not the beans) and banana skins (occasionally cooked as part of whole unripe bananas in a stew) must be avoided. Avocado pears have been reported to produce a reaction and should be avoided if possible.

● **Pizzas:**
Commercially available pizzas from large chain outlets seem safe, and even those with double orders of cheese appear safe. Gourmet pizzas from smaller outlets have higher tyramine contents, especially if mature cheeses are used.

● **Soy and Soybean:**
Some samples of Soy sauce and soy bean preparations may have very high tyramine levels. Either avoiding entirely or a 10ml maximum is recommended.
Soy sauce (Pearl River etc) — some have high quantities, ie. up to 3.4mg/15ml, and so double or triple helpings could be well above thresholds for a reaction.
Soybean curd (eg. Tofu) — some have high quantities, especially if kept refrigerated for 7 days or longer, ie. up to 5mg/300mg helping, and so double or triple helpings could be well above thresholds for reactions.

● **Yeast and meat extracts:**
Oxo®, Marmite®, Bovril® and other meat or yeast extracts must be avoided. Gravy made with Bisto® (ie. Original®, Powder®, Rich Gravy Granules®, Onion Gravy Granules® and Gravy Granules for Chicken®) is safe. Gravy made from juices of the roast or fresh meat should also be safe. Twiglets® are sprayed with 10% Marmite® and contain about 10mg of tyramine per 50g bag. This could be sufficient to cause a reaction and a 100g bag could be fatal.

Foods known to contain some tyramine where excessive consumption is not advisable, albeit unlikely:

Plums, spinach, Sauerkraut, matured pork.

Foods thought to contain only minute amounts of tyramine:

Aubergine, banana pulp (skins unsafe), chocolate (one anecdotal report of headache), Cottage cheese, cream or Dairylea® cheese, egg plant, octopus, raspberries, sausages, soy sauce, vinegar and yoghurt (commercial), Worcester sauce, Lee and Perrins etc.

Alcoholic drinks

Patient instructions usually state that all alcoholic and some non-alcoholic drinks must be avoided. Low or non-alcoholic beers may contain significant amounts of tyramine, shown by three reactions to less than 2/3 pint of alcohol-free and 'de-alcoholised' beer. There is a large variation in other beers, so use in moderation (ie. 1–2 bottles a day maximum), prefer canned beers from major brewers and take care with de-alcoholised beers. The maximum reported level in Chianti wine is 12 mg/l, likely to be dangerous only in overdose. The following may be of use where a particular patient wishes to drink:

1. Avoid	2. True moderation (eg. 1 unit)	3. Safest
Chianti	White wines	Gin
Home made beers and wines	Non-alcoholic beers and lagers	Vodka
Real ales		Other clear spirits
Red wines*		
*Red wines contain phenolic flavanoids which inhibit the enzymes which metabolise catecholamines, including tyramine.		

Over-the-counter medicines

Each patient should be warned about the possibility of interactions with over-the-counter medicines. The general advice for patients is:

1. Only buy medicines from a pharmacy. Do not use supermarkets, drug stores, newsagents etc, eg. Lemsip® contains phenylpropanolamine and is widely available. Do not take medicines given to you by friends or relatives. Do not take medicines taken before the MAOI was prescribed until advice has been sought.
2. Carry the MAOI card and show it to any doctor, dentist or pharmacist who may treat you.
3. Take special care over any medicines for coughs, colds, flu, hay fever, asthma and catarrh.

4.4 Lithium

ACE INHIBITORS + LITHIUM

Case reports of lithium toxicity with captopril and enalapril exist, with the elderly at greatest risk. Beta-blockers are preferable alternatives.

Alcohol + lithium

See alcohol (*4.7.1*).

Amfetamines + lithium

Lithium may suppress amfetamine 'highs'.

AMINOPHYLLINE + LITHIUM

See theophylline + lithium.

Amiodarone + lithium

The *BNF* notes an increased risk of hypothyroidism with the combination.

Antacids + lithium

See sodium + lithium.

Antidepressants + lithium

Generally considered a beneficial combination. Both can lower the seizure threshold which may be important.

ANTIPSYCHOTICS + LITHIUM

This is generally considered a useful combination but a few cases of mostly reversible neurotoxicity have been reported, particularly with **haloperidol**. **Chlorpromazine** levels may be lowered by up to 40% by lithium, a potentially important effect. Enhanced EPSEs and rarely neurotoxicity have been reported with lithium plus flupentixol, fluphenazine or thioridazine. With **clozapine** there is an increased risk of developing neuroleptic malignant syndrome and cases of diabetic ketoacidosis have been reported (monitor glucose carefully). Some cases of neurotoxicity and Neuroleptic Malignant Syndrome have been reported with **risperidone**. There appears no problem with **olanzapine**. Slightly increased lithium levels may occur with **quetiapine**. The QT prolongation potential with **sertindole** makes this combination a contraindication.

Baclofen + lithium

Two cases of aggravation of movement disorder in Huntington's disease exist.

Beta-blockers + lithium

A single case of bradycardia with propranolol and lithium has been reported, although propranolol has been used to treat lithium-induced tremor.

Benzodiazepines + lithium

There have been several anecdotal reports of reactions, eg. hypothermia, but extensive use of this usually beneficial combination suggests it to be safe.

BUMETANIDE + LITHIUM

Although studies have shown a minimal effect, bumetanide may occasionally cause lithium toxicity.

Calcium-channel blockers + lithium

Cases of enhanced effect and toxicity with unchanged lithium plasma levels have been reported with verapamil, as have reduced lithium levels. Acute parkinsonian side-effects and bradycardia have been reported with diltiazem.

Candesartan + lithium

Severe lithium toxicity has been reported with the combination.

Cannabis + lithium

See cannabis (*4.7.2*).

Carbamazepine + lithium

See carbamazepine (*4.5.1*).

Cisplatin + lithium

Reports exists of lithium levels reduced by 65%.

Citalopram + lithium

Lack of interaction has been reported.

Clonidine + lithium

Lithium may reduce the hypotensive effect of clonidine so monitor carefully.

Cocaine + lithium

See cocaine (*4.7.3*).

Corticosteroids + lithium

An isolated case exists of lithium reducing the effect of corticosteroids on the kidneys.

Co-trimoxazole + lithium

Two cases of enhanced toxicity with reduced lithium levels exist.

Digoxin + lithium

Lack of interaction has been shown.

Dipyridamole + lithium

Lack of interaction has been shown.

Disulfiram + lithium

See disulfiram (*4.6.6*).

Domperidone + lithium

An enhanced risk of EPSEs exists.

Escitalopram + lithium

Lack of interaction has been reported.

Fluoxetine + lithium

Lack of significant pharmacokinetic interaction has been shown, but there are rare cases of serotonin syndrome, absence seizures and acute confusion or lithium toxicity.

Fluvoxamine + lithium

See fluvoxamine (*4.3.2.3*).

FUROSEMIDE + LITHIUM

Although studies have shown a minimal interaction and furosemide to be the safest diuretic with lithium, isolated cases of toxicity have been reported so some vigilance is needed.

Gabapentin + lithium

Although both are exclusively eliminated by renal excretion, lack of interaction has been shown.

Herbal diuretics + lithium

A case of severe lithium toxicity has been reported.

Hypoglycaemics + lithium

Lithium has been used to improve glucose metabolism and assist the effects of oral hypoglycaemics and insulin.

Iodides + lithium

Enhanced antithyroid and goitre effects of lithium have been reported.

Ispaghula husk (eg. Fybogel®) + lithium

A single case exists of reduced lithium levels.

Lamotrigine + lithium

Lack of interaction has been shown.

Levodopa + lithium

Reversible Creutzfeldt-Jakob-like syndrome has been reported.

Levofloxacin + lithium

A case of rapidly developing lithium toxicity has been reported.

Losartan + lithium

A case has been reported of marked lithium toxicity five weeks after losartan 50 mg/d was added to stable therapy.

MAOIs + lithium

See MAOIs (*4.3.4*).

METOCLOPRAMIDE + LITHIUM

An enhanced risk of EPSEs and of neurotoxicity exists.

Metronidazole + lithium

Cases of toxic lithium levels induced by metronidazole exist.

Mirtazapine + lithium

See mirtazapine (*4.3.3.2*).

Neuromuscular blocking agents + lithium

Omitting the last dose or two of lithium before the use of an NMBA is recommended.

NSAIDS + LITHIUM

This is an important interaction (particularly now many NSAIDs are available over-the-counter) where lithium levels may rise, either slowly or quickly. Lithium levels should be monitored frequently (eg. monthly) if this combination is to be used. The general advice is:
- avoid: indometacin (good idea anyway)
- extra care: (eg. monthly lithium levels) with: **ibuprofen** (including over-the-counter and GSL purchases), **piroxicam** and **diclofenac**
- care with: **celecoxib, ketoprofen, ketorolac, mefenamic acid, meloxicam, naproxen, rofecoxib** and **tiaprofenic acid**
- drugs of choice: **sulindac** and **aspirin**.

Oxcarbazepine + lithium

See oxcarbazepine (*4.5.6*).

Phenytoin + lithium

Three cases of lithium neurotoxicity occurred without increased lithium levels but with care both drugs can be used together safely.

Potassium iodide + lithium

An additive effect may cause hypothyroidism.

SERTINDOLE + LITHIUM

See antipsychotics + lithium (*4.2.1*).

Smoking + lithium

See smoking (*4.7.4*).

Sodium + lithium

Excess sodium (eg. as bicarbonate in antacids) can reduce lithium levels and sodium restriction can lead to lithium intoxication so care with people on low-sodium diets.

Spironolactone + lithium

A rise in lithium levels has been reported, as indeed has synergism.

SSRIs + lithium

There are two cases of acute confusion or lithium toxicity caused by fluoxetine. Fluvoxamine might do similarly but no interaction has been seen with citalopram, escitalopram, paroxetine or sertraline.

Tetracyclines + lithium

Cases of lithium intoxication so monitor lithium regularly.

THEOPHYLLINE + LITHIUM

Theophylline and aminophylline may reduce lithium levels by 20–30%. An increased lithium dose can counteract this so monitoring of levels is essential, but care is needed if the theophylline is then stopped (or even missed). The interaction has even been made use of to treat lithium toxicity.

THIAZIDE DIURETICS + LITHIUM

This is a well-documented interaction where thiazides reduce the renal clearance of lithium and lithium levels rise within a few days, with potentially serious consequences. Thiazides should only be used where unavoidable and strict monitoring is used. The interaction has been shown with chlorthiazide, bendrofluazide, co-amilozide, hydroflumethiazide and triamterene. **Furosemide** (used with care) is a suitable alternative.

Topiramate + lithium

Elevated lithium levels have been reported with high-dose (800mg/d) but not low-dose lithium.

Tricyclics + lithium

See tricyclics (*4.3.1*).

Trimethoprim + lithium

Lithium toxicity has been reported with trimethoprim.

Triptans + lithium

The *BNF* notes an increased risk of CNS toxicity with sumatriptan.

Venlafaxine + lithium

See venlafaxine (*4.3.3.7*).

Warfarin + lithium

Lack of interaction has been reported.

4.5 Anticonvulsants

Anticonvulsants-anticonvulsants interactions

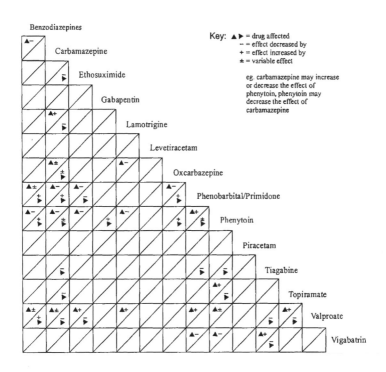

Key: ▲ ▶ = drug affected
− = effect decreased by
+ = effect increased by
± = variable effect

eg. carbamazepine may increase
or decrease the effect of
phenytoin, phenytoin may
decrease the effect of
carbamazepine

4.5.1 Carbamazepine (Tegretol®)

Carbamazepine is extensively plasma protein bound and induces its own and other drugs metabolism via CYP3A4. Auto-induction takes 1–4 weeks to occur although is virtually complete after a week.

Alcohol + carbamazepine

See alcohol (*4.7.1*).

ANTIPSYCHOTICS + CARBAMAZEPINE

Carbamazepine induces the metabolism of many antipsychotics, possibly reducing their effectiveness eg. with **haloperidol** (resulting in worsening psychiatric symptoms and possible lengthening of the QT interval), **risperidone, olanzapine** and **zotepine**. Lower levels of **quetiapine** and **aripiprazole** would be expected due to enzyme induction by carbamazepine so increased doses may be needed. Plasma carbamazepine metabolite levels may rise with **loxapine**, resulting in neurotoxicity, even with normal carbamazepine levels. Carbamazepine should **not** be used with **clozapine** (mandatory precaution in the UK SPC) as it increases the chances of drug-induced neutropenia. Antipsychotics also lower the seizure threshold, antagonising the anticonvulsant effects.

Benzodiazepines + carbamazepine

Slightly higher benzodiazepine doses may be needed, and raised carbamazepine levels (with toxicity) have been reported with clobazam.

Bupropion + carbamazepine

See bupropion (*4.6.4*).

Caffeine + carbamazepine

Carbamazepine induces the metabolism of caffeine via CYP1A2, so intake needs to be higher to achieve the desired effect.

CALCIUM-CHANNEL BLOCKERS + CARBAMAZEPINE

Carbamazepine levels may rise by 40–50% with diltiazem, isradipine and verapamil and there is a substantial risk of toxicity. Nifedipine is a safer alternative.

Charcoal, activated + carbamazepine

Carbamazepine absorption is almost completely stopped when activated charcoal is given 5 minutes after ingestion.

Chinese medicines + carbamazepine

Paeoniae Radix (a traditional Chinese medicine) may increase carbamazepine absorption.

CICLOSPORIN+CARBAMAZEPINE

Ciclosporin metabolism is accelerated by carbamazepine, to give reduced plasma levels.

Citalopram + carbamazepine

See citalopram (*4.3.2.1*).

Cocaine + carbamazepine

See cocaine (*4.7.3*).

CORTICOSTEROIDS + CARBAMAZEPINE

Corticosteroid CYP3A4 metabolism is accelerated by carbamazepine, giving a reduced effect.

Clarithromycin + carbamazepine

See erythromycin + carbamazepine.

DANAZOL + CARBAMAZEPINE

Danazol inhibits carbamazepine metabolism to give an increased effect. Monitor carbamazepine levels and look for side-effects.

DEXTROPROPOXYPHENE + CARBAMAZEPINE

Dextropropoxyphene (eg. in co-proxamol) enhances carbamazepine toxicity via enzyme inhibition and levels may rise 4-fold over 24 hours and lead to cerebellar dysfunction. Monitor carbamazepine closely if used together.

Disulfiram + carbamazepine

See disulfiram (*4.6.6*).

Diuretics + carbamazepine

Hyponatraemia may rarely occur with furosemide or hydrochlorothiazide.

DOXYCYCLINE + CARBAMAZEPINE

Doxycycline metabolism is accelerated by carbamazepine to give a much reduced effect. Other tetracyclines appear not to interact.

Enteral feeds + carbamazepine

Carbamazepine absorption is reduced so monitor levels carefully.

Escitalopram + carbamazepine

See citalopram (*4.3.2.1*).

Ethosuximide + carbamazepine

See ethosuximide (*4.5.2*).

Etretinate + carbamazepine

There is one case of a girl treated with etretinate and carbamazepine 200mg/d who only responded when carbamazepine was withdrawn.

ERYTHROMYCIN + CARBAMAZEPINE

A 100–200% rise in carbamazepine levels may occur and so the combination should only be used with great care. Monitor levels or use an alternative antibiotic. A single case exists of carbamazepine toxicity appearing within 3–4 hours of a 500mg dose of clarithromycin.

Fluconazole + carbamazepine

Fluconazole-induced carbamazepine toxicity has been reported several times.

Fluoxetine + carbamazepine

See fluoxetine (*4.3.2.2*).

Fluvoxamine + carbamazepine

See fluvoxamine (*4.3.2.3*).

Gabapentin + carbamazepine

No significant interaction occurs.

Grapefruit juice + carbamazepine

300ml grapefruit juice increased peak carbamazepine levels by 40% and trough levels by 39%, probably by CYP3A4 inhibition in the gut wall and liver.

Griseofulvin + carbamazepine

Reduced grisefulvin levels and effect have been suggested.

H2-BLOCKERS + CARBAMAZEPINE

Studies have shown a transient rise in carbamazepine levels with cimetidine. Monitor regularly or use ranitidine, antacids or sucralfate.

Influenza vaccine + carbamazepine

One study showed a transient 10% increase in carbamazepine levels.

ISONIAZID + CARBAMAZEPINE

Rapid carbamazepine toxicity may occur via enzyme inhibition by isoniazid, in this potentially serious interaction. Monitor carefully and assess for toxicity.

Isotretinoin + carbamazepine

A single case of reduced carbamazepine plasma levels exists.

Itraconazole + carbamazepine

Sub-therapeutic itraconazole levels may occur with carbamazepine so monitor for lack of efficacy.

Lamotrigine + carbamazepine

See lamotrigine (*4.5.4*).

Levetiracetam + carbamazepine

See levetiracetam (*4.5.5*).

Levothyroxine/thyroxine + carbamazepine

Levothyroxine metabolism is accelerated by carbamazepine and may increase the requirements in hypothyroidism.

Lithium + carbamazepine

This combination is often used for rapid-cycling bipolar mood disorder but neurotoxicity or lithium toxicity may occur without increased plasma levels. Risk factors include a history of lithium neurotoxicity or concurrent medical or neurological illness. Monitor carefully and regularly for signs of toxicity.

MAOIs + carbamazepine

See MAOIs (*4.3.4*).

Mefloquine + carbamazepine

Mefloquine may antagonise the anticonvulsant effect of carbamazepine.

Methadone + carbamazepine

See methadone (*4.6.8*).

Methylphenidate + carbamazepine

See methylphenidate (*4.6.9*).

Metoclopramide + carbamazepine

There is a single case of carbamazepine neurotoxicity occurring three days after metoclopramide 30mg/d was added.

Metronidazole + carbamazepine

There is a single case of toxic carbamazepine levels occurring when metronidazole was added.

Mianserin + carbamazepine

See mianserin (*4.3.3.1*).

Miconazole + carbamazepine

An isolated case report of an adverse response has appeared.

Mirtazapine + carbamazepine

See mirtazapine (*4.3.3.2*).

Nicoumalone + carbamazepine

The metabolism of nicoumalone is accelerated by carbamazepine to give a reduced effect.

ORAL CONTRACEPTIVE + CARBAMAZEPINE

The metabolism of OCs is accelerated by carbamazepine to give a reduced contraceptive effect. With Eugynon 50 no longer available in the UK, adequate contraception can be obtained from using a combination of Marvelon and Mercilon together, or two tablets of Ovranette. This is an interaction often overlooked, with disastrous consequences.

Orlistat + carbamazepine

Lack of interaction has been shown.

Oxcarbazepine + carbamazepine

See oxcarbazepine (*4.5.6*).

Paracetamol + carbamazepine

Paracetamol bioavailability may be reduced.

Paroxetine + carbamazepine

No significant interaction occurs.

Phenobarbital + carbamazepine

Phenobarbital induces carbamazepine metabolism, slightly reducing plasma levels. Carbamazepine may raise phenobarbital levels but not to a clinically significant amount.

PHENYTOIN + CARBAMAZEPINE

Phenytoin induces carbamazepine metabolism, reducing levels, often dramatically. Monitoring of levels is useful, although seizure control may not be affected. If stopping phenytoin, carbamazepine levels must be monitored during the de-induction stage to prevent toxicity developing. Additionally, carbamazepine may increase phenytoin levels by up to 100%, producing neurotoxicity. The clinical effect may be limited but it is certainly best to monitor the levels of both drugs.

Progabide + carbamazepine

Lack of interaction has been shown.

Protease inhibitors + carbamazepine

The *BNF* notes the possibility of reduced plasma indinavir and saquinavir levels with the combination, and raised carbamazepine levels with ritonavir.

PROTON-PUMP INHIBITORS + CARBAMAZEPINE

Carbamazepine induces the CYP3A4 metabolism of omeprazole, and multiple dose omeprazole may decrease carbamazepine clearance by 40% and thus increase levels. Pantoprazole appears to have no effect on carbamazepine levels.

Rifampicin + carbamazepine

Rapid CYP3A4 induction may lower carbamazepine levels.

Sertindole + carbamazepine

See sertindole (*4.2.7*).

Sertraline + carbamazepine

See sertraline (*4.3.2.5*).

Smoking + carbamazepine

See smoking (*4.7.4*).

St. John's wort + carbamazepine

See anticonvulsants + St John's wort (*4.3.3.8*).

Theophylline + carbamazepine

Theophylline metabolism may be accelerated by carbamazepine to give a reduced effect.

Tiagabine + carbamazepine

See tiagabine (*4.5.10*).

Tibolone + carbamazepine

The UK SPC notes that carbamazepine may reduce the activity of tibolone.

Topiramate + carbamazepine

See topiramate (*4.5.11*).

Tramadol + carbamazepine

The UK SPC notes that carbamazepine may reduce the activity of tramadol.

Trazodone + carbamazepine

Raised carbamazepine levels have been reported with trazodone.

TRICYCLICS + CARBAMAZEPINE

Studies have shown the metabolism of imipramine, doxepin and amitriptyline to be accelerated by carbamazepine to give plasma levels reduced by 42–50%. This is a common combination and other evidence supports this to be a clinically significant interaction.

VALPROATE + CARBAMAZEPINE

Carbamazepine levels may fall by about 25% if valproate is added, a well documented interaction. This is probably a relatively minor effect but a mean 59% increase in valproate levels on carbamazepine withdrawal can occur. Valproate may also inhibit carbamazepine metabolism which has led to carbamazepine metabolite-induced psychosis, and so a close watch must be kept for carbamazepine toxicity.

Venlafaxine + carbamazepine

See venlafaxine (*4.3.3.8*).

Vigabatrin + carbamazepine

See vigabatrin (*4.5.13*).

Vincristine + carbamazepine

Carbamazepine significantly increases the clearance of vincristine.

WARFARIN + CARBAMAZEPINE

Carbamazepine accelerates the metabolism of warfarin, reducing its effect. Warfarin doses may need to be increased by up to 100% and then reduced if carbamazepine is discontinued.

ZALEPLON + CARBAMAZEPINE

See zaleplon (*4.1.4*).

4.5.2 Ethosuximide (Zarontin®)

Carbamazepine + ethosuximide

Ethosuximide levels may fall by about 17%, although this is probably of minor significance.

Phenobarbital + ethosuximide

See phenobarbital (*4.5.7*).

PHENYTOIN + ETHOSUXIMIDE

A large study showed that phenytoin significantly reduces ethosuximide plasma levels.

Valproate + ethosuximide

Valproate increases ethosuximide plasma levels by up to 50%, although this may only be a transient effect and so the usual regular monitoring will probably suffice.

Zotepine + ethosuximide

See anticonvulsants + zotepine (*4.2.8*).

4.5.3 Gabapentin (Neurontin®)

Antacids + gabapentin

No significant interaction is thought to occur.

Benzodiazepines + gabapentin

No significant interaction occurs.

Carbamazepine + gabapentin

No significant interaction occurs.

Cimetidine + gabapentin

No significant interaction occurs.

Levetiracetam + gabapentin

See levetiracetam (*4.5.5*).

Lithium + gabapentin

See lithium (*4.4*).

Oral contraceptives + gabapentin

No change in the kinetics of norethindrone and ethinyloestradiol (as in Norlestrin 2.5/

50) were seen with gabapentin in one study.

Phenobarbital + gabapentin

No significant interaction occurs.

Phenytoin + gabapentin

No significant interaction was seen in one study but a trend towards an increase in phenytoin levels was observed elsewhere and there is a single reported case of phenytoin toxicity with gabapentin.

Valproate + gabapentin

No significant interaction occurs.

Zotepine + gabapentin

See anticonvulsants + zotepine (*4.2.8*).

4.5.4 Lamotrigine (Lamictal®)

Benzodiazepines + lamotrigine

No significant interaction occurs.

Bupropion + lamotrigine

A small study showed no significant interaction occurs.

Carbamazepine + lamotrigine

Lamotrigine has no effect *on* carbamazepine but carbamazepine reduces the half-life of lamotrigine from 29 hrs to about 15 hrs via enzyme induction so increased doses may be needed. Increased CNS side-effects have been reported, especially if lamotrigine is added to a higher dose of carbamazepine.

Clozapine + lamotrigine

See clozapine (*4.2.3*).

Fosphenytoin + lamotrigine

See phenytoin + lamotrigine.

Levetiracetam + lamotrigine

See levetiracetam (*4.5.5*).

Lithium + lamotrigine

See lithium (*4.4*).

Oral contraceptives + lamotrigine

No loss of contraceptive effect occurs but a 45% reduction in lamotrigine levels has been reported.

Oxcarbazepine + lamotrigine

See oxcarbazepine (*4.5.6*).

Phenobarbital + lamotrigine

No significant interaction occurs.

Phenytoin + lamotrigine

Lamotrigine has no effect on phenytoin but phenytoin reduces the half-life of lamotrigine from 29 hrs to about 15 hrs via enzyme induction so increased doses may be needed.

Sertraline + lamotrigine

Sertraline may double lamotrigine levels, with two cases reported.

Topiramate + lamotrigine

Lack of interaction has been shown.

VALPROATE + LAMOTRIGINE

Lamotrigine has no significant effect on valproate, but valproate inhibits lamotrigine metabolism and doubles it's half-life to about 59 hrs. Doses of lamotrigine should thus start at *half* the usual dose when used with valproate. The interaction has been used to enhance the effect of both drugs with striking responses in adults and children with intractable epilepsy. Disabling postural and action tremor in 3 patients on both has been reported, as has an increased incidence of rash.

Zotepine + lamotrigine

See anticonvulsants + zotepine (*4.2.8*).

4.5.5 Levetiracetam (Keppra®)

Levetiracetam has, as yet, no demonstrable drug interactions. It is not bound to plasma proteins, is not extensively metabolised and does not inhibit nor induce P450 and UGT enzymes.

Alcohol + levetiracetam

No data is available (MI).

Carbamazepine + levetiracetam

Lack of pharmacokinetic interaction has been shown, although some cases of carbamazepine toxicity (with unchanged levels) have been reported.

Digoxin + levetiracetam

Lack of interaction has been shown.

Food + levetiracetam

Levetiracetam absorption is slightly slowed by food, but total absorption remains unchanged.

Gabapentin + levetiracetam

Lack of interaction has been shown.

Lamotrigine + levetiracetam

Lack of interaction has been shown.

Oral contraceptives + levetiracetam

Lack of interaction has been shown.

Phenobarbital + levetiracetam

Lack of interaction has been shown.

Phenytoin + levetiracetam

Lack of interaction has been shown.

Probenecid + levetiracetam

Lack of significant interaction has been shown.

Valproate + levetiracetam

Lack of interaction has been shown.

Warfarin + levetiracetam

Lack of interaction has been shown.

Zotepine + levetiracetam

See anticonvulsants + zotepine (*4.2.8*).

4.5.6 Oxcarbazepine (Trileptal®)

Oxcarbazepine does not appear to have a significant effect on liver enzymes at lower doses, but some enzyme induction has been suggested at higher doses.

Alcohol + oxcarbazepine

Additive sedation can occur.

Antipsychotics + oxcarbazepine

Since carbamazepine reduces the plasma levels of many antipsychotics, substitution with oxcarbazepine may lead to plasma levels of some antipsychotics increasing by 50–200% over 2–4 weeks.

Carbamazepine + oxcarbazepine

Lack of significant interaction has been shown.

Ciclosporin + oxcarbazepine

Slightly reduced ciclosporin levels have been reported.

Cimetidine + oxcarbazepine

Lack of interaction has been shown.

Citalopram + oxcarbazepine

Carbamazepine may induce the plasma levels of citalopram, and when oxcarbazepine is substituted, citalopram plasma levels may rise.

Erythromycin + oxcarbazepine

Lack of significant interaction has been shown.

Escitalopram + oxcarbazepine

See citalopram above.

Felodipine + oxcarbazepine

Repeated doses of oxcarbazepine might slightly reduce the clinical effect of felodipine.

Fosphenytoin + oxcarbazepine

See phenytoin + oxcarbazepine.

Lamotrigine + oxcarbazepine

Oxcarbazepine induces the metabolism of lamotrigine, and so plasma levels fall by 29%. Reduced doses may be necessary if oxcarbazepine is discontinued.

Lithium + oxcarbazepine

The combination of lithium and oxcarbazepine might theoretically cause enhanced neurotoxicity (UK SPC).

MAOIs + oxcarbazepine

A theoretical risk of interaction exists (UK SPC).

ORAL CONTRACEPTIVES + OXCARBAZEPINE

Oxcarbazepine can produce significant reductions in some OC plasma levels, with some breakthrough bleeding. Increased doses of ethinylestradiol and levonorgestrel or additional non-hormonal contraception are recommended with oxcarbazepine. With Eugynon 50 no longer available, adequate contraception can be obtained from using a combination of Marvelon and Mercilon together, or two tablets of Ovranette, or Depot Provera given every 10 weeks rather than 12 weeks.

Phenobarbital + oxcarbazepine

Slightly increased phenobarbital levels and reduced oxcarbazepine levels have been reported.

Phenytoin + oxcarbazepine

Doses of oxcarbazepine above 1200mg/d have been reported to increase phenytoin levels by up to 40% (less than 10% for doses below 1200mg/d) and so close monitoring of phenytoin is essential, especially at higher doses.

Propoxyphene + oxcarbazepine

Lack of significant interaction has been shown.

St. John's wort + oxcarbazepine

See anticonvulsants + SJW (*4.3.3.8*).

Valproate + oxcarbazepine

Valproate levels may rise if oxcarbazepine is substituted for carbamazepine.

Verapamil + oxcarbazepine

Verapamil can produce a 20% reduction in oxcarbazepine's metabolite levels, which could be clinically significant (US SPC).

Warfarin + oxcarbazepine

Lack of significant interaction has been shown.

Zotepine + oxcarbazepine

See anticonvulsants + zotepine (*4.2.8*).

4.5.7 Phenobarbital (phenobarbitone)

Alcohol + phenobarbital

See alcohol (*4.7.1*).

ANTICOAGULANTS + PHENOBARBITAL

A well-documented and clinically significant reduction in anticoagulant levels and effects with barbiturates occurs. Doses of the anticoagulant may need to be raised by up to 60% if a barbiturate is started or lowered if stopped.

ANTIPSYCHOTICS + PHENOBARBITAL

See antipsychotics (*4.2.1*).

Benzodiazepines + phenobarbital

See benzodiazepines (*4.1.1*).

Beta-blockers + phenobarbital

Blood levels of metoprolol and propranolol (but not timolol, atenolol and nadolol) are reduced by barbiturates.

Bupropion + phenobarbital

See bupropion (*4.6.4*).

CALCIUM-CHANNEL BLOCKERS + PHENOBARBITAL

Phenobarbital may induce the CYP3A4 metabolism of verapamil, diltiazem, isradipine, nicardipine and nifedipine, reducing efficacy and so some care may be needed.

Carbamazepine + phenobarbital

See carbamazepine (*4.5.1*).

Charcoal, activated + phenobarbital

If given within 5 minutes, charcoal can almost completely prevent barbiturate absorption and can be an effective adjunct in overdose treatment.

Chloramphenicol + phenobarbital

Chloramphenicol metabolism is accelerated by barbiturates to give a reduced oral chloramphenicol effect.

Ciclosporin + phenobarbital

Even low dose phenobarbital induces the metabolism of ciclosporin.

Cimetidine + phenobarbital

Reduced actions of both can occur but is of limited clinical significance.

Clozapine + phenobarbital

See clozapine (*4.2.3*).

Corticosteroids + phenobarbital

Enzyme induction reduces the effect of some corticosteroids.

Digoxin + phenobarbital

Lack of interaction has been shown.

Disopyramide + phenobarbital

Reduced disopyramide plasma levels can occur with barbiturates.

Doxorubicin + phenobarbital

Doxorubicin clearance may be increased by barbiturates and so doses may need to be increased.

Doxycycline + phenobarbital

Doxycycline metabolism is accelerated by barbiturates, reducing it's effect, with a halved half-life. Other tetracyclines appear not to interact.

Ethosuximide + phenobarbital

A large study showed that ethosuximide levels may fall if primidone is added. Reduced phenobarbital effectiveness may also occur.

Fenoprofen + phenobarbital

Phenobarbital may slightly increase fenoprofen elimination and reduce it's efficacy.

Furosemide + phenobarbital

One study showed no significant interaction.

Gabapentin + phenobarbital

See gabapentin (*4.5.3*).

Glyceryl trinitrate + phenobarbital

A reduced nitrate effect via enzyme induction may occur.

Griseofulvin + phenobarbital

Cases of griseofulvin levels reduced by up to 45% by phenobarbital have been reported.

Indinavir + phenobarbital

Plasma levels of indinavir may be reduced by barbiturates via CYP3A4 induction.

Influenza vaccine + phenobarbital

A transient 20% rise in barbiturate levels occurred in one study.

Ketoconazole + phenobarbital

A single case of reduced ketoconazole levels with phenobarbital exists.

Lamotrigine + phenobarbital

No significant interaction occurs.

Levetiracetam + phenobarbital

See levetiracetam (*4.5.5*).

Levonorgestrel + phenobarbital

There is a case of levonorgestrel implant (Norplant) failing twice in a woman also taking phenobarbital.

Levothyroxine/thyroxine + phenobarbital

Levothyroxine metabolism is accelerated by barbiturates to give a reduced effect and this may increase requirements in hypothyroidism.

Lidocaine + phenobarbital

Serum lidocaine levels may be reduced by barbiturates.

MAOIs + phenobarbital

See MAOIs (*4.3.4*).

Methadone + phenobarbital

See methadone (*4.6.8*).

Metronidazole + phenobarbital

Metronidazole metabolism is accelerated by barbiturates, giving levels reduced by a third.

NICOUMALONE + PHENOBARBITAL

Nicoumalone metabolism is accelerated by barbiturates, giving a reduced anti-coagulant effect.

ORAL CONTRACEPTIVES + PHENOBARBITAL

Contraceptive failure via enzyme induction has been reported many times. With

Eugynon 50 no longer available, adequate contraception can be obtained from using a combination of Marvelon and Mercilon together, or two tablets of Ovranette, or Depot Provera given every 10 weeks rather than 12 weeks.

Oxcarbazepine + phenobarbital

See oxcarbazepine (*4.5.6*).

Paracetamol + phenobarbital

An isolated case of enhanced hepatotoxicity exists.

Paroxetine + phenobarbital

See paroxetine (*4.3.2.4*).

Pethidine + phenobarbital

A single case of severe CNS sedation on the combination has been reported.

Phenylbutazone + phenobarbital

Reduced levels of phenylbutazone may occur.

Phenytoin + phenobarbital

See phenytoin (*4.5.8*).

Pyridoxine + phenobarbital

High dose pyridoxine (eg. 200mg/d) can reduce phenobarbital levels by up to 40–50%, as well as being a danger in itself.

Quetiapine + phenobarbital

See quetiapine (*4.2.5*).

Quinidine + phenobarbital

Enzyme induction may reduce quinidine levels by up to 50%.

Rifampicin + phenobarbital

Rifampicin has been shown to induce barbiturate metabolism and so a decreased efficacy might be predicted.

Smoking + phenobarbital

See smoking (*4.7.4*).

St. John's wort + phenobarbital

See anticonvulsants + St John's wort (*4.3.3.8*).

Sulphonamides + phenobarbital

No reports of interaction exist.

Testosterone + phenobarbital

A reduced steroid effect via enzyme induction can occur.

THEOPHYLLINE + PHENOBARBITAL

Theophylline metabolism is accelerated by barbiturates, giving a reduced effect.

Tiagabine + phenobarbital

See tiagabine (*4.5.10*).

Topiramate + phenobarbital

See topiramate (*4.5.11*).

TRICYCLICS + PHENOBARBITAL

See tricyclics (*4.3.1*).

Tropisetron + phenobarbital

Phenobarbital reduces the plasma levels of tropisetron (*BNF*).

Valproate + phenobarbital

Valproate may increase phenobarbital plasma concentrations by up to 25%, increasing sedation and other side-effects. This may only be transient but dose reduction by a third or a half may be possible without loss of seizure control.

Vigabatrin + phenobarbital

See vigabatrin (*4.5.13*).

WARFARIN + PHENOBARBITAL

See anticoagulants + barbiturates.

Zaleplon + phenobarbital

See zaleplon (*4.1.6*).

Zotepine + phenobarbital

See anticonvulsants + zotepine (*4.2.8*).

4.5.8 Phenytoin

Phenytoin is a potent hepatic enzyme inducer and extensively bound to plasma proteins. It can be displaced, giving an increased proportion of free active phenytoin, significant where plasma level monitoring just measures **total** phenytoin rather than the proportion of free (hence active) phenytoin.

Acetazolamide + phenytoin

Acetazolamide may enhance the osteomalacia secondary to anticonvulsant use in a few patients.

ALCOHOL + PHENYTOIN

See alcohol (*4.7.1*).

Allopurinol + phenytoin

There is an isolated case report of phenytoin intoxication.

AMIODARONE + PHENYTOIN

Two studies show raised phenytoin levels so reduce the phenytoin dose by at least 25% and monitor carefully.

Antacids + phenytoin

Antacids may reduce phenytoin levels and seizure control could be impaired. Best to separate doses by about three hours or use ranitidine.

ANTIPSYCHOTICS + PHENYTOIN

Antipsychotics/neuroleptics lower the seizure threshold and may antagonise the anticonvulsant effect. A single case exists of reduced phenytoin levels with **loxapine**. Serum concentrations of **clozapine** may be markedly reduced by phenytoin and a large study suggested that phenytoin may reduce **haloperidol** levels by 40–75%. **Chlorpromazine** may increase phenytoin levels by up to 50%. Overall this is a variable effect so observe for toxicity or lack of efficacy. Severe EPSEs have been reported with **risperidone**. **Zotepine** may increase phenytoin plasma levels, so more frequent monitoring is required.

Benzodiazepines + phenytoin

Diazepam, clonazepam and chlordiazepoxide have been reported in some (but not all) studies to potentiate phenytoin, leading to toxicity. Monitor plasma levels regularly. Conversely, phenytoin may reduce clonazepam levels by up to 50%.

Bupropion + phenytoin

See bupropion (*4.6.4*).

Buspirone + phenytoin

See buspirone (*4.1.2*).

CALCIUM-CHANNEL BLOCKERS + PHENYTOIN

The effects of isradipine and nicardipine can be reduced. This may not occur with nifedipine as lack of interaction has been noted although one case exists of tremor, headache and restlessness three weeks after nifedipine was added to phenytoin. Phenytoin levels were tripled and fell to normal after the nifedipine was discontinued. Cases of inhibition of phenytoin metabolism and complete lack of verapamil absorption exist.

CARBAMAZEPINE + PHENYTOIN

See carbamazepine (*4.5.1*).

Charcoal, activated + phenytoin

Phenytoin absorption is almost completely (98%) prevented if activated charcoal is taken within 5 minutes.

Chinese medicines + phenytoin

Phenytoin toxicity has been reported after using Chinese proprietary medicines.

Chloral + phenytoin

Chloral might theoretically reduce phenytoin levels.

CHLORAMPHENICOL + PHENYTOIN

Phenytoin toxicity may occur with oral chloramphenicol. This is an uncommon combination but a well documented and serious interaction. Monitor very carefully if the combination has to be used.

Chlorphenamine + phenytoin

Two isolated cases exist of phenytoin intoxication and so care may be needed.

CICLOSPORIN + PHENYTOIN

Ciclosporin levels can be reduced by 80% by phenytoin.

CIPROFLOXACIN + PHENYTOIN

Phenytoin toxicity would be expected to occur via enzyme inhibition. Best to monitor very carefully, with more frequent phenytoin levels.

CLOZAPINE + PHENYTOIN

See clozapine (*4.2.3*).

CORTICOSTEROIDS + PHENYTOIN

Steroid metabolism is accelerated by phenytoin, reducing its effect and so higher doses may be needed. Hydrocortisone may be less affected than other steroids. Phenytoin levels may also alter.

Co-trimoxazole + phenytoin

There is a single case of increased phenytoin levels and toxicity, plus an enhanced antifolate effect.

Cytotoxics + phenytoin

There is a single case of reduced phenytoin levels.

DEXAMETHASONE + PHENYTOIN

Phenytoin levels may be halved by dexamethasone and (very) high doses of phenytoin may thus be needed, with regular and frequent monitoring.

Dextropropoxyphene + phenytoin

See propoxyphene.

DIAZOXIDE + PHENYTOIN

Reduced phenytoin levels may occur so monitor carefully.

DICOUMAROL + PHENYTOIN

Phenytoin levels may rise rapidly by over 100% so avoid the combination if at all possible by using warfarin or monitor very carefully.

Digoxin + phenytoin

Phenytoin reduces digoxin half-life by 30%, so monitor levels of both.

DISOPYRAMIDE + PHENYTOIN

Phenytoin may reduce the plasma levels of disopyramide to sub-therapeutic levels.

DISULFIRAM + PHENYTOIN

Phenytoin toxicity may occur via enzyme inhibition.

DOXYCYCLINE + PHENYTOIN

Doxycycline metabolism is accelerated by phenytoin to give a reduced effect, with a halved half-life. Other tetracyclines appear not to interact, so make dosage adjustments or use an alternative.

Ethosuximide + phenytoin

See ethosuximide (*4.5.2*).

FLUCONAZOLE + PHENYTOIN

Oral fluconazole inhibits phenytoin metabolism producing rapid and severe toxicity. It is recommended that continuous phenytoin plasma monitoring be carried out with doses of fluconazole at 200mg/d or above.

Fluorouracil + phenytoin

Toxic phenytoin levels have been reported 11 weeks after adding fluorouracil to phenytoin.

FLUOXETINE + PHENYTOIN

Phenytoin levels raised by 66% have been reported, and loss of phenytoin efficacy as a result of fluoxetine discontinuation has been reported.

FLUVOXAMINE + PHENYTOIN

Fluvoxamine may triple phenytoin levels.

Folic acid + phenytoin

Folic acid is often used to correct folate deficiency with phenytoin; plasma phenytoin levels are occasionally reduced by folic acid. Levels of both should be monitored and changes in seizure activity looked for. Folate supplements used at the start of phenytoin therapy can reduce phenytoin levels later in therapy, so care is needed.

Furosemide + phenytoin

The diuretic effect may be reduced by up to 50% by phenytoin so larger doses may be needed.

Gabapentin + phenytoin

See gabapentin (*4.5.3*).

Glucagon + phenytoin

Patients on phenytoin may get false negatives with glucagon stimulation tests.

Glucocorticoids + phenytoin

A reduced steroid effect is possible.

Griseofulvin + phenytoin

Reduced griseofulvin levels may occur, via enzyme induction.

H2-BLOCKERS + PHENYTOIN

Phenytoin levels may be increased by 30% by cimetidine and so toxicity is likely to occur. The effect is rapid and can occur within two days. Ranitidine, nizatidine and famotidine do not interact so use them as alternatives.

Indinavir + phenytoin

The *BNF* notes the possibility of reduced plasma indinavir level with phenytoin.

Influenza vaccine + phenytoin

Influenza vaccine is reported to reduce phenytoin levels although one study showed a transient 60% increase in levels.

Irinotecan + phenytoin

Phenytoin may decrease plasma levels of irinotecan.

ISONIAZID + PHENYTOIN

Phenytoin toxicity may occur so reduce phenytoin doses if necessary.

KETOCONAZOLE + PHENYTOIN

Phenytoin toxicity may occur and ketoconazole's effect may be reduced.

Lamotrigine + phenytoin

See lamotrigine (*4.5.4*).

Levetiracetam + phenytoin

See levetiracetam (*4.5.5*).

Levodopa + phenytoin

Levodopa can be completely antagonised by phenytoin and so increased levodopa doses may be necessary.

Levothyroxine/thyroxine + phenytoin

Levothyroxine metabolism is accelerated by phenytoin to give increased levothyroxine requirements.

Lidocaine + phenytoin

CNS effects may be enhanced if used concurrently. The mechanism is probably enhanced cardiac depression so beware of possible toxicity.

Lithium + phenytoin

See lithium (*4.4*).

Losartan + phenytoin

Losartan levels may rise with phenytoin.

Memantine + phenytoin

See memantine (*4.6.7*).

Methadone + phenytoin

See methadone (*4.6.8*).

Methotrexate + phenytoin

An increased antifolate effect with phenytoin may occur.

Methylphenidate + phenytoin

See methylphenidate (*4.6.9*).

Metronidazole + phenytoin

Mild phenytoin toxicity is possible but this does not usually cause problems.

MEXILITINE + PHENYTOIN

Mexilitine levels are reduced by up to 50% via enzyme induction and so dosage adjustments may be necessary.

MICONAZOLE + PHENYTOIN

Two cases of phenytoin toxicity have been reported.

Mirtazapine + phenytoin

See mirtazapine (*4.3.3.2*).

Nasogastric feeds + phenytoin

Reduced phenytoin levels have been reported with nasogastric feeds, with absorption patterns significantly different. Phenytoin dosage should be spaced to one hour before feeding or two hours after feeding (tube may need to be clamped). Monitor plasma levels frequently.

Neuromuscular blocking agents + phenytoin

Phenytoin reduces the effects of most NMBAs, eg. pancuronium, but not atracurium.

NICOUMALINE + PHENYTOIN

The metabolism of nicoumalone is normally accelerated by phenytoin, reducing its effect, although enhancement has also been reported.

Nitrofurantoin + phenytoin

There is a single case of a stable epileptic developing seizures when nitrofurantoin was added, requiring increased phenytoin dosage.

NSAIDs + phenytoin

There is a case report of plasma phenytoin levels being increased by aspirin but transient toxicity may be the only outcome. Plasma phenytoin levels may be increased by azapropazone. One study showed no interaction with ibuprofen, but a single case of toxicity has been reported.

ORAL CONTRACEPTIVES + PHENYTOIN

Contraceptive failure via enzyme induction has been reported many times so use higher dose OCs or alternative contraceptive methods. With Eugynon 50 no longer available, adequate contraception can be obtained from using a combination of Marvelon and Mercilon together, or two tablets of Ovranette, or Depot Provera given every 10 weeks rather than 12 weeks.

Oxcarbazepine + phenytoin

See oxcarbazepine (*4.5.6*).

Paroxetine + phenytoin

See paroxetine (*4.3.2.4*).

Pethidine + phenytoin

Attenuation of pethidine's effect via enzyme induction, with increased metabolite levels, is possible.

Phenobarbital + phenytoin

Phenytoin may increase phenobarbital levels by up to 100%, enhancing sedation, so monitor levels regularly. Additionally, phenytoin levels are increased by very high dose barbiturates, but decreased by lower or moderate dose barbiturates. The clinical effect may be minimal but care is needed if phenobarbital is stopped, as phenytoin levels may rise.

PHENYLBUTAZONE + PHENYTOIN

Phenytoin toxicity may occur via enzyme inhibition and plasma protein displacement so dosage adjustment may be necessary.

PROGABIDE + PHENYTOIN

Phenytoin levels may rise by up to 40%.

Propoxyphene + phenytoin

Large doses of propoxyphene may produce elevated phenytoin levels but normal doses have little or no effect.

Proton-pump inhibitors + phenytoin

Lack of interaction has been shown with omeprazole, as has a mild rise in phenytoin levels. The UK SPC for omeprazole states that patients should be monitored on this combination and doses adjusted if necessary, or use pantoprazole.

Pyrimethamine + phenytoin

There is an increased risk of an antifolate effect.

Pyridoxine + phenytoin

Large doses of pyridoxine (eg. 200mg/d) can reduce phenytoin levels by up to 50% so monitoring levels would be wise.

Quetiapine + phenytoin

See quetiapine (*4.2.5*).

QUINIDINE + PHENYTOIN

A reduced quinidine effect may occur.

RIFAMPICIN + PHENYTOIN

Significant reductions in phenytoin levels may occur via enzyme induction.

Sertindole + phenytoin

See sertindole (*4.2.7*).

Sertraline + phenytoin

See sertraline (*4.3.2.5*).

Shankhapushpi + phenytoin

It has been recommended to avoid the Ayurvedic herbal mixture shankhapushpi, as decreased plasma phenytoin levels may occur.

Statins + phenytoin

There is a case of phenytoin reducing the therapeutic effect of simvastatin and atorvastatin, probably via 3A4 induction.

St. John's wort + phenytoin

See anticonvulsants + St. John's wort (*4.3.3.8*).

SUCRALFATE + PHENYTOIN

One study showed a small reduction in phenytoin absorption. This can be avoided by giving phenytoin 2 hours or more after sucralfate.

Sulphonamides + phenytoin

Phenytoin toxicity is possible via enzyme inhibition so monitor plasma levels and reduce phenytoin doses if necessary.

Theophylline + phenytoin

Phenytoin produces a 45% increase in clearance of theophylline and phenytoin absorption may also be reduced. Separating the doses by 1–2 hours may help but adjust doses and monitor as necessary.

Tiagabine + phenytoin

See tiagabine (*4.5.10*).

Ticlopidine + phenytoin

Ticlopidine 500mg/d inhibits phenytoin clearance and dose adjustment and careful monitoring should be considered, especially as toxicity can be delayed by several weeks.

Tolbutamide + phenytoin

Mild phenytoin toxicity may occur via increased free phenytoin levels. Tolazamide may also interact.

Topiramate + phenytoin

See topiramate (*4.5.11*).

Trazodone + phenytoin

There is an isolated case of phenytoin toxicity developing when relatively high dose trazodone was added.

TRIMETHOPRIM + PHENYTOIN

Plasma phenytoin levels and the anti-folate effect may be increased by trimethoprim.

TRICYCLICS + PHENYTOIN

Phenytoin levels may be raised by imipramine (but not nortriptyline or amitriptyline). Phenytoin levels need to be monitored frequently. Tricyclics may also lower the seizure threshold.

VALPROATE + PHENYTOIN

Valproate inhibits phenytoin metabolism and competes for its binding sites. If enzyme saturation has not occurred then this displacement of phenytoin leads to decreased bound, but increased free, phenytoin. More phenytoin is then metabolised so the net result is reduced total and bound concentrations. The free concentration will, however, remain about the same and so lower plasma levels will still contain about the same amount of active/free phenytoin. Thus, beware of raising the dose of phenytoin to bring the total plasma concentration (which is what standard UK blood tests measure) into the 'therapeutic range' as the person could then become toxic with high free phenytoin levels. Alternatively, if the enzyme is saturated, then displacement may lead to a stable total concentration but decreased bound and increased free phenytoin. This could lead to **toxic effects within the therapeutic range**. In practice, phenytoin levels tend to fall initially, by up to 50%, then return to normal over about five weeks. Toxicity is possible if levels were higher at the start. Careful monitoring of seizures, toxic effects and plasma levels is thus essential. **Care** is also needed if switching to Epilim Chrono® as phenytoin levels can rise by up to 30%.

VIGABATRIN + PHENYTOIN

Vigabatrin produces a 20–30% reduction in phenytoin levels and this has been thought to compromise seizure control.

Vincristine + phenytoin

Phenytoin significantly increases the clearance of vincristine, probably by CYP3A4 induction.

WARFARIN + PHENYTOIN

Warfarin metabolism is accelerated by phenytoin, reducing its effect and one death has been reported.

Zinc + phenytoin

An isolated case exists of reduced phenytoin levels probably caused by zinc.

Zotepine + phenytoin

See anticonvulsants + zotepine (*4.2.8*).

4.5.9 Piracetam (Nootropil ®)

Warfarin + piracetam

There is a single case of prolonged prothrombin time.

4.5.10 Tiagabine (Gabitril®)

Tiagabine appears to be metabolised by CYP3A4.

Alcohol + tiagabine

Lack of interaction has been shown, although some caution is still advised.

Benzodiazepines + tiagabine

Lack of interaction has been shown.

Carbamazepine + tiagabine

Tiagabine clearance is 60% greater in people also taking carbamazepine, with plasma levels reduced by a factor of 1.5–3. There is no effect on carbamazepine.

Cimetidine + tiagabine

Lack of interaction has been shown.

Digoxin + tiagabine

Lack of interaction has been shown.

Erythromycin + tiagabine

Lack of significant interaction has been shown.

Fosphenytoin + tiagabine

See phenytoin + tiagabine.

Oral contraceptives + tiagabine

Lack of interaction has been shown.

Phenobarbital + tiagabine

Tiagabine clearance is 60% greater in people also taking phenobarbital, with plasma levels reduced by a factor of 1.5–3. There is no effect on phenobarbital.

Phenytoin + tiagabine

Tiagabine clearance is 60% greater in people also taking phenytoin and plasma levels are reduced by a factor of 1.5–3. There is no effect on phenytoin.

Theophylline + tiagabine

Lack of interaction has been shown.

Valproate + tiagabine

Tiagabine causes a 10–12% reduction in steady-state valproate levels whilst valproate increases free tiagabine levels by about 40%.

Warfarin + tiagabine

Lack of interaction has been shown.

Zotepine + tiagabine

See anticonvulsants + zotepine (*4.2.8*).

4.5.11 Topiramate (Topamax®)

Topiramate *in vitro* data suggests that effects on hepatic enzyme metabolism are small and interactions with antipsychotics, tricyclics, antidepressants, caffeine, theophylline and coumarin are unlikely via this mechanism. Concomitant use with drugs predisposing to nephrolithiasis (renal stone formation) is not recommended. Such drugs include acetazolamide and triamterene, with many other drugs implicated, eg. allopurinol, megadose ascorbic acid, furosemide, methyldopa, phenolphthalein abuse, steroids and, of all things, a Worcester Sauce overdose.

Acetazolamide + topiramate

There may be an increased risk of renal stone formation in susceptible patients.

Carbamazepine + topiramate

Topiramate has no effect on carbamazepine but topiramate plasma levels are reduced by about 40% by carbamazepine, important if carbamazepine is withdrawn.

Digoxin + topiramate

Topiramate may decrease digoxin levels slightly.

Lamotrigine + topiramate

See lamotrigine (*4.5.4*).

Lithium + topiramate

See lithium (*4.4*).

ORAL CONTRACEPTIVES + TOPIRAMATE

Estrogen levels are reduced by topiramate in patients taking combined estrogen/ progesterone oral contraceptives. With Eugynon 50 no longer available, adequate contraception can be obtained from using a combination of Marvelon and Mercilon together, or two tablets of Ovranette, or Depot Provera given every 10 weeks rather than 12 weeks.

Phenobarbital + topiramate

No interaction noted yet.

Phenytoin + topiramate

Phenytoin levels may rise slightly. Topiramate levels may fall, which could be important if phenytoin is withdrawn.

Triamterene + topiramate

There may be an increased risk of renal stone formation in susceptible patients.

Valproate + topiramate

Topiramate produces a small but significant reduction in valproate plasma levels, although *enhanced* valproate adverse effects have been reported. Topiramate plasma levels are increased by about 15% by valproate, which could be important if valproate is withdrawn.

Zotepine + topiramate

See anticonvulsants + zotepine (*4.2.8*).

4.5.12 Valproate (sodium valproate/valproic acid/ valproate semisodium) (Epilim®, Convulex®, Depakote®)

Antacids + valproate

A small, insignificant decrease in valproate absorption with antacids has been noted.

ANTIDEPRESSANTS + VALPROATE

Many antidepressants lower the seizure threshold and may antagonise valproate's anticonvulsant effect. A case of status epilepticus with the combination of valproate and clomipramine has been reported, with valproate possibly elevating clomipramine to toxic levels.

ANTIPSYCHOTICS + VALPROATE

Chlorpromazine may inhibit the metabolism of valproate so monitoring valproate levels may be appropriate. Valproate has no significant effect on haloperidol levels. There are cases of dose-related generalised oedema with risperidone and valproate. Valproate produces a nonsignificant rise in clozapine (but lower norclozapine) levels, although valproate is often used as anticonvulsant cover for high dose clozapine. No interaction occurs with **aripiprazole**. Antipsychotics lower the seizure threshold and may antagonise the anticonvulsant effect of valproate.

Aspirin + valproate

Valproate's clinical effect and toxicity may be enhanced by repeated high-dose aspirin, so monitor carefully.

Benzodiazepines + valproate

See benzodiazepines (*4.1.1*).

Bupropion + valproate

See bupropion (*4.6.4*).

CARBAMAZEPINE + VALPROATE

See carbamazepine (*4.5.1*).

Charcoal, activated + valproate

Activated charcoal has been shown to reduce the absorption of valproate by 65%, but another study failed to replicate this finding.

Erythromycin + valproate

A single case exists of valproate levels rising 300% when erythromycin was started, resulting in CNS toxicity.

Ethosuximide + valproate

See ethosuximide (*4.5.2*).

Fluoxetine + valproate
See fluoxetine (*4.3.2.2*).

Fluvoxamine + valproate
See fluvoxamine (*4.3.2.3*).

Gabapentin + valproate
See gabapentin (*4.5.3*).

H2-blockers + valproate
One study showed that cimetidine reduces the clearance and prolongs the half-life of valproate. Ranitidine is a suitable alternative.

Isoniazid + valproate
An isolated case exists of enhanced hepatotoxicity.

LAMOTRIGINE + VALPROATE
See lamotrigine (*4.5.4*).

Levetiracetam + valproate
See levetiracetam (*4.5.5*).

Methylphenidate + valproate
See methylphenidate (*4.6.8*).

Oral contraceptives + valproate
A reduced contraceptive effect has not been reported with valproate, unlike carbamazepine, phenytoin and phenobarbital.

Oxcarbazepine + valproate
See oxcarbazepine (*4.5.6*).

Paroxetine + valproate
See paroxetine (*4.3.2.4*).

PHENYTOIN + VALPROATE
See phenytoin (*4.5.8*).

PHENOBARBITAL + VALPROATE
See phenobarbital (*4.5.7*).

Tiagabine + valproate
See tiagabine (*4.5.10*).

Tricyclics + valproate
See antidepressants + valproate.

Topiramate + valproate
See topiramate (*4.5.11*).

Vigabatrin + valproate
See vigabatrin (*4.5.13*).

Warfarin + valproate
Rapidly raised INR (to 3.9) has been reported after a single dose of valproate. Care is thus needed.

Zidovudine + valproate
Valproate produces a dose-dependent rise in zidovudine levels, possibly by up to 3-fold. This is a new UK SPC warning.

4.5.13 Vigabatrin (Sabril®)

Carbamazepine + vigabatrin
A small rise in carbamazepine levels has been reported with the addition of vigabatrin.

Oral contraceptives + vigabatrin
One study showed that vigabatrin is unlikely to consistently affect the efficacy of steroid oral contraceptives.

Phenobarbital + vigabatrin
Lack of significant interaction has been shown.

PHENYTOIN + VIGABATRIN
See phenytoin (*4.5.8*).

Valproate + vigabatrin
Lack of significant interaction has been shown.

Zotepine + vigabatrin
See anticonvulsants + zotepine (*4.2.8*).

4.6   Other drugs

4.6.1 Acamprosate (Campral EC®)

Acamprosate probably has a very low liability for drug-drug interactions.

Alcohol + acamprosate

See alcohol (*4.7.1*).

Benzodiazepines + acamprosate

Lack of interaction has been shown.

Disulfiram + acamprosate

Lack of interaction has been shown.

Food + acamprosate

Food reduces the oral absorption of acamprosate.

Naltrexone + acamprosate

Lack of clinically significant interaction has been shown.

Tricyclics + acamprosate

Lack of interaction with imipramine has been shown.

4.6.2 Anticholinergic (antimuscarinic) agents

Anticholinesterases + anticholinergics

Some antagonism would be expected.

Antipsychotics + anticholinergics

See antipsychotics (*4.2.1*).

Benzodiazepines + anticholinergics

See benzodiazepines (*4.1.1*).

Beta-blockers + anticholinergics

Propantheline increases the effect of atenolol, but not metoprolol.

Betel nut + anticholinergics

Heavy betel nut consumption has resulted in severe EPSEs, possibly by antagonising the effect of procyclidine.

H2-blockers + anticholinergics

A single dose study showed possible reduced cimetidine absorption, but not with ranitidine nor nizatidine.

Levodopa + anticholinergics

Anticholinergics may reduce the peak blood levels of levodopa and reduce total absorption so higher doses may be necessary.

MAOIs + anticholinergics

See MAOIs (*4.3.4*).

Memantine + anticholinergics

See memantine (*4.6.7*).

Nitrofurantoin + anticholinergics

Nitrofurantoin blood levels and bioavailability may be increased by anticholinergics.

Olanzapine + biperiden

See olanzapine (*4.2.4*).

Paracetamol + anticholinergics

Propantheline delays the absorption of paracetamol.

SSRIs + anticholinergics

There are many cases of the combination causing delirium, probably via CYP2D6 inhibition.

Thiazide diuretics + anticholinergics

Thiazide bioavailability may be enhanced.

TRICYCLICS + ANTICHOLINERGICS

See tricyclics (*4.3.1*).

Zotepine + anticholinergics

See zotepine (*4.2.8*).

4.6.3 Anticholinesterases

4.6.3.1 Donepezil (Aricept®)

Donepezil is metabolised slowly by a P450 enzyme to multiple metabolites, only one of which appears to be pharmacologically active.

Anticholinergics + donepezil

See anticholinergics (*4.6.2*).

Antipsychotics + donepezil

Lack of interaction has been reported, although there are a few case reports of NMS and EPSEs. Severe EPSEs have been reported with donepezil and risperidone.

Cimetidine + donepezil

Lack of interaction has been reported.

Digoxin + donepezil

Lack of interaction has been reported.

Ketoconazole + donepezil

Donepezil levels may rise by around 25% over a week.

Memantine + donepezil

See anticholinesterases + memantine (*4.6.7*).

NSAIDs + donepezil

The donepezil SPC recommends additional monitoring of patients at risk of developing ulcers, eg. if taking concomitant NSAIDs.

SSRIs + donepezil

Lack of interaction has been shown.

Theophylline + donepezil

Lack of interaction has been reported.

Warfarin + donepezil

Lack of significant interaction reported.

4.6.3.2 Galantamine (Reminyl®)

Galantamine is metabolised by CYP2D6 and CYP3A4, and any interaction with potent inhibitors may result in increased side effects initially eg. nausea and vomiting. Reduced maintenance doses might be appropriate (SPC).

Anticholinergics + galantamine

See anticholinergics (*4.6.2*).

Antipsychotics + galantamine

Lack of interaction has been reported with risperidone.

Beta-blockers + galantamine

As galantamine may cause bradycardia, the UK SPC recommends care with drugs that significantly reduce heart rate eg. beta-blockers.

Digoxin + galantamine

As galantamine may cause bradycardia, the UK SPC recommends care with drugs that significantly reduce heart rate eg. digoxin. Galantamine has no effect on digoxin.

Erythromycin + galantamine

A small increase in galantamine plasma levels has been reported (SPC).

Ketoconazole + galantamine

A 30% in increase galantamine plasma levels has been reported (SPC). A reduced maintenance dosage might be appropriate.

Memantine + galantamine

See memantine (*4.6.7*).

Paroxetine + galantamine

A 40% increase in galantamine plasma levels has been reported (SPC). A reduced maintenance dosage might be appropriate.

Warfarin + galantamine

Lack of significant interaction has been shown.

4.6.3.3 Rivastigmine (Exelon®)

Anticholinergics + rivastigmine

See anticholinergics (*4.6.2*).

Benzodiazepines + rivastigmine

Lack of interaction has been shown.

Digoxin + rivastigmine

Lack of interaction has been shown.

Fluoxetine + rivastigmine

Lack of interaction has been shown.

Memantine + rivastigmine

See memantine (*4.6.7*).

Warfarin + rivastigmine

Lack of interaction has been shown.

4.6.4 Bupropion (Zyban®)

Alcohol + bupropion

There is an increased risk of seizures, so alcohol should be avoided or minimised. Extreme care is needed in overdose, chronic use and in alcohol withdrawal states.

Antipsychotics + bupropion

Caution is necessary due to the enhanced risk of seizures, especially with single bupropion doses above 200mg/d and daily doses of 350mg/d or more.

Carbamazepine + bupropion

Carbamazepine induces bupropion metabolism, markedly decreasing bupropion plasma levels.

Ciclosporin + bupropion

A life-threatening decrease in ciclosporin levels with bupropion has been reported.

Cimetidine + bupropion

Cimetidine may inhibit the metabolism of bupropion, and increase adverse effects.

Clonidine + bupropion

Lack of interaction has been shown.

Fluoxetine + bupropion

Panic disorder has been reported with the combination, but bupropion has no effect on fluoxetine plasma levels.

Fosphenytoin + bupropion

See phenytoin + bupropion.

Lamotrigine + bupropion

See lamotrigine (4.5.4).

Levodopa + bupropion

An increased incidence of side-effects has been reported with the combination.

MAOIs + bupropion

The combination is contraindicated as animal studies suggest toxicity may occur.

Moclobemide + bupropion

See MAOIs + bupropion.

Paroxetine + bupropion

There are no significant changes in paroxetine levels but the CSM recommends caution.

Phenobarbital + bupropion

Phenobarbital may induce the metabolism of bupropion, which would reduce bupropion efficacy.

Phenytoin + bupropion

Phenytoin may induce the metabolism of bupropion, which would reduce bupropion efficacy.

Pseudoephedrine + bupropion

There is a case of acute myocardial ischaemia with the combination.

Ritonavir + bupropion

Ritonavir may decrease the metabolism of bupropion, which would increase side-effects.

Selegiline + bupropion

See MAOIs + bupropion.

Smoking + bupropion

Lack of interaction has been shown.

Tricyclics + bupropion

Bupropion may increase tricyclic levels, and seizures and nortriptyline toxicity have been reported.

Valproate + bupropion

Lack of significant interaction has been shown.

Venlafaxine + bupropion

Bupropion significantly increases venlafaxine levels, so increase doses carefully.

Zolpidem + bupropion

There are some reported cases of antidepressants and zolpidem causing short-lived hallucinations.

4.6.5 Clomethiazole (Heminevrin®)

Alcohol + clomethiazole

See alcohol (4.7.1).

Cimetidine + clomethiazole

Cimetidine inhibits the metabolism of clomethiazole, raising plasma levels.

Methadone + clomethiazole

See methadone (*4.6.8*).

4.6.6 Disulfiram (Antabuse®)

Acamprosate + disulfiram

See acamprosate (*4.6.1*).

ALCOHOL + DISULFIRAM

See disulfiram under 'Alcohol dependence' (*1.3*) and disulfiram + alcohol (*4.7.1*).

Antipsychotics + disulfiram

There is a single case of psychotic relapse when disulfiram was started in a person stable on an antipsychotic.

Benzodiazepines + disulfiram

Disulfiram may inhibit the metabolism of diazepam, temazepam and chlordiazepoxide (but not oxazepam) leading to lengthened half-lives and possible toxicity.

Caffeine + disulfiram

Disulfiram may reduce caffeine clearance from the body by a half, increasing levels.

Cannabis + disulfiram

See cannabis (*4.7.2*).

Carbamazepine + disulfiram

Lack of significant interaction has been shown.

Isoniazid + disulfiram

CNS toxicity has been reported in patients taking isoniazid who then took disulfiram.

Lithium + disulfiram

These appear compatible, with no known reasons why an interaction should occur.

MAOIs + disulfiram

There is a single case of delirium occurring with tranylcypromine.

Methadone + disulfiram

See methadone (*4.6.8*).

Metronidazole + disulfiram

Psychotic reactions have been reported.

NICOUMALONE + DISULFIRAM

An enhanced anticoagulant effect is possible.

Omeprazole + disulfiram

An isolated case of confusion and disorientation has been reported.

PHENYTOIN + DISULFIRAM

See phenytoin (*4.5.8*).

Theophylline + disulfiram

Theophylline levels may be increased by disulfiram so monitor and reduce the theophylline dose if necessary.

Tricyclics + disulfiram

See tricyclics (*4.3.1*).

WARFARIN + DISULFIRAM

Prothrombin time can fall by about 10%, with one study showing a marked effect with reduced warfarin doses sometimes necessary.

4.6.7 Memantine (Ebixa®)

Amantadine + memantine

Both are NMDA-antagonists and the combination should be avoided as central ADRs may be more frequent (SPC). The same may be true of ketamine and dextromethorphan (SPC).

Anticholinergics + memantine

Anticholinergic's effects may be enhanced by memantine (SPC).

Anticholinesterases+memantine

Lack of interaction has been suggested.

Antipsychotics + memantine

Antipsychotic effects may be reduced by memantine (SPC).

Antispasmodic agents + memantine

The effects may be modified by memantine and dose adjustment may be necessary (SPC).

Baclofen + memantine

The effects may be modified by memantine and dose adjustment may be necessary (SPC).

Barbiturates + memantine

Barbiturate's effects may be reduced by memantine (SPC).

Dantrolene + memantine

Dantrolene's effects may be modified by memantine and dose adjustment may be necessary (SPC).

Dextromethorphan + memantine

See amantadine + memantine.

Dopamine agonists + memantine

Dopamine antagonists such as bromocriptine may be enhanced by memantine (SPC).

H2-blockers + memantine

There is the unproven potential for increased H2-plasma levels (SPC).

Hydrochlorothiazide + memantine

There is a theoretical possibility of reduced diuretic effect (SPC).

Levodopa + memantine

The effects of levodopa may be enhanced by memantine (SPC).

Phenytoin + memantine

There is one case report of interaction.

Procainamide + memantine

A theoretical interaction between smoking (nicotine) and memantine via competition for cationic transport system exists and there is the potential for increased plasma levels (SPC).

Quinidine/quinine + memantine

There is the unproven potential for increased memantine plasma levels (SPC).

Smoking + memantine

There is the unproven potential for increased memantine plasma levels (SPC).

4.6.8 Methadone (eg. Physeptone®)

Alcohol + methadone

See alcohol (*4.7.1*).

Ascorbic acid + methadone

Vitamin C and other urine acidifiers (eg. ammonium chloride) can decrease plasma levels via increased renal excretion if the pH is less than 6. Methadone's half-life can be halved to around 19–20 hrs.

Barbiturates + methadone

Enhanced sedation and respiratory depression may occur, as well as reduced methadone levels.

Benzodiazepines + methadone

Additive sedation can occur.

Buprenorphine + methadone

An antagonistic effect would be predicted. Enhanced sedation and respiratory depression may occur.

Carbamazepine + methadone

Reduced methadone levels can occur through CYP3A4 induction.

Chloral + methadone

Additive sedation can occur.

Cimetidine + methadone

Raised methadone levels can occur.

Clomethiazole + methadone

Additive sedation can occur.

Cyclizine + methadone

There are rare reports of hallucinations with the combination.

Didanosone + methadone

Serum levels of didanosone can be reduced by about 40%.

Diphenhydramine + methadone

There are rare reports of additional CNS effects with the combination.

Disulfiram + methadone

Lack of kinetic interaction has been shown.

Domperidone + methadone

Increased absorption has been reported.

Efavirenz + methadone

Efavirez can induce CYP3A4 and produce withdrawal symptoms from reduced methadone levels.

Erythromycin + methadone

Raised methadone levels through CYP3A4 inhibition could occur.

Fluconazole/ketoconazole + methadone

Methadone levels can rise by a mean of 27% through CYP3A4 inhibition.

Fluoxetine + methadone

Lack of significant interaction has been shown.

Fluvoxamine + methadone

Fluvoxamine may inhibit methadone metabolism leading to raised methadone levels. Severe hypoventilation has been reported.

Fosphenytoin + methadone

See phenytoin + methadone.

Grapefruit juice + methadone

Raised methadone levels through CYP3A4 inhibition could theoretically occur.

Hypnotics + methadone

Enhanced sedation can occur.

Indinavir + methadone

Slightly raised methadone levels have been reported (MI).

MAOIs + methadone

See MAOIs (*4.3.4*).

Metapyrone + methadone

Metapyrone can cause a withdrawal-like syndrome with methadone.

Naloxone + methadone

This opiate antagonist would block the effect of methadone within 5–10 minutes.

Naltrexone + methadone

This opiate antagonist would block the effect of methadone.

Nevirapine + methadone

Reduced methadone levels through CYP3A4 induction can occur, inducing a withdrawal state.

Phenytoin + methadone

Phenytoin may reduce methadone levels through enzyme induction. Withdrawal symptoms may occur within 4 days so dosage adjustment may be needed.

Paroxetine + methadone

See paroxetine (*4.3.2.4*).

Reboxetine + methadone

See reboxetine (*4.3.3.5*).

Rifampicin + methadone

Methadone levels reduce by 30–65% within 4–5 days in 70% patients given rifampicin, through CYP3A4 induction.

Risperidone + methadone

There is a report of possible interaction, resulting in irritability and aches.

Ritonavir + methadone

Ritonavir may decrease methadone levels slightly, although ritonavir/saquinavir has been used without dose adjustment in AIDS patients.

Sodium bicarbonate + methadone

Sodium bicarbonate and other urinary alkalinisers can increase plasma levels via decreased renal excretion.

Tricyclics + methadone

Additive sedation might occur and raised tricyclic levels have been reported.

Zidovudine + methadone

Raised zidovudine levels have been reported.

4.6.9 Methylphenidate (Concerta®, Ritalin® etc)

Carbamazepine + methylphenidate

There is a report of carbamazepine causing an extreme reduction of methylphenidate levels.

Ciclosporin + methylphenidate

Raised ciclosporin levels has been reported with methylphenidate.

MAOIs + methylphenidate

See MAOIs (*4.3.4*).

Modafinil + methylphenidate

See modafinil (*4.6.10*).

Phenytoin + methylphenidate

Phenytoin toxicity has been reported.

Tricyclics + methylphenidate

Raised tricyclic levels, and mood and cognitive deterioration have been reported.

Valproate + methylphenidate

Rapid onset and severe dyskinesia and bruxism has been reported with the combination.

4.6.10 Modafinil (Provigil®)

Modafinil is moderately bound to plasma proteins (62%), essentially to albumin. Renal excretion is the main route of elimination.

Amfetamines + modafinil

Lack of significant interaction has been shown.

Benzodiazepines + modafinil

Benzodiazepine plasma levels may be reduced slightly by modafinil.

Dexamphetamine + modafinil

Lack of significant interaction has been shown.

Ethinylestradiol + modafinil

Ethinylestradiol levels may be reduced by modafinil.

Methylphenidate + modafinil

Lack of significant interaction has been shown.

Oral contraceptives + modafinil

Higher dose oral contraceptives containing 50mcg ethinylestradiol should be used (MI).

Tricyclics + modafinil

Possible tricyclic toxicity may occur.

Warfarin + modafinil

Lack of significant interaction has been shown.

4.7 Non-prescribed drugs

4.7.1 Alcohol (various brands and manufacturers)

Alcohol/ethanol-psychotropic drug interactions can occur frequently and with varied outcome, depending upon:

- alcohol usage (eg. chronic and/or acute, altered enzymes etc.)
- consumption (amount, time span)
- type of interaction (eg. additive sedation, antagonism or cross-tolerance)
- what the individual then tries to do (eg. sleep, drive etc)
- comorbidity (eg. asthma etc).

These variables need to be taken into consideration when assessing the effect or potential effect of the interaction.

Acamprosate + alcohol

Continued alcohol consumption has been stated to negate the therapeutic effect of acamprosate. There is no detectable pharmacokinetic interaction.

ANTIPSYCHOTICS + ALCOHOL

Enhanced CNS depression resulting in impaired concentration, coordination and judgement, drowsiness and lethargy, as well as hypotension and respiratory depression is well known. Alcohol-related drowsiness may be less with **haloperidol**, **amisulpride** and **sulpiride**. Enhanced CNS sedation would be expected with **olanzapine**, and raised heart rate and increased postural hypotension have been reported. **Zotepine** should not be used in people with alcohol intoxication (UK SPC). No significant difference in performance or gross motor skills has been shown with **aripiprazole** and alcohol. There is no published evidence that alcohol reduces antipsychotic effectiveness. Overall, this is a potentially important interaction, especially in the community. Accidental alcohol overdosage, especially in people with asthma, respiratory depression or chest infections, could prove fatal if combined with antipsychotics.

BENZODIAZEPINES + ALCOHOL

Alcohol can enhance the sedation caused by benzodiazepines by 20–30%, a well-established, documented and entirely predictable interaction. Larger quantities of alcohol may inhibit benzodiazepine metabolism, especially in those with impaired or borderline hepatic function.

Beta-blockers + alcohol

Alcohol may slightly reduce propranolol absorption and increase excretion.

Bupropion + alcohol

See bupropion (*4.6.4*).

Buspirone + alcohol

A minimal interaction has been reported in two studies.

Cannabis + alcohol

See cannabis (*4.7.2*).

Carbamazepine + alcohol

Nothing is published but an additive sedative effect would be expected.

CHLORAL + ALCOHOL

Additive (or more) CNS depressant effects occur when alcohol is taken with chloral, with tachycardia, impaired concentration, disulfiram-like effects and profound vasodilation also reported.

Clomethiazole + alcohol

Alcohol increases the bioavailability of oral clomethiazole.

Citalopram + alcohol

Lundbeck state that (es)citalopram does not enhance the sedation caused by alcohol.

Cocaine + alcohol

See cocaine (*4.7.3*).

DISULFIRAM + ALCOHOL

Disulfiram inhibits the aldehyde dehydrogenase enzyme, leading to accumulation of acetaldehyde from incomplete alcohol metabolism, producing flushing, sweating, palpitations, hyperventilation, increased pulse, hypotension, nausea and vomiting (often in that order). Arrhythmias and shock can follow. Patients should be warned that reactions can occur with disguised sources of alcohol eg. 'Listerine' mouth-wash, sauces, pharmaceuticals (eg. cough mixtures) and topical preparations (eg. shampoos).

Escitalopram + alcohol

See citalopram above.

Fluoxetine + alcohol

Alcohol has no additional significant effect on drowsiness, sedation or task performance tests with fluoxetine 40mg/d.

Fluvoxamine + alcohol

There may be a moderately enhanced sedation with fluvoxamine.

Levetiracetam + alcohol

See levetiracetam (*4.5.5*).

Lithium + alcohol

Impaired driving skills have been suggested.

MAOIs + alcohol

As well as an interaction occurring with alcoholic and low alcoholic drinks (see *4.3.4.4*), MAOIs may inhibit alcohol dehydrogenase, potentiating alcohol's effect.

Methadone + alcohol

Increased sedation can occur.

MIANSERIN + ALCOHOL

Mianserin causes drowsiness, enhanced considerably by alcohol.

Mirtazapine + alcohol

Mirtazapine may cause drowsiness, considerably enhanced by alcohol.

Moclobemide + alcohol

Some potentiation of alcohol sedation has been noted, but less than with trazodone and clomipramine.

Olanzapine + alcohol

Enhanced sedation would be expected.

Oxcarbazepine + alcohol

See oxcarbazepine (*4.5.6*).

Paroxetine + alcohol

Lack of interaction has been shown.

PHENYTOIN + ALCOHOL

Alcohol usually decreases phenytoin levels but, if alcohol intake is heavy, increases them via enzyme induction. Higher doses may be needed initially in alcoholics. The half-life of phenytoin can be up to 50% shorter in an abstaining alcoholic than in a non-drinker.

PHENOBARBITAL + ALCOHOL

Prolonged CNS and respiratory depression can occur, seriously impairing concentration and performance. The lethal dose of barbiturates is up to 50% lower when alcohol is also present, mainly due to additive respiratory depression.

Quetiapine + alcohol

Additive sedation would be expected.

Reboxetine + alcohol

No potentiation of alcohol's cognitive effects has been reported (UK SPC).

Sertraline + alcohol

Lack of interaction has been noted.

Tiagabine + alcohol

See tiagabine (*4.5.10*).

TRAZODONE + ALCOHOL

Alcohol enhances the sedation caused by trazodone.

TRICYCLICS + ALCOHOL

Enhanced sedation with most tricyclics is known, but little has actually been published. Most studies refer to the effect on driving performance. Sedation caused by amitriptyline and doxepin is enhanced by alcohol, but less, or minimally so, with nortriptyline, clomipramine and amoxapine, which are less sedating. Both alcohol and tricyclics lower the seizure threshold and care is needed in patients susceptible to seizures.

Venlafaxine + alcohol

Lack of enhanced psychomotor impairment has been reported.

Zaleplon + alcohol

Any enhanced sedation would be short-lived.

Zolpidem + alcohol

There is no published information available indicating an interaction.

Zopiclone + alcohol

No significant interaction.

4.7.2 Cannabis (tetrahydrocannabinol)

Cannabis/marijuana is a frequently (and usually secretively) used drug but, with the exception of perhaps tricyclics, has few known important adverse drug interactions.

Alcohol + cannabis

Decreased ethanol metabolism may occur, with enhanced CNS depression. Cannabis may reduce peak alcohol levels.

Antidepressants + cannabis

Mental state changes consistent with delirium and tachycardia and other clinically significant adverse events have been reported following use of marijuana and tricyclic antidepressants. Increased heart rate has been reported, eg. marked sinus tachycardia. There is a case report of mania with cannabis and fluoxetine.

Antipsychotics + cannabis

Chlorpromazine clearance has been shown to be slightly increased by cannabis smoking, and additive drowsiness has been reported. Stopping cannabis has led to clozapine toxicity by removal of CYP1A2 induction. Cannabis will increase dopamine levels in the mesolimbic system, which will increase the risk of psychosis.

Benzodiazepines + cannabis

Additive drowsiness with benzodiazepines and hypnotics has been reported.

Cocaine + cannabis

See cocaine (*4.7.3*).

CNS depressants + cannabis

The combination of cannabis and other CNS depressants has resulted in additive drowsiness, eg. antidepressants, anticholinergics, benzodiazepines, lithium, barbiturates etc.

Disulfiram + cannabis

There have been two reported reactions: a hypomanic episode and an acute confusional state.

Lithium + cannabis

Single cases exist of toxic lithium levels and additive drowsiness.

4.7.3 Cocaine

Alcohol + cocaine

Simultaneous cocaine and alcohol may produce changes in heart rate and blood pressure, increasing the risk of cardiovascular toxicity.

Antidepressants + cocaine

Desipramine may reduce, fluoxetine has no significant effect, trazodone has minor physiological effects and MAOIs probably augment the pressor effect of cocaine.

Antipsychotics + cocaine

Flupenthixol may reduce cocaine craving and haloperidol may moderate the stimulant effects. Clozapine increases cocaine levels but reduced cocaine "high", and some cardiac events (near-syncopal episode) have been reported, so caution is necessary.

Carbamazepine + cocaine

Cocaine may enhance the cardiac effects of carbamazepine.

Cannabis + cocaine

Enhanced cardiotoxicity (eg. increased heart rate) may occur.

Lithium + cocaine

Lithium probably has little effect on cocaine.

4.7.4 Cigarette smoking

Many people with mental health problems smoke. There are over 3000 different known chemicals in cigarette smoke, but which ones are significant is not fully known. Only a few cigarette-drug interactions are important, and only brief details of the more significant ones are included here.

Antipsychotics + smoking

Reduced **haloperidol** and **chlorpromazine** levels in smokers have been shown, but the significance is unclear, although smoking schizophrenics tend to receive higher doses of antipsychotics than non-smokers. **Clozapine** levels are lowered by smoking, so stopping smoking could be dangerous for someone taking clozapine. **Olanzapine** clearance may be 33% lower and half-life 21% longer in non-smokers compared to smokers (MI), probably via CYP1A2 induction. There appears no interaction with **aripiprazole** or **zotepine**.

Benzodiazepines + smoking

Benzodiazepine levels are unchanged in smokers.

Bupropion + smoking

See bupropion (*4.6.4*).

Carbamazepine + smoking

No significant interaction.

Fluvoxamine + smoking

Fluvoxamine levels are lower in smokers.

Lithium + smoking

Smoking induces CYP1A2 and caffeine is metabolised by CYP1A2. Theoretically, ceasing smoking could raise xanthine levels, which could increase lithium excretion (as with theophylline), lowering levels.

Memantine + smoking

See memantine (*4.6.7*).

Phenobarbital + smoking

Smoking has been shown not to effect the drowsiness caused by phenobarbital.

Propranolol + smoking

Steady-state propranolol levels may be reduced in smokers, via 1A2 induction.

Tricyclics + smoking

Although serum levels of tricyclics fall in smokers, free levels rise, minimising the clinical significance.

Zolpidem + smoking

See zolpidem (*4.1.5*).

5.
Drug-induced psychiatric disorders

The drugs listed in each section have been reported to cause that condition in some context (eg. standard dose, high dose, prolonged courses etc). The drugs are listed without qualification and no indication of frequency or status of reports can be given as this information is not readily available, except where a side-effect is well recognised. The CSM requests reports of all side-effects of new drugs and severe reactions to established drugs.

Consult your local (psychiatric) hospital pharmacy for more information if required.

5.1 Agitation, anxiety and nervousness

Psychotropics, anticonvulsants etc
Benzodiazepine withdrawal
Bromocriptine
Bupropion
Carbamazepine
Citalopram (a few cases)
Clomethiazole
Clonazepam
Dexamfetamine
Ethosuximide
Fluoxetine (9% incidence)
Gabapentin (inc. withdrawal)
Lamotrigine
Moclobemide (5–10% incidence)
Olanzapine
Paroxetine (11%? incidence)
Phenobarbital and other barbiturates
Risperidone
Rivastigmine
Temazepam
Tricyclics (eg. amitriptyline, lofepramine at
    < 2% incidence)
Valproate
Vigabatrin

Anti-Parkinsonian drugs
Atropine eye drops (case in child)
Levodopa (common)

Gastrointestinal
H2-blockers (rare, *BNF*)
Mesalazine (SPC)
Omeprazole (SPC)

Cardiovascular
Doxazosin (2.4% incidence)
Hydralazine
Methyldopa (rare)
Nicardipine (rare)

NSAIDs and analgesics
Ibuprofen (several cases)
Indometacin (a few cases)
Mefenamic acid
Naproxen
Nefopam
Pentazocine

Miscellaneous
Amantadine (SPC)
Aminophylline
Baclofen
Bismuth intoxication
Botulinum toxin A injection
Caffeine OD
Co-trimoxazole (rare cases)
Dexamethasone and other
    glucocorticoids
Fentanyl transdermal
Flumazenil (SPC)
Flunisolide (SPC)
Ganciclovir
Ginseng
Granisetron (unconfirmed)
Isoniazid
Levamisole (rare)
Levothyroxine/thyroxine
Mefloquine
Misoprostol (SPC).
Morphine
Naltrexone
Neostigmine (rare cases)
Octreotide (SPC)
Phenylephrine (rare)
Phenylpropanolamine OD
Piperazine

Prednisone (especially in children)
Pseudoephedrine (rare cases)
Pyridostigmine (obscure case)
Salbutamol
Sibutramine
Streptokinase
Theophylline
Yohimbine

5.2 Aggression incl. hostility and violence

Alcohol withdrawal
Amantadine (rare cases)
Amphetamine withdrawal
Anabolic steroids
Anabolic steroid withdrawal
Barbiturate withdrawal
Benzodiazepines eg.
   Chlordiazepoxide (increased hostility)
Carbamazepine
Dapsone
Donepezil
Gabapentin
Lamotrigine
Naloxone IV (2 cases)
Olanzapine
Omeprazole (SPC)
Paroxetine withdrawal
Tricyclics (rare)
Vigabatrin

5.3 Behavioural toxicity

Behavioural changes

Anabolic steroids
Barbiturates
Benzodiazepines eg. clonazepam
Bismuth
Carbamazepine
Donepezil
Levodopa
Levodopa + carbidopa
Lithium + neuroleptics
Prednisone withdrawal
Theophylline (disputed)

5.4 Delirium (acute organic psychosis) and confusion

Usually an acute reaction and always with fluctuating levels of awareness of self and environment. Most frequent in the elderly, drug misusers and with pre-existing organic brain disease.

Psychotropics etc

Alcohol + disulfiram
Amfetamines
Anticholinergics
Barbiturates
Benzodiazepines
Bupropion (some cases reported)
Butyrophenones (eg. haloperidol)
Cannabis
Chloral
Clomethiazole
Clozapine
Cocaine
Disulfiram
Donepezil
Fluoxetine
Lithium
MAOIs
Mianserin
Mirtazapine
Paroxetine and benzatropine
Phenelzine
Phenothiazines
Risperidone
Rivastigmine
Solvent intoxication
Trazodone
Tricyclics (especially in the elderly)
Zolpidem

Drug withdrawal

Alcohol cessation
Baclofen withdrawal
Barbiturate withdrawal
Benzodiazepine withdrawal
Clomethiazole withdrawal
Clozapine withdrawal
Dextropoxyphene withdrawal
Nicotine withdrawal

Anticonvulsants

Barbiturates (dose-related)
Carbamazepine (esp. on initiation)
Ethosuximide
Phenytoin (dose-related)
Topiramate
Valproate (high doses)

Anti-parkinsonian drugs

Amantadine

Anticholinergics
Bromocriptine
Levodopa
Lysuride
Methixene
Pergolide withdrawal
Selegiline

Cardiovascular drugs
Amiloride
Amiodarone
Beta-blockers eg. atenolol
Clonidine
Digoxin
Disopyramide
Diuretics (via severe K+ loss)
Hydralazine
Lidocaine
Methyldopa
Mexiletine
Spironolactone

NSAIDs and analgesics
Aspirin toxicity
Fenoprofen
Ibuprofen
Indometacin (inc. overdose)
Nalbuphine
Naproxen
Narcotics
Papaveretum
Sulindac
Tramadol

Anti-infections
May occur indirectly via diarrhoea and
    dehydration.

Acyclovir
Cephalosporins
Chloramphenicol
Chloroquine
Cicloserin
Ciprofloxacin
Clarithromycin
Isoniazid
Mefloquine
Penicillins
Rifampicin
Streptomycin
Sulphadiazine

Miscellaneous
Aminophylline

Baclofen
Caffeine
Cimetidine
Corticosteroids (11% incidence)
Doxapram
Ergotamine
Famotidine
Gancyclovir
Hydroxychloroquine
Hypoglycaemics (oral)
Iodoform gauze
Interferon alpha
Mentholatum
Misoprostol
Nabilone
Nalbuphine
Phenylpropanolamine OD
Piperazine
Ranitidine
Theophylline
Triamcinolone

5.5 Depression
Occurs mainly in patients with a history of
depression.

Psychotropics etc
Benzodiazepines (especially resistant dep-
    ression) eg: alprazolam, bromazepam,
    lorazepam
Benzodiazepine withdrawal
Buspirone (3% incidence?)
Disulfiram (rare cases)
Flumazenil (< 1% incidence, SPC)
Fluoxetine (intense suicidal ideation -
    disproven)
Fluphenazine depot (cases)
MDMA ('Ecstasy')
Nortriptyline
Smoking cessation, especially if person has
    previously had depression
SSRIs (no association with suicidal beha-
    viour — *Curr Prob* 2000, **26**, 11–12)
Tetrabenazine
Zuclopentixol

Anticonvulsants
Carbamazepine
Clobazam
Clonazepam
Ethosuximide
Lamotrigine (rare)

Levetiracetam
Phenobarbital
Topiramate
Vigabatrin (< 10% incidence)

Anti-parkinsonian drugs
Amantadine
Anticholinergics
Levodopa (well known)

Cardiovascular drugs
Amiodarone (a few cases)
Beta-blockers lipophilic drugs may be more likely: atenolol, nadolol (low lipid solubility), labetalol, oxprenolol, timolol, acebutol (low/moderate), pindolol (moderate), metoprolol (moderate/high), propranolol (high).
Calcium-channel blockers (no increase in risk of suicide compared to other antihypertensives)
Diltiazem
Felodipine
Nicardipine (some cases)
Nifedipine
Clonidine (1% incidence)
Enalapril (rare case)
Hydralazine
Inositol
Lisinopril (rare, SPC)
Methyldopa
Prazosin
Procainamide
Quinapril
Quinidine (several cases)
Streptokinase (some cases)

Gastrointestinal
H2-blockers (*BNF*)
Metoclopramide
PPIs (*BNF*)
Sulphasalazine (SPC)

NSAIDs and analgesics
Diflunisal (<1% incidence, SPC)
Etodolac (rare, SPC)
Flurbiprofen (>1% incidence?, SPC)
Ibuprofen (uncommon)
Indometacin (4% incidence?)
Nabilone
Nalbuphine
Naproxen (rare)
Pentazocine
Sulindac
Tramadol

Anti-infection
Anti-TB drugs
Cefradine (rare case)
Chloramphenicol (rare mild cases)
Ciprofloxacin (very rare)
Clotrimazole – oral
Co-trimoxazole (rare but severe cases)
Dapsone
Griseofulvin (as part of psychosis)
Mefloquine
Metronidazole (rare cases)
Piperazine (some cases)
Primaquine (rare cases)
Sulphonamides

Respiratory
Aminophylline
Ephedrine (as part of a psychosis)
Flunisolide (inhaled, 1–3% incidence, SPC)
Theophylline

Cytotoxics etc
Interferon alfa
Mesna
Octreotide (rare, SPC)
Tamoxifen — **no** increased risk of depression
Triamcinolone (up to 8%)

Steroids
Dexamethasone (up to 40% incidence)
Methyltestosterone (rare)
Prednisolone
Prednisone
Stanozolol

Miscellaneous
Allopurinol
Astemizole (debatable)
Baclofen (rare cases)
Botulinum toxin A injection
Caffeine withdrawal
Cinnarizine
Clomifene
Codeine use (long-term)
Danazol (rare cases)
Diphenoxylate (SPC)
Ethinylestradiol (UK SPC)
Etretinate
Fentanyl (transdermal)

Hydroxyzine (some reports)
Isotretinoin (very rare)
Ondansetron
Oral contraceptives, combined (16–56% incidence)
Organophosphates
Phenylpropanolamine
Progestogens
Roaccutane
Simvastatin (low cholesterol may be a risk factor for attempted suicide)
Trimeprazine/alimemazine
Xylometazoline (case in child)

5.6 Hallucinations (including visual disturbances)

Psychotropics etc
Alcohol
Amfetamines
Benzodiazepines
Carbamazepine
Fluoxetine (rare cases)
Gabapentin
Imipramine
LSD
Maprotiline
Methadone
Midazolam IV
Phenelzine
Tricyclics
Valproate
Zolpidem
Zopiclone

Anti-parkinson drugs
Amantadine (rare cases)
Anticholinergics
Bromocriptine (< 1% incidence)
Levodopa (< 26% incidence in elderly)
Pergolide (in up to 13%)
Pergolide withdrawal

Cardiovascular drugs
Beta-blockers
Clonidine (3 cases)
Digoxin
Diltiazem
Disopyramide
Procainamide
Streptokinase (rare reports)
Timolol

NSAIDs and analgesics
Buprenorphine (rare, < 1%)
Celecoxib (case)
Fenbufen
Indometacin (rare)
Nefopam
Oxycodone
Pentazocine
Salicylates
Tramadol

Anti-infections
Amoxicillin
Ciprofloxacin
Gentamicin
Itraconazole (one case)

Miscellaneous
Corticosteroids
Decongestants
Dextromethorphan
Erythropoetin (5 cases)
Ginseng
H2-blockers (*BNF*)
Ketamine
Khat chewing
Mefloquine
Phenylephrine
Phenylpropanolamine
Promethazine
Pseudoephedrine
Radio contrast media
Salbutamol (nebulised)
Sulphasalazine
Tolterodine

5.7 Mania, hypomania or euphoria

The most common symptoms of drug-induced mania are increased activity, rapid speech, elevated mood and insomnia. The main risks are prior history, family history or concurrent mood disorder. Steroids, levodopa, triazolobenzodiazepines and hallucinogens are most commonly associated.

Hallucinogens
LSD

CNS stimulants
Amfetamine withdrawal

Dexamfetamine
Ephedrine
Methylphenidate
Phenylephrine
Phenylpropanolamine
Pseudoephedrine

Antidepressants

Induction of hypomania by antidepressants is well known, as is the spontaneous swing to hypomania from depression in bipolars.

Amitriptyline
Amitriptyline withdrawal
Bupropion
Citalopram + sibutramine
Clomipramine
Fluoxetine
Flupentixol
Fluvoxamine
Imipramine
Imipramine withdrawal
Isocarboxazid (3 cases)
Isocarboxazid withdrawal (2 cases)
Maprotiline (some cases)
Mianserin
Mirtazapine
Mirtazapine withdrawal
Paroxetine
Phenelzine
Quetiapine
Reboxetine
Sertraline (some cases)
St. John's wort
Trazodone
Trazodone withdrawal
Tryptophan + MAOI
Venlafaxine

Other psychotropics etc

Alprazolam
Benzodiazepine withdrawal
Bupropion
Buspirone
Disulfiram
Lithium + tricyclic
Lithium toxicity
Lorazepam withdrawal
Midazolam (euphoria possible)
Olanzapine (some documented cases)
Risperidone (some documented cases)
Risperidone withdrawal

Anticonvulsants

Carbamazepine
Carbamazepine withdrawal
Clonazepam
Ethosuximide (SPC)
Gabapentin
Phenobarbital
Topiramate
Valproate
Vigabatrin

Anti-Parkinsonian drugs

Amantadine (some cases)
Bromocriptine
Levodopa (some cases)
Levodopa + carbidopa (Madopar)
Procyclidine

Cardiovascular drugs

Captopril (a few cases)
Clonidine
Clonidine withdrawal
Digoxin
Diltiazem
Hydralazine
Methyldopa withdrawal
Procainamide
Propranolol
Propranolol withdrawal

NSAIDs and analgesics

Buprenorphine (up to 1%)
Codeine + paracetamol
Indometacin
Nefopam IM (euphoria reported)
Pentazocine

Gastrointestinal

Cimetidine
Metoclopramide (one case)
Ranitidine IV (one case)

Steroids

ACTH
Beclomethasone aerosol
Beclomethasone nasal spray
Corticosteroids
Cortisone
Dexamethasone (up to 31% incidence)
Hydrocortisone
Prednisone
Testosterone patches
Triamcinolone (rare cases)

Anti-infection
Anti-TB drugs
Chloroquine
Clarithromycin
Dapsone
Efavirez overdose (case)
Isoniazid
Mepacrine
Zudovudine

Miscellaneous
Alimemazine/trimeprazine
Aminophylline
Baclofen
Baclofen withdrawal
Calcium IV
Ciclosporin
Cyclizine (SPC)
Cyproheptadine (rare)
Decongestants
Dextromethorphan abuse
Ginseng
Herbal remidies
Interferon-alpha
Levothyroxine/thyroxine
Nicotine withdrawal
Omega-3 fatty acids
Procarbazine
Salbutamol
Silbutramine+citalopram (case)
Tramadol (one case)
Triiodothyronine
Triptorelin (one case)
Yohimbine?

5.8 Movement disorders

5.8.1 Extra-pyramidal disorders
Four distinct types of drug-induced extra-pyramidal disorders are common, especially by antipsychotics. These are the acute onset dystonias, akathisias and pseudoparkinsonism, and the later onset tardive dyskinesia. The majority are reversible on discontinuation of the drug or on dose reduction.

5.8.1.1 Pseudoparkinsonism
Characterised by akinesia, tremor and rigidity, generally occurring within a month of the start of treatment.

Psychotropics etc
Amoxapine
Antipsychotics (see *2.1.4*)
Bromocriptine
Bupropion
Clozapine
Cocaine abuse
Dexamfetamine
Donepezil
Fluoxetine (many cases)
Fluoxetine withdrawal
Fluvoxamine
Lithium (long and short-term)
MAOIs
Olanzapine overdose
Paroxetine (cases reported)
Prochlorperazine
Risperidone (a few cases)
Rivastigmine (SPC)
Sertraline (cases)
Trazodone
Tricyclics

Anticonvulsants
Carbamazepine (in up to 20%?)
Lamotrigine (SPC)
Valproate

NSAIDs and analgesics
Fenoprofen
Flurbiprofen
Ibuprofen
Indometacin
Mefenamic acid (single case)
Nabilone
Pethidine & other opioids
Sulindac (single case)

Cardiovascular drugs
Amiodarone
Diazoxide (6 cases)
Diltiazem
Metirosine
Mexiletine
Nifedipine
Tocainide

Gastrointestinal
Cimetidine (possible cases)
Domperidone (rare)
Metoclopramide (2–30% incidence)
Prochlorperazine (common)

Anti-infection
Aciclovir
Cephaloridine
Chloroquine

Respiratory drugs
Brompheniramine
Cinnarizine
Diphenhydramine
Orciprenaline
Promethazine
Salbutamol
Terbutaline

Hormones
Medroxyprogesterone

Cytotoxics
Ciclosporin
Interferons

Miscellaneous
Cyclizine
Levodopa
Ondansetron (rare cases)
Prednisolone (increases incidence with neuroleptics)
Tetrabenazine

5.8.1.2 Akathisia
Characterised by restlessness, it can occur early or later on in treatment and has been implicated with all antipsychotics, but especially with the high potency ones.

Psychotropics etc
Antipsychotics (trifluoperazine and haloperidol more likely than less potent drugs, eg. chlorpromazine or thioridazine)
Alimemazine/trimeprazine (SPC)
Alprazolam (SPC)
Buspirone (rare cases)
Citalopram (cases)
Clozapine (6% incidence?)
Fluoxetine
Fluvoxamine
Haloperidol
Imipramine (cases)
Lithium
Lorazepam (cases)
Mianserin

Mirtazapine
Olanzapine
Paroxetine
Pipothiazine
Prochlorperazine
Promazine (SPC)
Risperidone
Risperidone withdrawal (few cases)
Sertraline (rare cases)
Tricyclics
Venlafaxine withdrawal
Zuclopentixol

Others
Diltiazem (case)
Interferon-alpha
Levodopa
Melatonin withdrawal
Metoclopramide (case)
Ondansetron (rare cases)
Prochlorperazine
Verapamil

5.8.1.3 Dystonias
Includes oculogyric crisis, trismus and torticollis. May occur within 72 hours of start of therapy. Occurs more frequently with high-potency antipsychotics, where the incidence may be as high as 10%.

Psychotropics etc
Amoxapine
Benzatropine (cases)
Bupropion (case)
Buspirone (possible cases)
Carbamazepine (cases)
Clozapine (rare)
Clozapine withdrawal
Cocaine
Cocaine withdrawal
Disulfiram (cases)
Fluoxetine
Flupentixol decanoate (cases)
Loxapine (SPC)
Midazolam
Mirtazapine
Olanzapine (case)
Paroxetine
Phenelzine (cases)
Risperidone (several cases)
Sertraline (SPC)

Tiagabine
Tricyclics
Venlafaxine (SPC)
Zuclopentixol

Others

Alimemazine/trimeprazine (SPC)
Amiodarone (isolated case)
Azapropazone (rare cases)
Diphenhydramine
Domperidone
Ergotamine
Indometacin (rare cases)
Metoclopramide (3% incidence)
Nifedipine
Penicillamine
Prochlorperazine (many cases)
Promethazine (case)
Propranolol
Sumatriptan (case)
Verapamil

5.8.1.4 Tardive dyskinesia

TD is a potentially irreversible EPSE with some relationship to drug, dose and duration (see separate section).
Amoxapine
Bupropion
Buspirone?
Clomipramine
Cocaine (case)
Diphenhydramine (cases)
Donepezil (case)
Doxepin (10% incidence)
Fluoxetine
Fluoxetine + low dose neuroleptics
Fluvoxamine
Gabapentin
Lithium?
Metoclopramide (*BNF*)
Neuroleptics eg:
    Clozapine (case)
    Clozapine withdrawal
    Flupentixol decanoate
    Haloperidol (many cases)
    Olanzapine
    Pimozide (35% incidence reported)
    Quetiapine (cases)
    Risperidone (many cases)
    Sulpiride
Phenytoin
Venlafaxine

5.8.2 Other movement disorders

5.8.2.1 Catatonia

Allopurinol (case)
Baclofen (cases)
Benzodiazepine withdrawal (cases)
Bupropion (case)
Cicloserin
Cocaine
Disulfiram
Fluphenazine (rare case)
Morphine epidural
Phenelzine + haloperidol (case)
Piperazine
Prochlorperazine (cases)

5.8.2.2 Choreas

Psychotropics etc
Amoxapine
Amfetamines (chronic abuse)
Anticonvulsants (see also phenytoin)
Antipsychotics eg:
    Chlorpromazine (cases)
    Haloperidol (many cases)
    Risperidone (case)
    Sulpiride (cases)
Benzhexol/trihexyphenidyl
Cocaine (cases)
Donepezil (case)
Fluoxetine
Lamotrigine + phenytoin
Methadone
Methylphenidate
Mianserin (cases)
Paroxetine
Phenytoin
Valproate

Others

Anabolic steroids
Cimetidine (possible case)
Cyclizine (cases)
Dienestrol (SPC)
Metoclopramide
Oral contraceptives (cases)
Ranitidine

5.8.2.3 Tics (inc. Tourette's Syndrome)

Amfetamines
Androgenic steroids (eg. stanozolol, methandrostenolol, testosterone)

Carbamazepine
Clozapine (case)
Cocaine (cases)
Dexamfetamine
Fluoxetine (cases)
Haloperidol
Lamotrigine (cases)
Methylphenidate
Ofloxacin (case)
Risperidone withdrawal
Thioridazine (case with methylphenidate)

5.9 Neuroleptic malignant syndrome

See *1.21* for treatments.

Antidepressants

Amoxapine (possible cases)
Clomipramine (SPC)
Phenelzine (many cases)
Trimipramine (rare cases)

Antipsychotics

Clozapine (rare)
Chlorpromazine
Flupentixol (possible case)
Fluphenazine
Haloperidol (many cases)
Loxapine
Olanzapine (many cases)
Promazine
Quetiapine (cases)
Risperidone (many cases)
Thioridazine (several cases)
Zuclopentixol (cases)

Others

Alimemazine/trimeprazine
Amantadine
Amantadine withdrawal
Anticholinergic withdrawal
Carbamazepine (may also complicate symptoms)
Carbamazepine withdrawal
Ganciclovir
Iron (low levels)
Levodopa
Levodopa withdrawal (3 cases)
Lithium (possible cases)
Methylphenidate
Metoclopramide (several cases)
Oral contraceptives (possible case)

5.10 OCD (Obsessive compulsive disorder)

See *1.21* for treatments.
Clozapine (several cases)
Gabapentin withdrawal (case)
Methylamphetamine (cases)
Olanzapine (rare cases)
Risperidone (dose-dependent)
Stimulants (case)

5.11 Panic disorders

See *1.22* for treatments.

Psychotropics

Alprazolam
Amfetamines (cases)
Buspirone (case)
Cannabis (case)
Citalopram (case)
Clobazam withdrawal
Cocaine
Flumazenil
Fluoxetine (unless initial doses kept low)
Fluoxetine + bupropion
Naltrexone
Olanzapine (case)
Topiramate (case)
Trazodone

Others

Aspartame?
Carvedilol (case)
Co-trimoxazole
Lactate (oral, case)
Oxymetazoline abuse
Phenylephrine
Sibutramine
Smoking cessation (cases)
Steroids
Sumatriptan (7% incidence?)
Yohimbine

5.12 Paranoid or schizophrenic-like psychoses

Characterised by paranoid delusions and hallucinations in a person with little clouding of consciousness.

Hallucinogens (major cause)

Cannabis (at higher doses is a risk factor for the development or relapse of

schizophrenia, acute onset, usually
resolves in 2–7 days)
Dimethoxy-methylamphetamine (DOM)
Lysergic acid diethylamide (LSD)
Khat chewing
Mescaline
MDMA/Ecstasy
Petrol
Phencyclidine (angel dust)
Psilocybin (magic mushrooms)
Volatiles

CNS stimulants (major cause)
Amfetamines
Cocaine
Ephedrine
Methylamphetamine
Phenylephrine
Phenylpropanolamine
Pseudoephedrine (many cases)
Solvent abuse

CNS depressants
Alcohol
Antihistamines
Barbiturates
Benzodiazepines:
  Alprazolam
  Lorazepam
  Midazolam
  Triazolam
Benzodiazepine withdrawal
Bromides
Bupropion (many cases)
Buspirone
Chloral
Chlorpromazine (rare case)
Clozapine withdrawal (ie. rebound
  psychosis)
Codeine OD (cases)
Disulfiram (cases)
Fluoxetine
Fluvoxamine (case)
Haloperidol
Imipramine
Methadone withdrawal
Modafinil (case)
Morphine (rare)
Paroxetine
Phenelzine
Promethazine (rare but possible)
Zolpidem

Zopiclone (some cases reported)

Anticonvulsants
Carbamazepine toxicity
Clonazepam (rare cases)
Ethosuximide
Gabapentin
Phenytoin
Tiagabine (cases)
Topiramate
Valproate (isolated cases)
Vigabatrin (2% incidence)
Vigabatrin withdrawal

**Anti-parkinsonian drugs
(excess DA)**
Amantadine
Anticholinergic withdrawal
Benzhexol/trihexyphenidyl
Bromocriptine (< 1% chance)
Levodopa (especially hallucinations)
Lisuride (a few cases)
Pergolide (especially hallucinations, in up
  to 13%)
Selegiline (a few cases)

NSAIDs and analgesics
Aspirin
Ibuprofen ?
Indometacin (rare)
Pentazocine (especially hallucinations)
Sulindac

Cardiovascular drugs
Amyl nitrate
Beta-blockers (see under depression for
  differentials) eg:
Atenolol (rare cases)
Propranolol (well known)
Clonidine (rare case)
Clonidine withdrawal
Digoxin toxicity (rare)
Diltiazem (cases)
Disopyramide (isolated cases)
Doxazosin (rare cases)
Enalapril (rare cases)
Hydralazine
Lidocaine IV (6 cases)
Methyldopa
Mexiletine (case)
Nifedipine (possible case)
Procainamide
Tocainide

Anti-infection
Amphotericin B IV (case)
Antituberculous drugs
Cefuroxime
Cefalexin (cases)
Chloroquine (cases)
Ciprofloxacin (cases)
Clarithromycin (cases)
Colistin (especially with large doses)
Dapsone
Erythromycin
Ganciclovir
Isoniazid (rare)
Ketoconazole
Mefloquine (many cases)
Metronidazole
Nalidixic acid (many cases)
Primaquine (cases)
Procaine Penicillin G (several cases)
Sulphonamides
Tobramycin (a few cases)

Steroids
Adrenocorticotrophin
Clomiphene
Cortisone
Methylprednisolone
Methyltestosterone
Prednisone (usually > 40 mg/d)
Triamcinolone (possible but no specific
    reports)

Miscellaneous
Anti-diarrhoeals (OTC)
Atropine (oral, IV, eye drops. Many cases)
Baclofen
Carbaryl (case)
Carbimazole
Chlorphenamine OD (cases)
Cimetidine
Desmopressin (cases)
Dextromethorphan (case)
Dicyclomine (SPC)
Diphenhydramine
Disulfiram
Estrogen withdrawal (cases)
Hyoscine-transdermal
Insulin abuse
Interferon alpha
Isotretoin (case)
Lactate oral (eg. in calcium lactate)
Lariam (rare but can be severe)

Melatonin
Nabilone
Nicotine abrupt withdrawal
Oxymetazoline (several cases)
Phenylephrine
Phenylpropanolamine
Pyridostigmine (case)
Quinine
Quinidine
Salbutamol
Scopolamine (transdermal)
Sibutramine
Yohimbine?

5.13 Seizures
These are rare at normal doses and occur
mostly where seizure threshold is reduced,
in at-risk patients or in overdose. The list
of drugs which could induce seizures is
enormous and so a literature search would
be needed to clarify the current situation
for any one drug.

Psychotropics etc
Alcohol
Amitriptyline
Amoxapine
Bupropion (CSM warning)
Citalopram (case)
Clozapine (especially above 600 mg/d. May
    be due to hyponatraemia)
Donepezil
Fluoxetine (cases)
Fluvoxamine (case)
Imipramine
Levomepromazine
Lithium
MAOIs
Maprotiline (esp. in higher dose)
Mianserin
Neuroleptics (esp. phenothiazines)
Olanzapine (cases, including one fatal)
Sertraline (case)
Venlafaxine overdose
Zolpidem

Drug withdrawal
Alcohol?
Anticonvulsants (ie. non- compliance)
Barbiturates
Benzodiazepines eg. alprazolam

Carbamazepine
Zolpidem (case)

CNS stimulants
Cocaine
Ephedrine

Anticonvulsants
Carbamazepine (case)
Carbamazepine overdose (cases)
Ethosuximide
Phenobarbital
Phenytoin
Tiagabine (cases)
Valproate

NSAIDs and analgesics
Dextropoxyphene
Fentanyl
Indometacin (rare)
Mefenamic acid
Penicillamine
Pentazocine
Pethidine
Salicylate overdose
Sulindac
Tramadol (rare, but cases)

Cardiovascular drugs
Beta-blockers, eg:
    Oxprenolol
    Propranolol
Digoxin toxicity (rare)
Disopyramide
Enoximone infusion
Lidocaine
Metolazone
Mexiletine
Thiazides
Tocainide

Anti-infection
Ampicillin?
Benzylpenicillin
Carbenicillin
Cefazolin
Ceftazidime
Cefalexin (cases)
Cefalosporins (high dose in renal failure)
Chloroquine
Ciprofloxacin
Gentamicin
Imipenem

Isoniazid
Mefloquine
Metronidazole
Nalidixic Acid
Niridazole
Ofloxacin (cases)
Penicillins
Piperazine
Piperacillin
Pyrimethamine
Zudovudine

Respiratory drugs
Aminophylline
Doxapram
Phenylpropanolamine
Terbutaline
Theophylline
Theophylline toxicity

Hormones
Glucocorticoids
Insulin
Oral contraceptives (exacerbate
    pre-existing)
Oxytocin
Prostaglandins

Cytotoxics
Alprostadil
Busulfan
Chlorambucil
Ciclosporin
Cisplatin
Methotrexate
Vinblastine
Vincristine

Anaesthetics
Alfentanil
Enflurane
Ether
Halothane
Ketamine
Local anaesthetics:
    Bupivacaine
    Lidocaine
    Etidocaine
    Procaine
Propofol (many cases, can be delayed by
    up to 6 days)
Propofol withdrawal

Miscellaneous
Allopurinol withdrawal
Aluminium toxicity?
Amantadine?
Baclofen withdrawal
Caffeine
Camphor
Clomiphene (case)
Colchicine OD
Cyclopentolate eye drops
Diphenhydramine
Diptheria-tetanus-pertussis vaccine
Flumazenil
Fluorescin IV
Ginkgo biloba (anecdotal)
Hepatitis B vaccine
Interferon (case)
Ketamine
Ketotifen (cases)
Levodopa
Levothyroxine/thyroxine
Lindane, topical
Measles/mumps/rubella vaccine
Naftidrofuryl
Naloxone (rare)
Ondansetron
Pertussis vaccine
Phenylpropanolamine
Pyridoxine (cases)
Pyrimethamine
Radiographic contrast media (eg. metrizamide)
Sodium bicarbonate
Steroids, eg:
    Dexamethasone
    Hydrocortisone
    Prednisolone
Sulphasalazine
Sulphonylureas
Yohimbine (unproven)

5.14 Serotonin syndrome

Individual drugs
Amitriptyline (case)
Clomipramine (many cases)
Citalopram (even low dose)
Dothiepin/dosulepin overdose
Ecstasy
Fluoxetine (cases)
Fluvoxamine (cases)
Mirtazapine (isolated case)

Paroxetine (cases)
Sertraline (even low dose, and overdose)
Trazodone (cases)
Venlafaxine (cases, plus in overdose)

Combinations
There are many listed cases of serotonin syndrome with a combination of two or more of the following:

SSRIs (citalopram, escitalopram, fluoxetine, fluvoxamine, paroxetine, sertraline) *plus:* buspirone, carbamazepine, dolasetron, erythromycin, linezolid, lithium, loxapine, MAOIs, mirtazapine, moclobemide, OTC cold remedies, Parstelin, risperidone, tramadol, tricyclics or venlafaxine.

MAOIs (isocarboxazid, tranylcypromine and phenelzine) *plus:* tricyclics, dextromethorphan or venlafaxine

Combinations of any two or more of the above, plus dexamphetamine, metoclopramide, olanzapine, pethidine, selegiline or St. John's wort.

5.15 Sleep problems

5.15.1 Sleep disturbances

Psychotropics etc
Benperidol
Bupropion (11% incidence)
Chlorpromazine
Donepezil (cases)
Fluoxetine
Fluspirilene
Lamotrigine (dose-related)
Levetiracetam
Lorazepam
MAOIs
Methylphenidate
Phenytoin
Rivastigmine (< 5% incidence)
SSRIs (somnambulism and may disturb sleep architecture)
Sulpiride
Trazodone
Tricyclics

Anti-parkinsonian drugs
Amantadine (4% incidence)
Bromocriptine
Pramipexole (cases)
Ropinirole

Cardiovascular drugs

Amiodarone (frequent)
Beta-blockers (very common especially with propranolol, plus atenolol and carvedilol)
Clonidine
Digoxin
Diltiazem
Isradipine (up to 3%)
Nifedipine

NSAIDs and analgesics

Diclofenac
Diflunisal
Fenoprofen
Indometacin
Naproxen
Nefopam
Sulindac

Respiratory drugs

Aminophylline
Brompheniramine
Pseudoephedrine
Theophylline

Anti-infection

Cinoxacin
Ciprofloxacin (case)

Miscellaneous

Bismuth toxicity

Clomifene
Dexamethasone
Ginseng
Lovastatin (case)
Nicotine (many cases)
Propantheline
Ranitidine
Sibutramine
Simvastatin
Sulphasalazine
Tolazamide
Triamcinolone

5.15.2 Vivid dreams and nightmares

Antihypertensives (eg. methyldopa, clonidine)
Baclofen
Beta-blockers (esp. atenolol, propranolol)
Digoxin toxicity
Famotidine (case)
Indometacin (rare)
Nalbumetone
Pergolide
Nicotine patches
Stanozolol (SPC)
Verapamil
Withdrawal from barbiturates, benzodiazepines, narcotics etc

6.
Other useful information

6.1 Fitness to drive

It is against the law to drive, attempt to drive or be in charge of a vehicle when unfit, either through illness or from the side effects of medication. Under UK law, it is the drivers responsibility to let the DVLA and insurance company know they may be "unfit" to drive. If they do not, and have an accident, it could effect their insurance cover.

Doctors should advise patients accordingly. For up-to-date advice, you may wish to access the UK Driver and Vehicle Licensing Agency (DVLA) guidelines website (see below), which has the current guidance on anxiety, depression, psychotic disorders, mania, epilepsy and other conditions.

Confidentiality

If you advise a patient not to drive, and they continue to do so, a doctor can inform the DVLA directly, as he or she could be lawfully responsible were the patient to have an accident.

To quote from the website "When a patient has a condition which makes driving unsafe and the patient is either unable to appreciate this, or refuses to cease driving, GMC guidelines advise breaking confidentiality and informing DVLA. [GMC Confidentiality Handbook]".

Once told, the DVLA may wish to carry out an enquiry, but the person may be entitled to drive until a decision is made.

The DVLA website to consult is:

www.dvla.gov.uk/at_a_glance/content.htm

Index

All the main psychotropic drugs are indexed according to their BNF or other main indications in chapter one, but obviously may appear elsewhere. In order to keep the index down to a manageable size, you are then referred to the index listing for that drugs chemical or therapeutic group. Individual drugs should be looked up under their drug group.

Abbreviations used

AAPCD = American Academy of Pediatrics Committee on Drugs
ACh = Acetylcholine
ADHD = Attention Deficit Hyperactivity Disorder
ADD = Attention Deficit Disorder
ADR = Adverse Drug Reaction
AFP = alpha-fetoprotein
AIMS = Abnormal Involuntary Movement Scale
APE = Acute psychiatric emergency
APA = American Psychiatric Association
AWS = Alcohol withdrawal syndrome

BDZ = Benzodiazepine(s)
BMA = British medical Association
BNF = British National Formulary
BPD = Borderline Personality Disorder
BPRS = Brief Psychiatric Rating Scale
bp = Blood pressure
BP = British Pharmacopoeia

CBZ = Carbamazepine
CGI = Clinical Global Impression
CNS = Central nervous system
CPZ = Chlorpromazine
CSM = Committee on the Safety of Medicines
CVA = Cardiovascular accident

D1 = Dopamine-1 (receptor)
D2 = Dopamine-2 (receptor)
DA = Dopamine
d/b = double-blind

DSM-III-R = Diagnostic Statistical Manual III (Revised)
DT = Delirium Tremens

e/c = enteric-coated
ECG = Electrocardiogram
ECT = Electroconvulsive therapy
EEG = Electroencephalogram
EMS = Eosinophilia-myalgia syndrome
EPSE = extra-pyramidal side effects

FBC = Full blood count

GABA = Gamma-amino-butyric acid
G/I = Gastro-intestinal
GFR = Glomerular filtration rate
GTC = Generalised tonic-clonic (seizure)

5-HT = 5-hydroxytryptamine
HD = High dose

IV = Intra-venous
IM = Intra-muscular
ISE = Ion-selective electrode

L/A = Long-acting
LD = Low dose
LFT = Liver function tests

MAOI = Mono-amine oxidase inhibitor
MHA = Mental Health Act (1983)

NA = Noradrenaline
N/K = Not known
NMS = Neuroleptic malignant syndrome

OCD = Obsessive-compulsive disorder
O/C = Oral contraceptive
OD = Overdose

OTC = Over-the-counter (medicine)
PD = Personality Disorder, Parkinson's Disease, Pro-drug
PG = Prostaglandin
PMH = Previous medical history
PMS = Pre-menstrual syndrome
pt = patient
PTSD = Post-traumatic stress disorder

REM = Rapid eye movement
RIMA = Reversible Inhibitor of Monoamine-A
RPSGB = Royal Pharmaceutical Society of Great Britain
RT = Rapid tranquillisation

SA = Short-acting
s/c = Sub-cutaneous
SF = Sugar-free
SIB = Self-injurious behaviour
SPC = Summary of Product Characteristics
SSRI = Serotonin-selective reuptake inhibitor

t1/2 = Half-life
TCA = Tricyclic anti-depressant
TD = Tardive dyskinesia
TDM = Therapeutic drug monitoring

U&E = Urea and electrolytes
UKPPG = United Kingdom Psychiatric Pharmacy Group
USP = United States Pharmacopoeia

Wt = Weight

yo = Year old

the complete guide to
Thailand

WITH COMPLIMENTS

C F W

COMPLIMENTARY | REVIEW

CFW GUIDEBOOKS
Hong Kong

CFW Guidebooks
Published by CFW Publications Limited
130 Connaught Road C Hong Kong

© CFW Publications Limited, 1981
Printed in Hong Kong

PHOTO CREDITS
Alain Evrard: Pages 33, 79
John Everingham: Pages 41, 42 (lower), 42/43, 84 (lower), 85 (top
right), 85 (lower), 86, 87 (lower), 88/89, 100, 100/101, 104/105.
Robin Moyer: Page 91.

ISBN 962 7031 04 6

the complete guide to
Thailand

by Juliellen Leyman

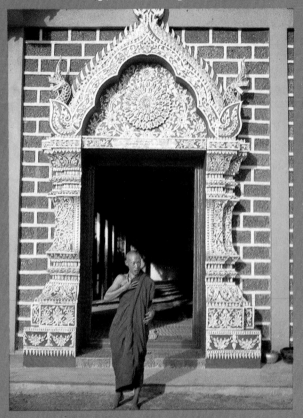

Photography: Dean Barrett

CFW GUIDEBOOKS
Hong Kong

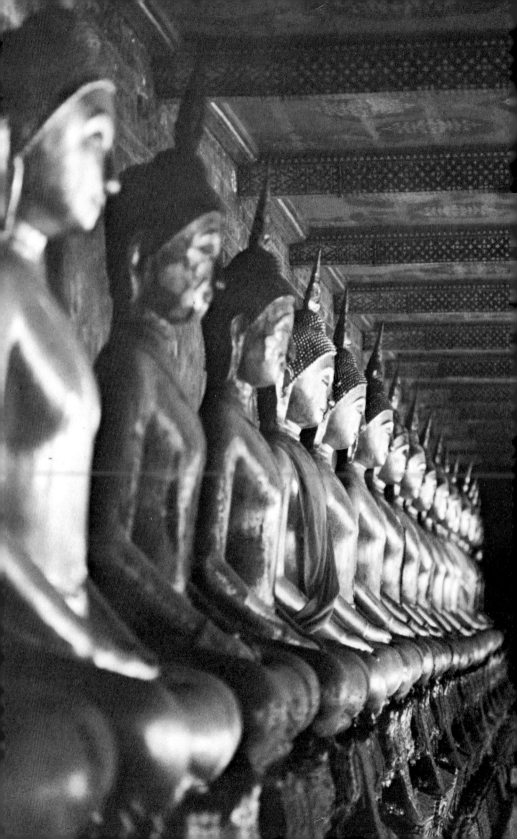

Contents

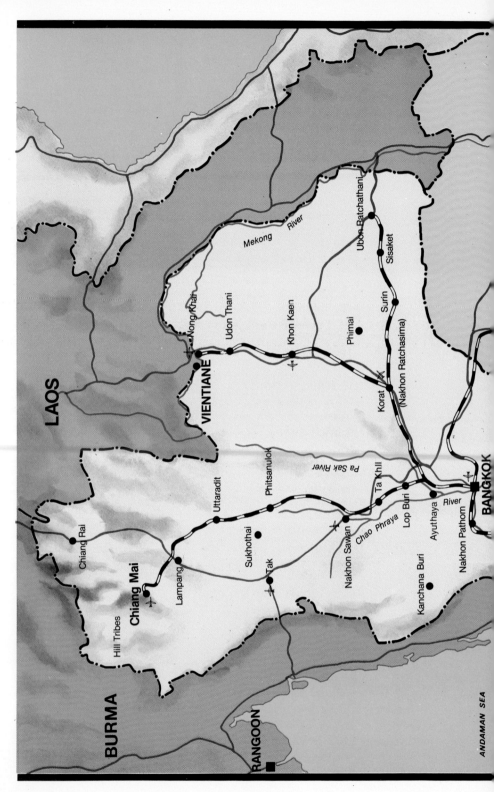

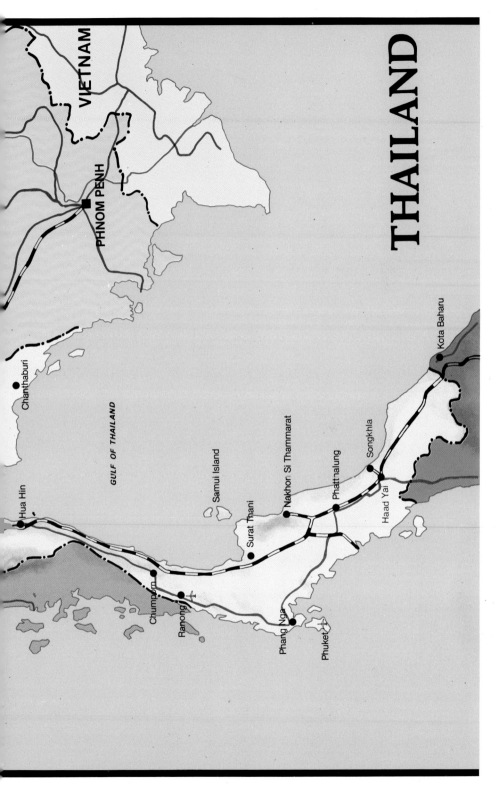

THAILAND

VIETNAM

PHNOM PENH

Kota Baharu

Chanthaburi

GULF OF THAILAND

Samui Island

Nakhon Si Thammarat

Phatthalung

Songkhla

Hua Hin

Surat Thani

Haad Yai

Chumporn

Ranong

Phang Nga

Phuket

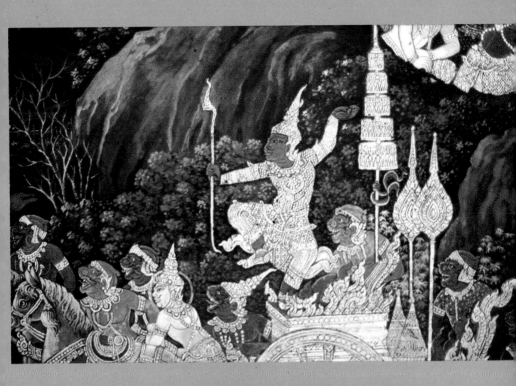

Siamese Heritage
The Physical and Historical Thailand

The Origins

Thailand as an independent nation has been moulded by over seven hundred years of social, cultural and economic conflict and triumph. From Siam's emergence as a unified kingdom in the 13th century, wise and imaginative rulers fostered the development of a strong national identity. A distinctively "Thai character" grew from the blending of a diversity of ethnic structures and a unique culture that is seen in language, beliefs, customs, food and artistic expression. Shrewd international diplomacy, a harmony of religion, and rich natural resources at a strategic location at the heart of Southeast Asia have all contributed to Thailand's remarkable success in maintaining her tradition as "Land of the Free."

The origins of the Thai people are clouded by myth and conjecture, but it is generally believed that the earliest Thais migrated from the Nanchao kingdom in southern China in the 11th century, seeking fertile lands and escape from the oppression of overlords.

Culturally-important groups were already well established. The *Khmers* and *Mons*, also from southern China, had arrived around the first century BC and were both to have an immense influence on the development of Thai culture. The Mons had established a strong seat of power at **Lopburi**, adopting Buddhism as a complement to the Brahmanism already practiced there, and the Khmers had settled deep into the area that is present-day Kampuchea (Cambodia), setting up magnificent cities under the control of Angkor, the empire's capital.

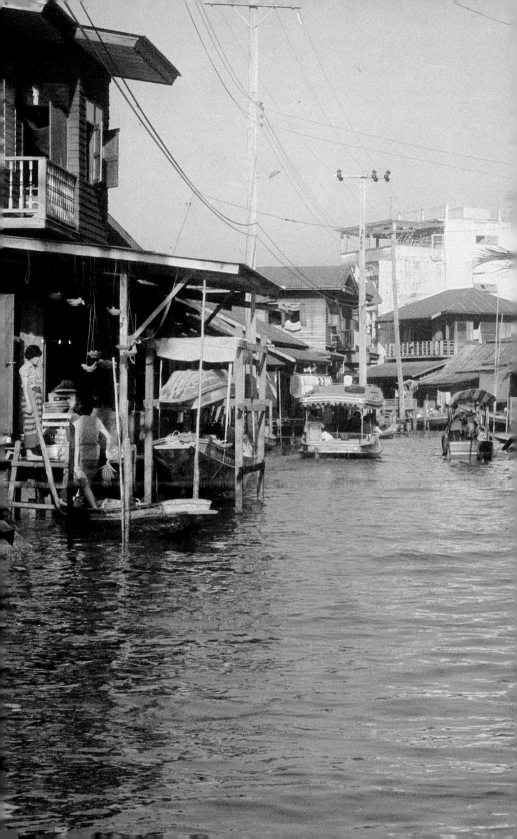

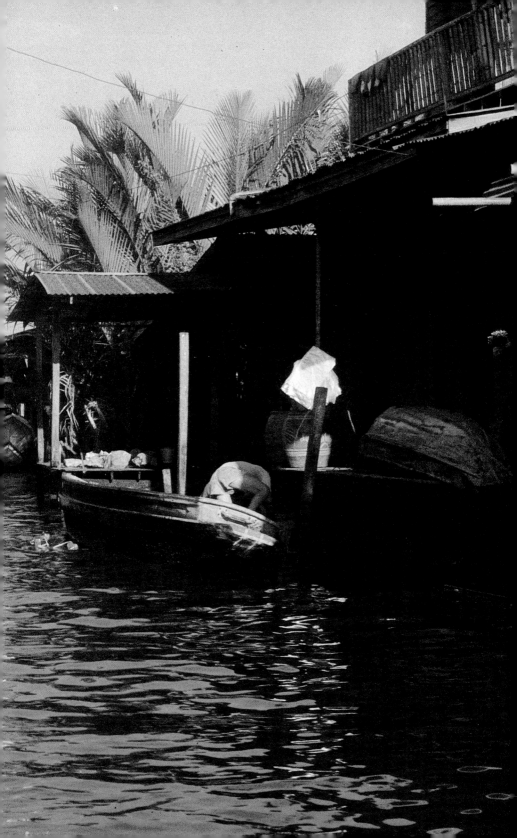

By the 13th century, many Thai settlements had a firm foothold on the fertile lands of the **Chao Phya River** basin, but each was powerless to defy the supremacy of the Khmers. The true beginning of Siam as an independent kingdom was in 1238 when the heads of two Thai "states" combined forces and defeated the local Khmer stronghold. Thus *Sukhothai*, the "dawn of Happiness," began — an era that was to last just 200 years but to have a tremendous cultural impact on the centuries to follow.

The third king, Ramkamhaeng the Great, brought Sukhothai to the height of its power. He ruled as an absolute monarch from 1275 till 1317 and is known as "the Father of Thailand." He created the Thai alphabet, which remains little changed today, uniting the ethnically diverse peoples with a common written language, beginning the outward surge of a uniquely Thai literary and educational style.

Theravada Buddhism was taught by monks brought by Ramkamhaeng from Ceylon, purifying the Khmer Buddhist ideas and inspiring a new freedom of artistic expression in paintings, sculpture and architecture. Ramkamhaeng brought Chinese artisans to Sukhothai to teach the art of pottery and porcelain. Great kilns produced the Sawankaloke celadon that was exported all around the region. The land was rich, the people were prosperous, creating a life-style that was both "elegant and harmonious."

The decline of Sukhothai began with the death of Ramkamhaeng. His successors were weak, and Ayuthaya, to the south, which had been founded by Ramathibodi, one of the Sukhothai princes, was becoming increasingly powerful. Ramathibodi needed men for his armies, to carry out ambitious plans of dominating the entire Chao Phya River basin and the Khmer empire to the east. The citizens of Sukhothai gradually abandoned their city, to be assimilated

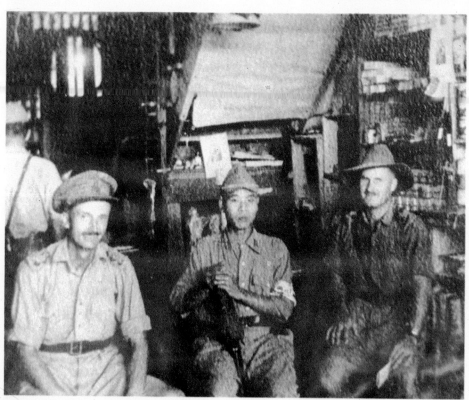

into the realm of **Ayuthaya**, which, by the middle of the 17th century, became the largest and most magnificent city in the region.

Destruction to Triumph

Ayuthaya ruled Siam for four centuries, with a succession of 33 kings, opening the first trade contacts with the West and establishing the policy of shrewd Thai diplomacy that has kept the country open to outside influence with very little loss of national prestige or identity. The strength of Ayuthaya waned in the 17th century, with its kings becoming increasingly ineffectual, while the Burmese kings grew stronger and more covetous of Siamese territory. A massive Burmese invasion overran the kingdom in 1767; Ayuthaya was looted, burnt, and its artistic treasures destroyed.

The Thais retreated south, setting up a new capital at **Thonburi**, across the Chao Phya River from the small trading town of **Bangkok**. Thonburi's first king, Taksin, reunited the fragmented Thai settlements, revived a centralised system of government and within 10 years succeeded in driving the Burmese out of the kingdom.

Taksin's successor was a leading general, Phya Chakri, who became King Rama I, the first monarch of the present Chakri dynasty. The Thai king today, King Bhumibol Adulyadej, is the ninth of the Chaki rulers. King Rama I moved the seat of power to Bangkok in 1782, feeling that Thonburi was too vulnerable to attack.

The modern phase of Thailand began in 1851 with Rama IV, King Mongkut, an imaginative monarch who opened the country to advantages of Western technology. He liberalised trade while managing to avoid the pressures of Western nations intent on colonising Southeast Asia. His successors, King Chulalongkorn, who ruled for over 40 years until 1910, and King Vajiravudh, carried on the work of modernisation in government, education, communications and social reform.

The absolute rule of the monarchy ended after 700 years in 1932, when a junta of army officers took over, giving Thailand a constitutional monarchy and a limited measure of democracy. There have been many Constitutions since the first, as well as *coups d'etat* and aborted struggles for power, but Thailand is now achieving a good measure of political stability, although the leaders frequently change, and is seeking internal prosperity and cooperation with its neighbours in action on regional problems.

Although there has been great social change down the centuries and a developed awareness of the theoretical value of democracy, outside the capital city the people remain basically apolitical. They have, however, kept their ancient reverence for the king, their pride in independence and their faith in the Buddhist religion.

The Land

Covering an area of around 515,000 square kilometres, Thailand is predominantly a country of small towns and villages, with 80 percent of the almost 50 million population involved in agriculture. Life outside the provincial centres basically revolves around the family, farm and community temple, and the most obvious signs of material progress are the television aerials stuck proudly atop the roofs of stilted teak houses.

Physically, the land presents an incredible array of contrasts, with the country divided by geography and climate into four distinct regions. The Thai people consider the shape of the country to be symbolic of its heritage — the shape of the head of an elephant, the animal most revered and honoured for its place in the shaping of history. The **North** of Thailand forms the crown, the **Northeast** the head and ear, the **Gulf of**

Opposite, *the real thing: life during World War II at the bridge on the River Kwai.*

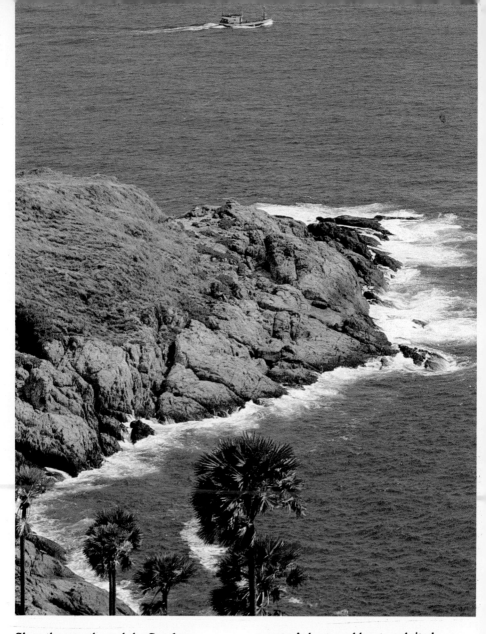

Siam the mouth, and the **Southern Peninsula** the trunk.

The prosperous heart of the country is the vast area of the Central Plains, rich in nature's most precious gifts, fruitful soil and plentiful water. Major rivers like the Chao Phya, which flows through capital Bangkok to the Gulf, along with sea keeps temperatures constant and moderate compared with the fluctuations of the centre and north. Some of the

country's best, and least exploited beaches are in the south, most notably along the bays of the island of **Phuket**, tributaries, streams and man-made channels feed the fields for the cultivation of rice, Thailand's top export commodity and staple diet of all its people. The landscape changes with the seasons in a timeless cycle of ploughing, planting, luxuriant growth and harvest — scenes which have altered little over the centuries. It is in this rich environment that the mighty ancient cities flourished, under constant threat of invasion by other regional powers seeking fertile lands for settlement.

Sukhothai and Ayuthaya, once splendid capitals of Siam, are now reclaimed by jungle and farmland, with only isolated reminders of their centuries of power. Modern Bangkok is a sprawling 6,000-square-kilometre home for 10 percent of Thailand's population and nearly 50 times larger than Chiang Mai, the second-largest city. It is Thailand's only city in international terms — the centre of almost all export/import activity, 90 percent of the country's motor vehicles, seat of government and industry and the focal point of aviation, railway and communications networks. But Bangkok merges gently with the rice fields of the Central Plains, thereafter having little effect on social harmony and the ordered ways of living off the land.

Thailand's northern mountains are part of the foothills of the Himalayan chain, giving rise to a landscape spectacular in natural wealth and vastly different ways of living than the ordered patterns of the plains. Here are teak forests with working elephants; thickly-forested hills and misty valleys that hide illicit poppy fields; strange mountain hilltribe people with multi-coloured costumes and quiet but tenacious resistance to the winds of progress; a climate that is kind to growing temperate as well as tropical fruit and flowers; and a history that has seen the rise and fall of powerful independent kingdoms.

Here, too, is Chiang Mai, traditional centre of handicrafts, claimed by Thais to have the country's prettiest girls. It is the country's second-largest city and northern centre for trading and tourism. Although the last few years have seen a phenomenal growth in Bangkok-style contributions to better living, the pace is still calm and pleasantly relaxed.

The northeastern areas of Thailand have a third of the country's population and the most severe of the agricultural problems. On the flat limestone plateau the soil is thin and infertile, with total dependence on the monsoons — which either bring too little rain or devastating floods. Life here is, in general, a struggle for subsistence, with the major farm production in cotton, jute and mullberry bushes — food plants for silk worms, creators of the lustrous fibre that is woven into the country's most beautiful exports. The provincial centres of Korat, Khon Kaen, and Ubon became boom towns during the years of American military presence but offer little for the visitor apart from being convenient bases for travelling around the spread-out sites of cultural and historical interest.

The well-watered coastal plains of the Eastern Gulf produce tapioca (identified by vile smells as it lies drying in the sun), rubber and a rich array of fruits; but the biggest attribute is Pattaya, one of the hottest pieces of beach-side real estate in Asia. Shorespace is crammed with resort hotels, nightclubs that match Bangkok standards of disco noise and whatever-you-want variety, and restaurants that specialise in seafood. Other resorts along the Eastern Gulf offer quieter pursuits of beach and sunshine, and the area of Chantaburi is rich in sapphires.

The southern peninsula, the elephant's trunk, is sandwiched between Burma and the Gulf of Siam, widening to form a wildly beautiful area between the Gulf and the Andaman Sea. Rich in natural resources, the southern provinces are the most prosperous after the Central Plains, and are widely different in terms of climate, culture and industry. Rubber and tin are big business in the south, the mosque is more familiar than the Buddhist temple, and the proximity to the and in the area of Songkhla. Historically, the south was governed by its own fierce rulers, only in the last century being integrated with the Kingdom of Thailand.

Opposite, *escape: the shoreline at Phuket.*

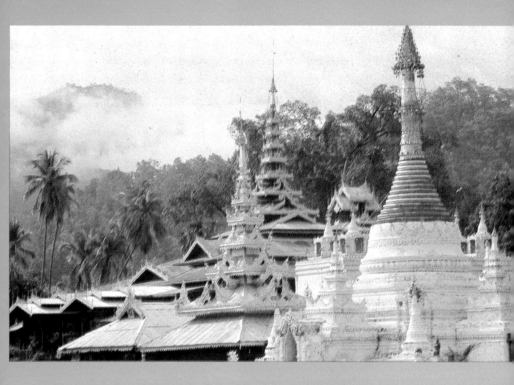

TV and Temple Bells
The Cultural Heritage

Faces of Buddhism

In Thailand, Buddhism is the dominant spiritual force, but its great flexibility, and tolerance towards change and adaptation, has inspired the development of a culture both complex and unique. Philosophies, superstitions, rituals, customs and beliefs embrace not only the precepts of Theravada Buddhism, but also refined ideas of Brahmanism and the worship of deities and spirits.

Buddhism was introduced by Indian missionaries to Thailand during the third century and was refined by Theravada monks from Ceylon during Ramkamhaeng's reign in Sukhothai during the late 1200s. The basic premise is that life does not begin with birth and end with death, but is part of a cycle of lives, each influenced by previous existences. Everyone is responsible for his own *karma*, the Buddhist idea of cause and effect, and individual initiative controls the achievement of happiness and well-being and the elimination of suffering.

Buddhism was readily adopted in Thailand because it offered an emotionally satisfying philosophy that did not conflict with the formalised rituals of Brahmanism or the animist customs that were already firmly established. Although Buddhism became the primary religion, the tolerance of the faith allowed a rich variety of other thoughts to develop. Buddhism answered most of the people's spiritual needs and the minority faiths in Thailand — Muslims, Hindu, Sikh, Confucian and Christian — today are followed by a total of less than 10 per cent of the population.

Buddhist practice in Thailand has changed little since Ramkamhaeng's time and the Brahman etiquette is still strong, particularly in various royal court rituals and ceremonies. The annual **Ploughing Ceremony**, presided over by the king at Bangkok's **Pramane Ground** in May, is a Brahman ritual. Rice seeds are blessed and sown and the success of the coming harvest is predicted by Brahman priests. The formal and traditional Thai wedding ceremony is also Brahman in origin.

The shrine outside Bangkok's **Erawan Hotel** is probably the most venerated image of Brahma in the country, worshipped primarily to ask for the granting of wishes and to give thanks when wishes are fulfilled.

Spirit worship, dating back to animist customs of placating evil spirits, is still very much a part of Thai life. Most houses will feature a "spirit house" in the garden — usually beautifully ornate and modelled on the style of a temple — built as homes for the spirits of the land. Thais believe there are spirits all around and a harmonious household can only be achieved if the spirits are happy. Roadside shrines are common, also, and motorists will stop, present flowers, food and lighted joss-sticks to ask for safety on the highways. Buddhist monks distribute *amulets*, which are tiny Buddha images worn on chains around the neck, to ensure good fortune and protect the wearer from evil spirits.

Astrology has a firm place in Thai beliefs, with a lunar system of months and days adopted centuries ago with the influence of China. Fortune-tellers play an essential role in most Thai lives, and again a mixture of folk-lore and various religious concepts forms an intricate pattern of superstition in harmony with Buddhism.

Personal milestones in life are marked by 12-year cycles, like the lunar months, a system that originated in China. Each year has its own "element" — water, earth, wood, gold, fire or iron — its own guardian spirit and its own type of being. The year of birth defines a person's basic character, represented by the rat, ox, tiger, rabbit, serpent, small snake, horse, goat, monkey, cock, dog or pig. The completion of each 12-year cycle and the beginning of another is an auspicious occasion for ceremony and celebration.

Thailand has nearly 30,000 Buddhist temples, most located in the rural areas, and a quarter of a million monks. Apart from the major role of guiding people toward nirvana, the temples provide a hub for village life, in the past being particularly important in the services of education and medicine.

Monks have daily contact with the people, particularly during the early morning collection of food offerings, and at religious ceremonies in the blessing of new homes and buildings, the anointing of new ships and aircraft, and at rituals associated with birth, marriage and death.

The majority of Thailand's national holidays are to mark the holiest of Buddhist occasions, such as the Lord Buddha's birth, enlightenment and death, the first sermon, and the beginning of Buddhist Lent, the monks' three-month period of retreat.

It is Thai custom for males to be ordained once they reach 20 years of age, for periods of from a few days up to three months. The ceremony of ordination is based on both Buddhist and Brahman ritual and considered one of the three most important events in a man's life, the others being his birth and marriage.

The Cities

In the rural communities, the central concepts of religion, family and village structure remain strong, but over recent years the effects of "Westernisation" have escalated. The cultural patterns of the capital city, Bangkok, in particular appear seriously eroded under the onslaughts of foreign trade, Western military presence during the Vietnam

Opposite: *portals of enlightenment: a temple in Northern Thailand.*

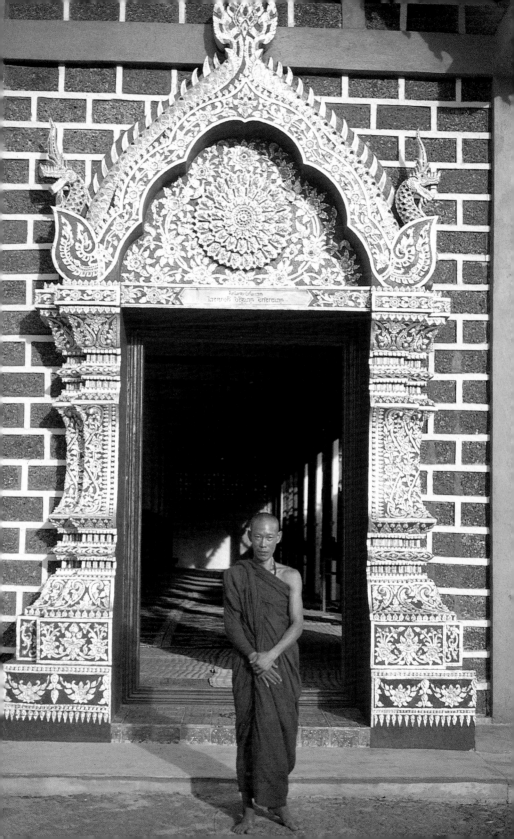

War years, and tourism. Bangkok now is Asia's most vivid illustration of tradition in collision with change, and to the casual visitor Thai culture may seem buried beneath the harsh surface of Western influence.

In Bangkok, East meets West with an awesome clash of materialism versus deep-rooted values; the conflict of preserving old concepts in the face of dazzling new enticements to prosperity. Fierce commercialism flourishes under traditions of the gentle Buddhist way and the pursuit of "sanuk" — the art of feeling good and at ease with one's environment. Bangkok, centre of government, monarchy and big business, with a population pushing five million, is frantically busy at one thing: Achievement. The temple spires that used to dominate the skylines have been challenged, and overpowered by the office blocks and plush hotels, each new edifice aimed higher than the last. The city canals have all but disappeared in the demand for wider roads, and the rows of

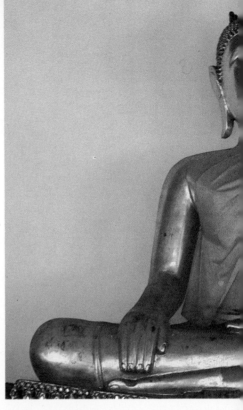

tatty shop-houses, crammed in fascinating disarray, are giving way to air-conditioned complexes, monotonous in their diligence to Western concepts of organised presentation.

On main streets the noise is astounding, with traffic demonstrating the competitive independence that has inspired Thai hearts for centuries. Taxis recreate the roaring charges of elephants into battle at every intersection. Motorcycles have mufflers removed to terrify opponents with 150cc bravado. Offensive tactics are known to win the right of way, with the horn more important than the brake in the achievement of motoring safety. For sheer volume and variety of vehicles, Bangkok undoubtedly outdoes any city in the world. The overall impression is chaos, with thunderous orchestration. Daunting for the visitor, but part of Bangkok's ebullient pace of progress to the true believer.

Bangkok's surface has indeed become highly Westernised, along with excesses

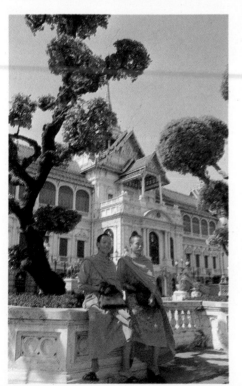

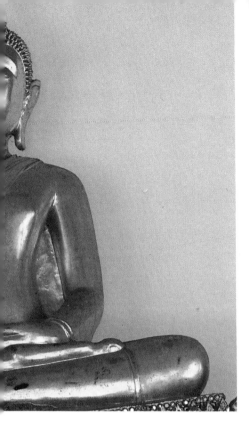

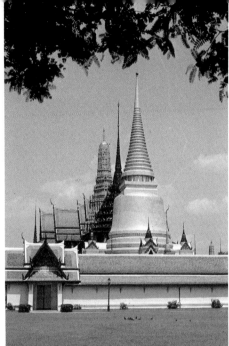

of noise and city-planning confusion, but underneath it all do lie the strong forces of traditional ways not yet eroded by the influences of dramatic modernisation. Fixed-price stores are still few, and bargaining is as avidly accepted in the fancy new shops as in the profusion of markets. The Bangkok Thai has adopted Western dress with a flair for fashion, and little regard for climate. The businessman in a hand-tailored suit will be amused, and disapproving, of his Australian visitor's cool dress shorts and long socks, but will tolerantly refrain from comment. An office girl will wear the new see-through fabrics but preserve total modesty with layer upon layer of underwear beneath. And trustworthiness in business is still often judged as much on the reading of a face as on the credentials presented.

And underneath the harried, hurried surface, Bangkok does preserve the calm of the Buddhist religion. In the midst of commercial fervour, the temples are surprising for their peace and serenity.

Showplaces of history, royal treasures and glorious architecture, and presented to the visitor in endless variations of style and importance, they retain their powerful religious significance and remain the centres of worship, meditation, merit, teaching and emotional guidance for the people they serve.

To the visitor, Bangkok will appear to have both greatly benefitted and sadly suffered from the influences of material and social change. The capital is still a gracious old lady, but with a plastic flower in her hair, retaining majesty and charm while flashing the tackier side of big-city tourism. The pleasures are found in the comforts of modern hotels, the broad scope of day-time and evening entertainment and the experiences of "old Thailand" still to be found, but the pleasures will undoubtedly be tempered by the pressures of a teeming metropolis and the somewhat impersonal approach that has been adopted to tourism.

The Middle Way of the Buddha: left, *relaxation near the Grand Palace, Bangkok;* centre, *Buddha image; above, the Temple of the Emerald Buddha, Bangkok.* Over, *meditation: a monk at Pathum Thani, Central Thailand.*

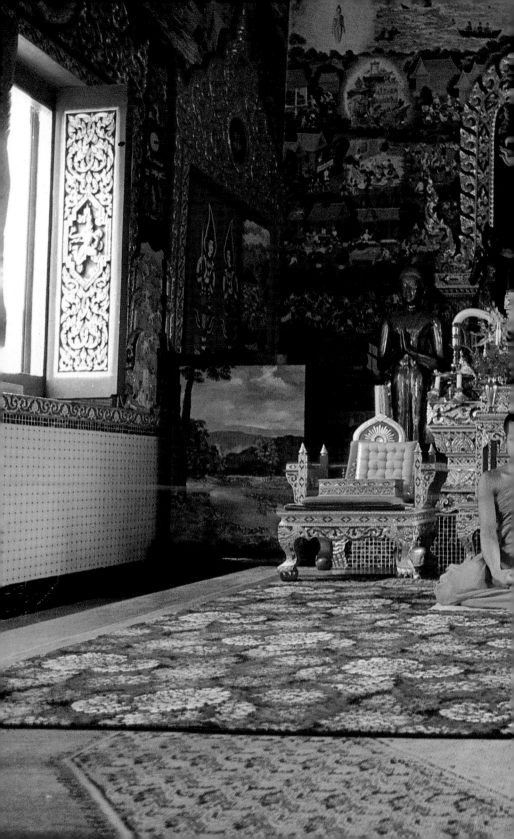

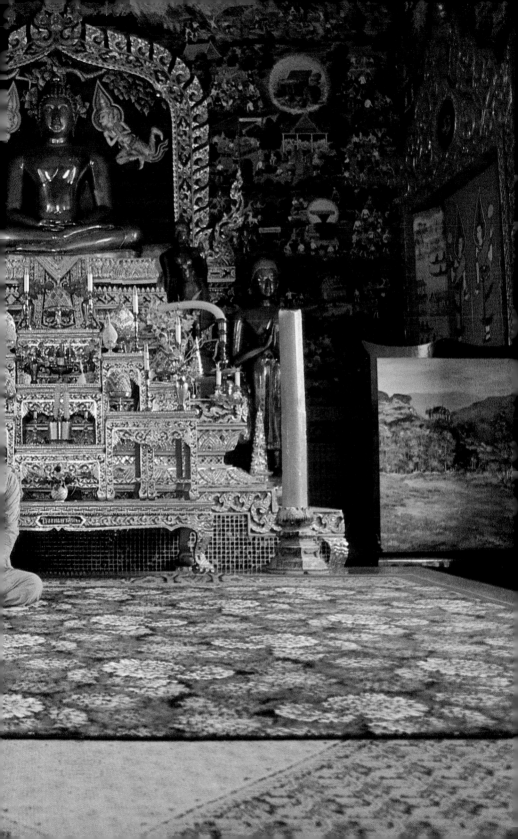

The Village Life

Today's Bangkok, however, is hardly a reflection of Thailand and it takes little effort to discover that the years of political upheaval and developing material awareness have had little effect on the traditional ways of living that have visibly endured outside the capital.

The village is the basic social and economic unit of the country and routine has remained comparatively unchanged since ancient times. Although there are regional variations in the styles of houses and the agriculture practices, each village is basically an extension of each family unit. The codes of behaviour taught in the home, related to family members, are applied outside in dealings with other villagers, and in the greater worlds of commerce and government.

Social values are in their purest forms in the villages, based on the importance of social harmony in communal life-styles. The Thai patterns of behaviour are therefore similar throughout the country. Even in the cities, where outside forces are having the most marked effects on life-styles, common characteristics can clearly be seen. These are often puzzling to the visitor, but all form part of the ordered social structure that has governed Thai attitudes for centuries.

The idea of "mai pen rai," usually translated as "never mind," is often considered by foreigners as a too-relaxed approach to situations. Its actual meaning is more complex, involving the acceptance of *karma* and the feeling that one should gracefully submit to forces that are beyond one's control. "Kreng jai" is equally confusing, but is defined as a reluctance to cause problems, a hesitation about disturbing anyone or his equilibrium. The manifestations can be exasperating, as a Thai will not willingly volunteer criticism, avoids confrontation on issues, and will rarely admit that an instruction is not understood.

To be "detached" is a major Thai virtue, defined as "choei choei," which is a state of no feeling for or against

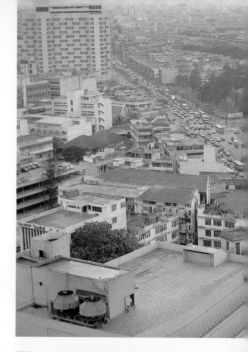

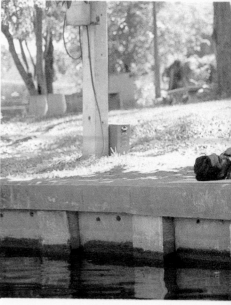

anything. It is therefore regarded as bad form to show strong displays of anger, displeasure, disapproval or extreme enthusiasm.

With regard to aquaintances and visitors, politeness predominates, based on the Buddhist concept of kindness to one's fellow beings. A stranger visiting a village will seldom feel an intruder. He is

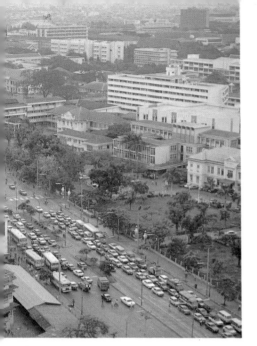

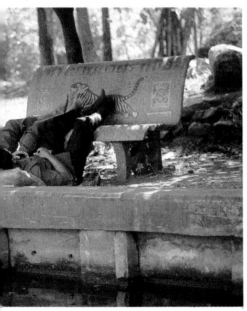

The Festive Life

Life in a Thai rural community follows three distinct cycles — a daily routine of tending to the land, a seasonal cycle of ploughing, planting and harvest, and the personal cycles of childhood, adolesence, maturity and old age. Ceremonies and annual festivals form an essential part of the cycles, most festivals centred around the Buddhist religion, and all involving whole villages in celebration. **Vissakha Bucha**, the most important religious holiday on the lunar calender, commemorating the Buddha's birth, enlightenment and death, falls usually in May. Ceremonies are held in every temple, with a candle-lit procession paying silent homage.

After the traditional Buddhist three-month retreat, ending in October, are the ceremonies of **Tod Krathin**, the presentation of new robes to monks. The day of ceremony is usually preceded by a village fair, with film-shows, folk-dances, plays and a carnival atmosphere.

During the 12th lunar month, usually November, there's the most spectacular of all Thai festivals, **Loy Krathong**. In honour of the "Mother of Water," the goddess Mae Kongkha, people float lotus-shaped *krathongs* on the rivers and canals, each holding a lighted candle, incense, a flower and a coin. It is believed that the krathongs carry away the sins of the past year and if the candle stays alight one's wishes will be fulfilled. In Bangkok, Loy Krathong is usually celebrated around the swimming pools of hotels and it is only in the rural areas that the true beauty of the festival can be appreciated.

The Thai New Year, the beginning of the Buddhist year, is in April, occurring during a time of relative leisure for many of the farming communities, **Songkhran** is therefore a three or four day festival, in temple fairs, merit-making, pilgrimages to

more likely to be welcomed as a friend, and this warmth of hospitality is the basis of Thailand's reputation as the "Land of Smiles." The Bangkok approach to visitors is, in general, more impersonal, through its familiarity with over 1.5 million travellers a year, but outside the capital the true Thai nature is much more in evidence.

Pace: Bangkok's awesome merger of 20th century commercial aggression and ancient submission to the inevitability of karma.

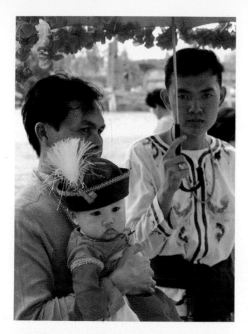

holy places, and a great splashing around of water.

Apart from the national celebrations there are a number of regional festivals, such as the northeast's annual plea to the gods for plentiful rain. Usually in May or June, the highspot of festivities comes when villagers fire home-made rockets, some enormous, into the sky.

The **Elephant Round-up**, in mid-November, turns the sleepy little northeastern town of **Surin** into a carnival of elephants, tourists, and village merry-makers. Over 200 elephants are gathered together to recreate the pageantry of ancient parades and battles, and there are demonstrations of elephant hunts and training, and elephants at work and at play. This is a show widely promoted by the Tourism Authority of Thailand, and all-inclusive tours by train from Bangkok to Surin are organised for around 1,600 Baht per person.

Village culture, in its forms of folk arts and festivals centres around a core of religion and the cycles of life. Classical culture, in art, sculpture, music and drama, originated in the ancient royal courts, under the patronage of kings. Classical art is Buddhist art, reflected in

temple architecture, intricate murals and images of the Buddha.

Classical drama, once only for the entertainment of royalty, centres around the stones of the Hindu epic *Ramayana*, which the Thais call "Ramakien". A complex web of plots and characters illustrate the triumph of good over evil, in two dramatically different styles. The *khon*, or masked play, is both formal and strenuous demanding great skill and years of practice. Players are always men, with jewelled masks to portray the personalities of the characters. In the *Lakhon* the more graceful form of dance and drama, the characters and costumes are the same as the khon, without the masks, and both male and female dancers enact not only the Ramakien but also tales from the life of the Buddha and fables from mythology. Much of the court-inspired culture was adapted into simpler forms and folk opera *Likay*, has long been one of the most popular styles of village entertainment. A burlesque of Lakhon, it combines pantomime and social satire, with players garishly costumed and embellishing traditional stories with bawdy local anecdotes.

In rural Thailand today, evening scenes of families gathered on the verandahs have been replaced by the glow of television sets, but village culture has lost little of its vibrancy. Classical art from the past remains, and is still fostered today, in the richness of temple decoration, towering golden spires, the revival of mural art and the classical dance, and the serenity of monuments to the Lord Buddha.

Thai culture is a complicated mosaic of countless ancient influences, blended together in a pattern that is distinctly Thai and a richly rewarding experience.

Tradition: above, the festival at Lopburi and right: Buddhist College near Pattaya.

26

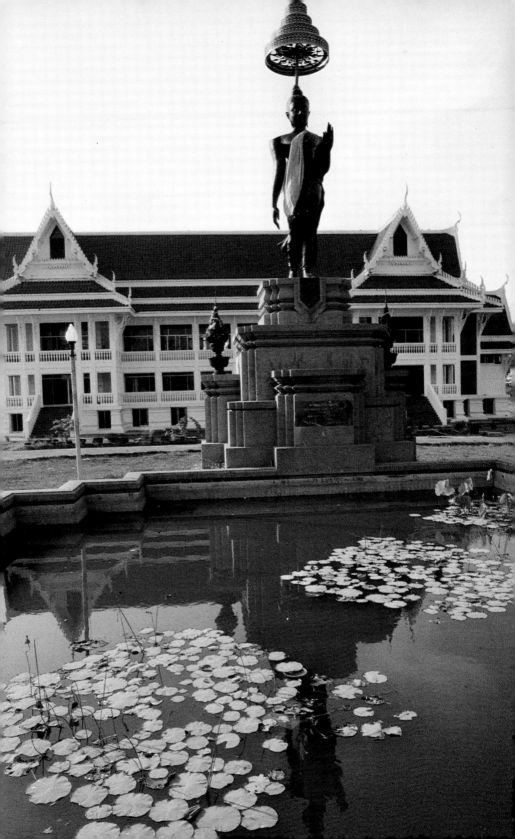

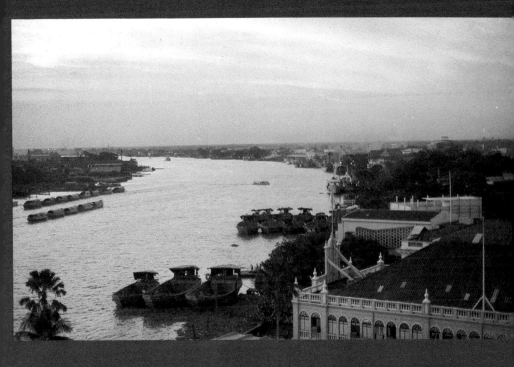

The Tourist Trail
On the Beaten Track

Bangkok

At first sight, Bangkok will be a shock to those whose imaginations have been inspired by the travel-poster images of brilliant colour and tranquility. In reality, the city appears a daunting experience — a bewildering mixture of East and West, gracious old and ugly new, in an atmosphere of chaos and clamour — and the serenity then seems hard to imagine let alone to find. But that's just a first impression, and, with little effort, the visitor will discover the fascinations that lie beneath the surface. With a good map and a blend of organised tours and plot-it-yourself excursions, Bangkok can live up to every expectation of traditional, and tranquil, Thailand.

The oldest part of the city and the area least touched by Bangkok's building boom is in the curve of the Chao Phya River where King Rama I set up the royal court in 1782. Here lies the magnificent **Grand Palace**, almost a city in itself, with towering spires and a collection of richly ornate royal buildings and treasures, started by King Rama I and added to by the following Chakri kings.

Main attractions in the areas open to visitors are the **Chakri Hall**, an impressive mixture of Thai and European architecture built during the reign of King Chulalongkorn in the late 1800s; the **Dusit Palace**, in classic Thai architecture which dates back to 1789; and the **Amarinda Vinichai Hall**, another of the palace's few original buildings. The present king moved the royal residence to **Chitralada Palace** in the late 1940s and the Grand Palace is now used only for important state banquets and royal ceremonies.

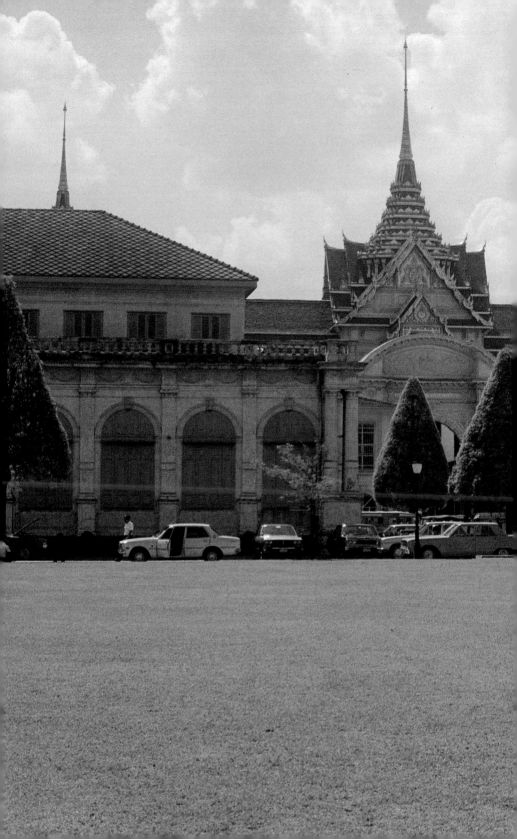

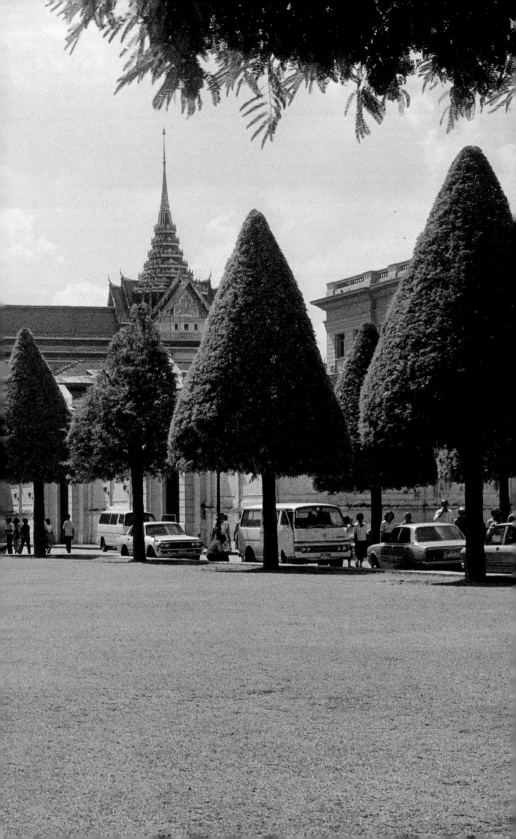

The Temple Trek

Within the Grand Palace compound is **Wat Phra Keo**, the Temple of the Emerald Buddha, which houses one of the world's most precious, and venerated, images of the Buddha. The chapel reveals the full spectacle of Buddhist art; a dazzling collection of golden spires, vividly-ornate pavilions and a lavish use of shimmering mother-of-pearl. Around the walls of the cloister that surrounds the temple are murals that illustrate the epic Ramakien, painted in the 1820s with many restorations since, some sadly lacking the inspired talent of the original artists. The Buddha image itself has its history shrouded in legend, but it is a 75 cm statue of translucent jade, which sits atop an 11 metre golden pedestal. Robes of the image are changed by the king according to the seasons.

Photography is permitted throughout the Grand Palace, but movie cameras are restricted to 8 mm and all photography is forbidden in the interior of the Emerald Buddha Chapel.

Nearby the Grand Palace is **Wat Po**, Thailand's oldest and largest temple complex, known as Thailand's first university. It dates back to before the founding of Bangkok as the Siamese capital. The temple is most famous for its gigantic reclining Buddha, 15 metres high and 46 metres long, representing the Buddha attaining nirvana.

The atmosphere of Wat Po is rather spoilt by hoards of souvenir hawkers, but time spent exploring is well rewarded as it has a splendid array of art and sculpture not seen in other temples. The compound is crammed with statues of the Buddha, *chedis* small and large (the four largest are memorials to the first Chakri kings), a charming series of stone animals and pagodas; and mural paintings depicting scenes of old Thai life, many of them needing restoration.

Although one hesitates to suggest buying anything from the hawkers at Wat Po, there are very good rubbings of the stone reliefs of the many scenes from the Ramakien that appear around the main chapel.

The old royal area of Bangkok also houses the **National Museum**, on Naprathat Road, which displays a fine collection of Buddhist art, in a series of beautiful old buildings. The collection ranges from the Davaravati era of Thai history up to the present Bangkok period, and there also exhibits of elephant battle-gear and *howdahs*, weapons, furnishings, ceramics and a prehistoric art collection, in particular of the earthenware jars and bronzes discovered in recent years at **Ban Chiang** in northeast Thailand. There are free guided tours conducted at the museum on specific subjects. These are in English on Tuesdays (Thai Culture), Wednesdays (Buddhism) and on Thursdays, alternating each week between Early Thai Art and Later Thai Art. All begin at 9.30 a.m. The museum is closed on Mondays, Fridays and public holidays, but is open, free of charge, on weekends. On other days, a small entrance fee is charged.

The Bangkok city stone is well worth a visit during an excursion around "old Bangkok". The small shrine is sandwiched between the **Law Courts** and the **Ministry** of **Defence**, opposite the entrance to Wat Phra Keo. **Lakmuang**, the somewhat phallic stone pillar, is covered with gold leaf and flower garlands, and there are frequent performances of classical dance. Here, people make merit by releasing birds from small bamboo cages and ask the old spirits for wishes to be fulfilled. This shrine, as well as the Brahman shrine outside the **Erawan Hotel**, is particularly well-favoured by devotees on the days before drawings of the government lottery, on the 1st and 16th of each month.

One of the most pleasant ways of getting to this area of Bangkok is by river, along the Chao Phya from the landing next to the **Oriental Hotel**. It

---

Opposite, *magnificence: the Temple of the Emerald Buddha.*

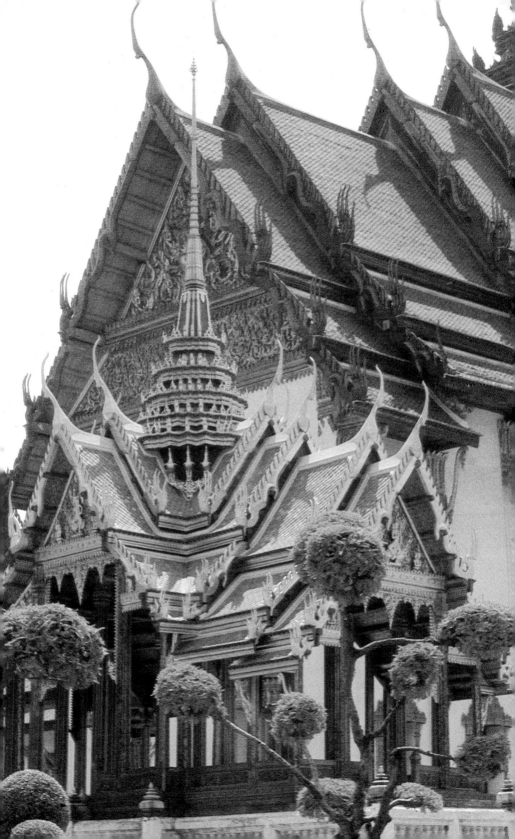

costs less than 5 Baht (US$0.25) for the trip by open-sided river bus, and it is much more relaxing than tackling the traffic through **Chinatown**.

Apart from the temples in the "old Bangkok" vicinity, there are many others worthy of attention. **Wat Trimitr**, on Charoen Krung Road where it intersects with Yaowaraj, appears insignificant and rather shabby but houses a Buddha image three metres high, cast in 5.5 tons of solid gold. Believed to have originated in the 13th century kingdom of Sukhothai, it was covered in stucco until 1953 when it fell from a crane. A delightful story has been woven around the discovery — how a storm was generated by the gods to soften the plaster and enable it to crack when the statue was "magically" dropped. The image remains in its humble surroundings, as the Thais believe that that's clearly the place the spirits intended it to be.

Wat Benchamaborpit, the Marble Temple, was built by King Chulalongkorn at the turn of the century. The name means "Temple of the Fifth King" and it is the newest of the royal temples in Bangkok, located on Sri Ayuthaya Road near **Chitralada Palace**. This temple is considered one of the most beautiful expressions of "modern" Thai religious architecture. The brilliantly coloured Chinese tiles of the curved roof make a stark contrast with the gleaming Carrara marble of the main building. Two enormous marble lions guard the entrance and in an enclosed courtyard are over fifty images of the Buddha in a variety of different styles and attitudes. Not only the classical Thai depictions of the Buddha are represented — there are examples of images from Tibet, Japan, India and China, but unfortunately most of the inscriptions are in Thai. Hundreds of pigeons flock around the compound and there's a rather smelly turtle pool.

To fully appreciate the **Golden Mount**, one must climb to the top of over 300 steps, but it's well worth it for the view. Located on **Rajdamnoen Avenue**, the

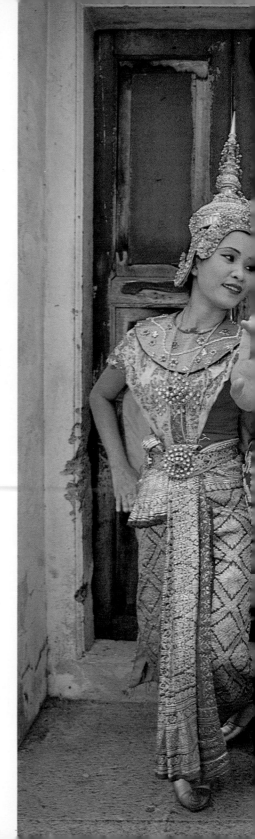

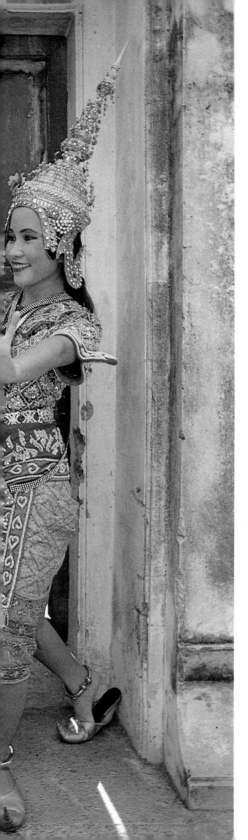

artificial hill was started in the reign of King Rama III and finished in the late 19th century by Rama V, originally intended to recreate an artificial hill that had been made during the Ayuthaya kingdom. The golden spire holds a relic of the Buddha, and the temple shrine, in **Wat Sakhe**t at the bottom of the Mount, displays one of the largest bronze Buddhas in Thailand. In November, a visit is especially entertaining, with the annual temple fair that draws pilgrims from all over the country to pay homage to the relic.

Water Tours

Bangkok's water tours, both along the river and her remaining negotiable "klongs," or canals, are among the city's most captivating attractions. The **Floating Market**, however, is now a disappointment. The sheer volume of tourists, hundreds every day, combined with the development of roads into an area once basically isolated by water, has made the local people who used the market for trading and commerce go elsewhere. The situation now is an unhappy scene of tour boats jockeying for positions outside souvenir shops. However, while the actual market has virtually disappeared, the canal trip to get there does offer fascinating glimpses of life on a residential klong. It can be done without the morning crowds, by hiring a private boat from the landing next to the Oriental Hotel, for around 150 Baht (US$7.50) an hour. Ask the boatman to follow the floating market route (he'll know it well), and stop on the way at **Wat Arun**, the glorious Temple of Dawn. The main spire is covered with shards of multi-coloured Chinese porcelain and pottery. There are Khmer-style pagodas, some interesting murals, and a possible climb about half way up the 87 metre tower which provides an excellent view of the river if you're keen enough to tackle

Cultivated grace: Thai classical dancing.

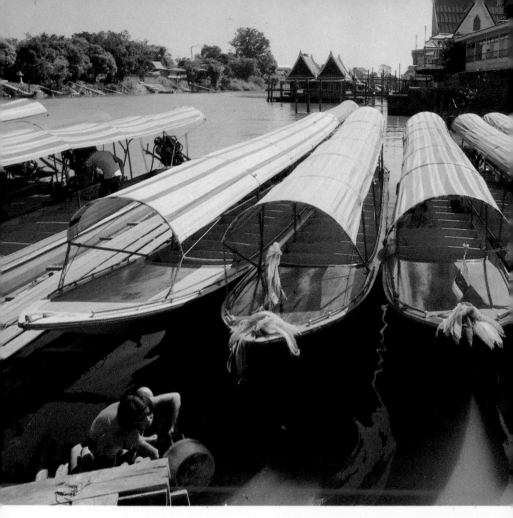

it. One can also visit the collection of royal barges, further along the river, until quite recently used for ceremonial occasions with much pomp and pageantry.

There is another floating market, much larger than the one in Bangkok ever was, which retains a little of the genuine charm. This is an hour's drive southwest of the city, to **Damnoen Saduak** in Rajburi, and is offered by agents as a full-day tour combined with the **Rose Garden Country Resort**.

Here is an afternoon "village show" of Thai music, dance and village living, rather staged and touristy but excellently presented. There are additional pleasures in a display of elephants and village handicrafts, and the river-side restaurant

is an ideal setting for lunch. The area is a popular retreat for Bangkok residents. The park is beautifully landscaped and overnight accommodation is provided in a good hotel and a number of Thai-style houses. There is also an 18-hole golf course.

One of the best canals for excursions within Bangkok itself is **Klong San Saep** which runs through the city and out into the rice fields beyond. East West Tours, on Soi Nana 3, Sukhumvit Road, operates a cruise by rice barge (around 250 Baht (US$12.50) per person) which is a gentle way to float through the afternoon. You can put together the same basic trip yourself by hiring a long-tailed boat at the small landings on Soi 63 or Soi 71, Sukhumvit Road. Cost, with

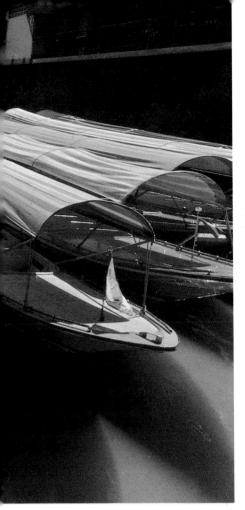

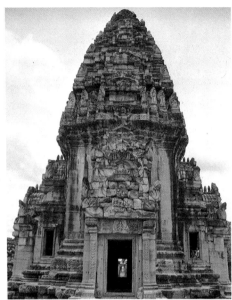

bargaining, is about 150 Baht an hour and it's best to make it a two-hour trip. Late afternoon, around 3.00 p.m., avoids the harshest sun of the day, but ladies would still feel more comfortable wearing a hat.

A more luxurious style of cruising is by the riverboat *Oriental Queen*, owned by the Oriental Hotel, which travels up-river to the old capital of **Ayuthaya**. One way of the tour is by road, visiting the old **Summer Palace** at Bang Pa-In which has a fabulous Chinese pavilion and numerous other buildings in a quaint mixture of European and Thai architecture. One of the highlights is a delicate Thai-style pavilion, sited in the middle of the lake. This is probably the most photographed piece of classical Thai architecture in the country.

Ayuthaya itself gets little attention on the tour, basically just a look at the most impressive ruins of **Wat Mahathat** and the royal palace, but perhaps only a dedicated historian would demand more. A Western buffet lunch is served on board the cruiser, and total cost is around 600 Baht (US$30). Bookings can be made at the Oriental Hotel or any **World Travel Service** counter.

A new riverboat, the *Orchid Queen*, also owned by the Oriental Hotel, travels down-river, to the crocodile farm and **Ancient City**. A common impression after the tour is that crocodiles are ugly, and they stink, but the farm is indeed a rare experience in animal husbandry.

Culture

The **Ancient City** is one man's fulfillment of a dream — a vast area of private parkland with replicas, many full size, of many of Thailand's most important landmarks. Billed as the "world's largest outdoor museum," it features reconstructions of some buildings that no

Sculpted lines: left, *river boats at Ayuthaya and* above, *stone at Pimai.*

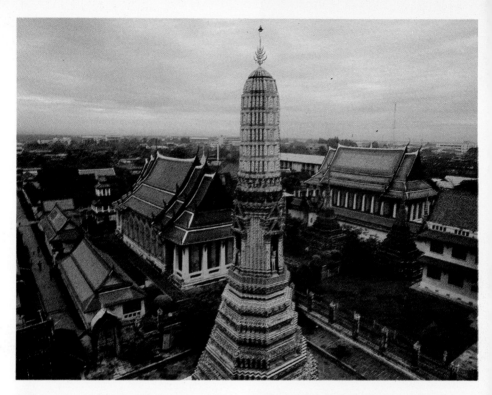

longer exist, and others that are now impossible to visit — such as **Khao Phra Viharn**, at the border of Kampuchea (Cambodia) and Thailand. The fact that this historic temple is Kampuchean is a sore point with Thais . . . the dispute over to whom it belonged was resolved by the world court in 1961, and the Thais were not happy with the decision. At the Ancient City there is also a model Thai village, complete with artisans working on native handicrafts. The full day Orchid Queen tour is one way by river and the other by road, around 500 Baht including lunch, but one can visit just the Ancient City by booking at the city office on Rajdamnoen Avenue, near the **Democracy Monument**. The tour is offered twice daily.

For lovers of tropical gardens, old wooden Thai houses and antiques, the places to explore are the **Suan Pakkard Palace** and the **Jim Thompson House**. The former is a beautiful private garden that is open to the public Monday through Saturday, for an entrance fee of 50 Baht (US$2.50). There are five traditional Thai houses, and an impressive collection of antiques, plus an exquisite lacquer pavilion that was brought from Ayuthaya and carefully restored and reassembled. The black and gold panels are fine examples of Thai classical decorative art. The palace is on Sri Ayuthaya Road, near the corner with Phya Thai.

The Jim Thompson House, at the end of Soi Kasemsarn 2, opposite the national stadium on Rama I Road, is open weekdays for a fee of 50 Baht. The millionaire silk king, who mysteriously disappeared in Malaysia in 1967, recreated several Thai houses on the present site and filled them with antiques and rare *objets d'art*. It's worth a visit to see how the cultured rich traditionally lived in Bangkok.

Roots: above, *around Wat Saket, the Temple of the Golden Mount and* right, *festive dress at the old capital of Lopburi.*

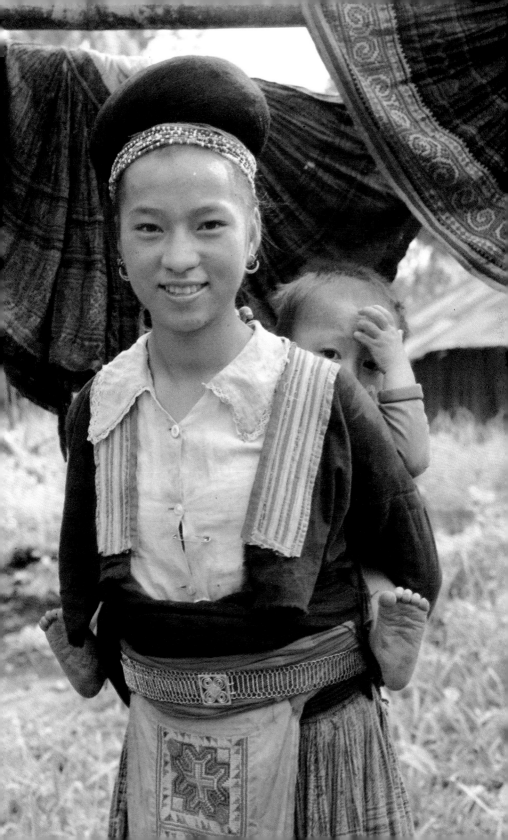

The **Siam Society** on Soi 21, Sukhumvit, also has an antique Thai house, once an ancestral home in Chiang Mai that was dismantled and brought to Bangkok as a museum for displays of folk art and other aspects of northern Thai culture. The society also has a fine reference library and books for sale on specific topics of Thai history and culture.

Another lovely garden area is the zoo, **Khao Din**, behind Chitralada Palace, which has a good collection of native and imported animals and birds. Here also are the revered white elephants, not white at all but sort of piebald and pinky-grey around the edges. The zoo is open daily from 8.30 a.m., admission 6 Baht.

For a close-up look at snakes, head for the **Red Cross** compound at the corner of Henri-Dunant and Rama IV Roads. Eleven in the morning on most days is feeding time, not recommended for the squeamish, of the cobras, kraits, vipers and other deadly nasties. (A recent report on the deadliness of Thai snakes indicated that after a bite from a krait one could live for up to two hours, but cobras are better because one lasts longer, maybe up to four hours). Anti-snake-bite serum is produced at the farm, and on Thursdays one can watch the poison being extracted.

Markets

No Bangkok experience is complete without exploration of some of the markets. Most famous, and frenetic, is **Sanam Luang**, the weekend market at the **Pramane Ground**, in the old Bangkok area of the Grand Palace and Wat Phra Keo. Every Saturday and Sunday, the grassy areas, with concrete walkways, are transformed with thousands of stalls selling literally everything. Food, household goods, gaudy souvenirs, clothes, pets, patent medicines, antiques and junk, with a weird array of smells that both delight and offend. (Steer clear of the dried fish and pig entrails sections if your stomach's not strong). The central

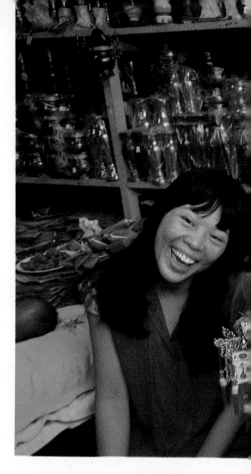

area gets rather icky in the rainy season, but is worth the sloshing about for the sight of brisk sales of multi-coloured mice, irridescent beetles, otters, squirrels, birds, fish and pedigree dogs and 5 Baht mongrels. Here, one also sees pure-bred Siamese cats; cats in the streets are more likely to resemble your tabby moggy at home. If you're lucky you'll find a medicine show, with props of snakes and mongooses. As a variation of man-swallows-sword, there's sometimes girl-swallows-snake, designed to entertain while flogging a new remedy for warts or fever.

Many other markets are in **Chinatown**, an ill-defined area stretching around Yaowaraj and the upper end of Charoen

Clutter: above, *a Chinese altar shop and* right: *pots for all purposes*

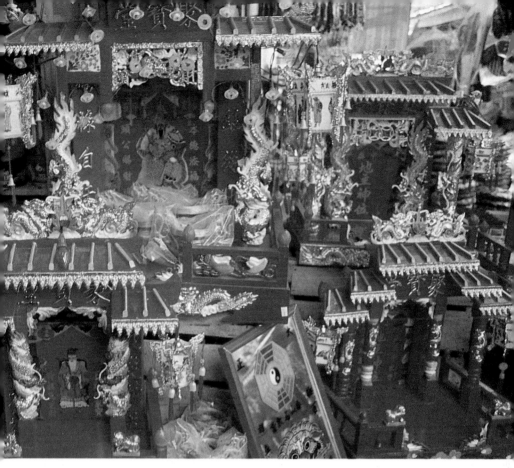

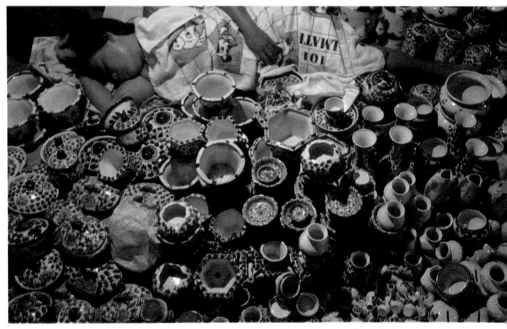

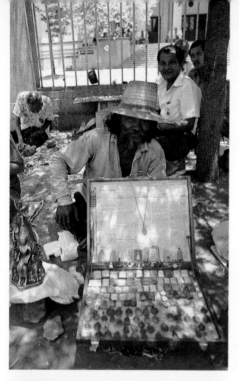

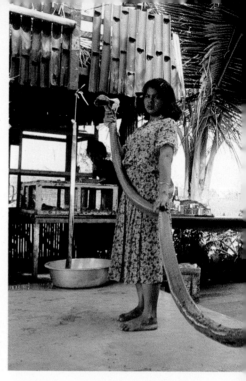

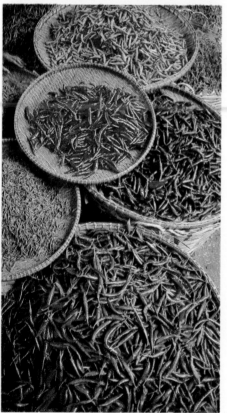

Krung Road. Off Mahachai Road is
Pahurat, the massive Indian market, and
Sampaeng Lane, which has been a busy
centre of commerce since the mid 1800s.
Main specialty is fabrics, in endless
variation, along with baskets, mats and
beautiful Chinese lanterns.

Off **Bamrung Muang Street** are the
shops specialising in religious objects —
Buddha images, the nine-tiered altars,
monk's bowls and bags, and hand-carved
caskets. Nearby is the square of the
Giant Swing, two soaring red poles joined
at the top by a carved beam, once used in
Brahman rituals. Facing the Giant Swing
is **Wat Suthat,** with a Buddha image that
was cast in 14th century Sukhothai, some
excellently-preserved murals, and bronze
figures of horses and stone pagodas.

Also in Chinatown is **Nakhon Kasem,**
the official name for what has long been
called the **Thieves Market,** a composite of
antiques and modern-day merchandise.
Fierce bargaining is needed, but best
finds are in Chinese porcelain, snuff
bottles and furniture inlaid with mother-
of-pearl. It's a good place also for copper
bells and lanterns.

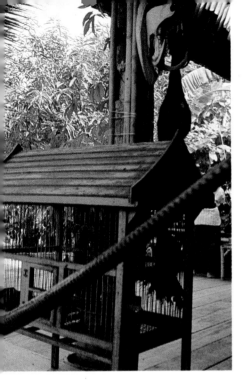

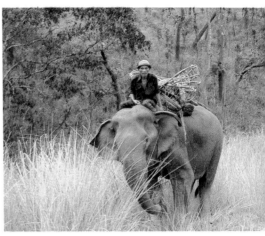

The Country Trail

Lying 130 kilometres away from Bangkok, **Kanchanaburi** is the site of the Bridge over the River Kwai and two cemeteries for the Allied prisoners of war who died during the construction of the bridge and "Death Railway" during World War II. Until recent years the bridge and the cemeteries were the major reasons that foreign visitors went to Kanchanaburi, usually on day-trips out of Bangkok. With the construction of a river-side lodge and bamboo-raft accommodation anchored at the river bank, the area has become a new destination for visitors keen to explore the more remote, but easily accessible, attractions of river and jungle.

There are trains and buses, some air-conditioned, out of Bangkok daily, but one of the best ways to visit Kanchanaburi is to join an organised programme. Diethelm Travel operates the **River Kwai Village**, and will arrange a package that includes just the transportation and accommodation, or include various trips along the river and to the bridge. The hotel costs around 540 Baht (US$27) for a twin room, per night,

And don't forget the gold shops. Yaowaraj has hundreds of them, selling gold in chains and ornaments, with a fixed cost for the weight of a one-Baht coin, almost half an ounce.

Nearer the "central city" is **Bangrak market**, on Charoen Krung Road between Silom and Sathorn, a general hubub of produce, flowers and clothing by day and an open-air dining place at night. Food is excellent, if spicy, but standards of hygiene are likely to make the fastidious squirm.

Pratunam, around Rajprarop Road where it links with Petchburi, is the other main city market, also for general produce, clothes, leather goods and economical tailoring. From here one can catch a water taxi along the San Saep Klong that parallels Petchburi Road. Cost, one Baht, and good value.

Bangkok is a haphazard sprawl of visual delights and eye-sores. A brash, bawdy, noisy city that offers moments of incredible calm. The heat may be trying, the confusion exasperating, and the traffic horrendous, but, above all else, Bangkok is never boring.

Marketing: left, amulets for safe travelling and below, chillies for dangerous eating. Centre, preparing snakes for rich Chinese gourmets. Above, safe travelling by elephant.

and a two-day package is 1,700 Baht (US$85) per person, three days 2,800 Baht (US$140). These programmes include trips by boat to the Kaeng Lava limestone cave, and along the "Death Railway". All meals also are included.

A more "exotic" way to enjoy Kanchanaburi is to stay on one of the river-rafts located in the area of the **Sai Yok Waterfall**. East West Tours, Floatel, and the River Kwai Farm (which has land-based bamboo cottages as well but is not so easy to reach by road) all cost in the region of 460 Baht (US$23) per person per day, inclusive of all meals. Adding the transportation from Bangkok, Floatel charges 1,500 Baht (US$75) for a two-day stay, 2,000 baht (US$100) for three.

From the rafts, or the River Kwai Village, one can take walks into the jungle (one brochure describes the "millions of butterflies" as "cheerful"); trips by boat and foot to the **Daowadung Caves**; visit the hot springs at **Hin Dat**, where the Japanese soldiers built pools fed by natural springs (not particularly interesting, but the river trip makes it worthwhile); walk along the remains of the railway line where it disappears into the jungle; or take an elephant ride. One of the prettiest waterfalls in the area is **Erawan**, a series of 15 large pools and several smaller ones, in a national park where the forest is particularly cool and peaceful.

One of the more lengthy tours, taking up a full day, is from the end of the existing railway back to **Lum Sum**, an elevated section of the line where a trestle bridge clings precariously, it seems, to a 30 metre cliff. It is also possible to spend overnights in the jungle, and take a six-day expedition by jeep, boat and foot up to the **Three Pagodas Pass** border with Burma.

Khao Yai

This national park and wild life reserve is just over 200 kilometres from Bangkok at an average of 800 metres above sea level. It covers 2,000 square kilometres, spreading into four provinces. The main attractions are the forest trails that wind out from the centre of the park, to waterfalls, fields of flowers and orchid groves. For extended hikes one should hire a guide from the office of the **Tourism Authority of Thailand** there, as it's quite easy to get lost. Camping grounds have been set up but you must bring all your own equipment and inform the park authorities.

The TAT operates a motor lodge with two-bedroom bungalows starting at 700 Baht (US$35) a night, and motel units for 450 Baht (US$22.50). The park is the home of wild elephant, bear, deer, boar, buffalo, porcupines, mongooses, civet cats and even tigers, and night safaris are arranged by jeep with spotlights. By day one sees a multitude of birds, squirrels, monkeys and every imaginable colour of tropical butterfly.

One of Khao Yai's biggest drawcards for Bangkok residents is the 18-hole golf course, with plenty of trees, streams, hills and the forest all around. A few years

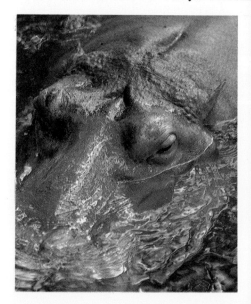

Imports: left, *a hippo at Bangkok Zoo* and opposite, *a Burmese-style temple in the north.*

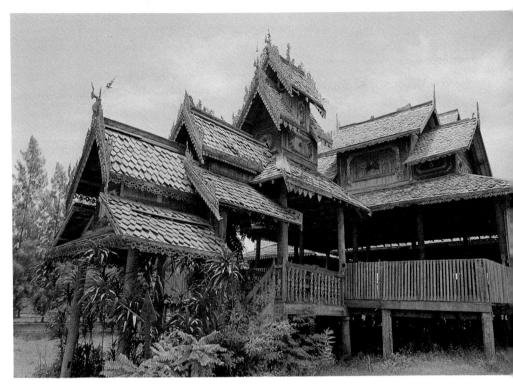

ago a tiger killed a deer and quiety ate it at the ninth hole, but park authorities give assurances that not one tourist has yet been eaten. Green fees at the course are 80 Baht (US$4); to hire clubs is 150 baht (US$2.50), and a caddy 50 Baht.

Easiest way to get to Khao Yai is to take an air-conditioned bus from the office of **Suranaree Tour**, near Bangkok's **Victory Monument**. This goes to **Pakchong** (for 55 Baht one way, 100 Baht round trip), and the TAT bus leaves Pakchong daily at 12 noon and 5.00 p.m. for the drive into the hills. Accommodation should be arranged ahead through the TAT's office on Rajdamnoen Nok Avenue.

Day tours are offered by train on weekends and public holidays, not the best time to visit Khao Yai as the main areas are rather crowded. The train leaves the Bangkok station, **Hualumpong**, at 6.50 a.m., and returns at 7.50 p.m., 120 Baht (US$6) pays for the train, the bus from Pakchong and back, and lunch. Book in advance at Hualumpong.

The Far Northeast

The ancient Khmer centre of **Phimai**, near the northeastern city of **Korat**, represents one of the world's richest periods of art and sculpture, the height of the Khmer empire in the 11th and 12th centuries. Now that Angkor, the old empire's enormous heart in Kampuchea, cannot be visited, Phimai offers one of the few opportunities to study the magnificent architecture and temple design of the period. The plan of the old town, once linked by road to Angkor, can still be traced and the central sanctuary has been reconstructed. Both Buddhist and Brahman influence can clearly be seen in the delicately-carved lintels and massive stone monuments.

Phimai is best reached out of Korat, but an easier and more comfortable way is to take an organised tour. Diethelm Travel offers a two-day programme which uses Korat or Khao Yai as the accommodation base. The tour also includes a visit to the giant banyan tree near Phimai and the return journey makes a stop at **Wat Phra Buddhabhat**, one of Thailand's most sacred shrines, built around a Buddha's footprint. The original temple was looted and destroyed during the Burmese invasion of Ayuthaya but reconstruction was begun by the first of the Bangkok kings and continued through the early part of the Chakri dynasty. The site has a magnificent main temple, outbuildings and **chedis**, and grounds full of beautiful bronze bells and gilded monuments. Price for the Phimai tour by private car, two persons, is 4,000 Baht (US$200) each.

Ban Chiang, a tiny village 500 kilometres from Bangkok, near the town of **Udon Thani**, has attracted archaeological scholars from all over the world. The site has revealed sophisticated bronzes and earthernware pots that have been dated back 6,000 years, pre-dating similar objects from China, long regarded as mankind's cradle of culture.

Ban Chiang can be disappointing for those who are expecting to see a major archaeological site. There are few excavations that actually still show relics — most have been removed for study and display in museums, like the **Khon Kaen Museum** and the **National Museum** in Bangkok which both have fine collections of the Ban Chiang pottery, bronzes and other artifacts.

For dedicated hikers, Thailand's northeast offers **Phu Kradung**, Bell Mountain, in the province of **Loei**. A five-kilometre trail and not an easy climb, leads to a 60-sq km tableland at an elevation of between 1,200 and 1,500 metres. You can arrange for porters to carry your gear. The plateau is beautiful for nature walks, along trails that lead to waterfalls and havens of birds and monkeys. The park provides bedding in cabins but it is best to take along some packaged foods as the catering service is very limited. Best time of year is October through January, at the end of the rains, when the plants and flowers are at their richest. The entrance to the park is around 50 kilometres from Loei, and this provincial centre is reached by a 12-hour train via Udon Thani.

One of the northeast's particularly delightful attractions is elephants. The Suay people, in the area of **Surin**, are the traditional elephant trainers and every year there's a lively festival of elephant action and entertainment. The small town of Surin is transformed with a carnival atmosphere as the elephants recreate the pageantry of the past. There are ceremonial parades of elephants in battle dress, demonstrations of the great elephant hunts and performances of local music and dances. The Tourism Authority of Thailand arranged a special tour by train, around 1,600 Baht (US$80) per person for a two-day programme.

The Far North

The powerful King Mengrai, who ruled the north of Siam in the 13th century, founded **Chiang Mai**, so the legend goes, because of the auspicious sighting of a group of rare white animals. The walls were constructed "by 90,000 men," establishing a fortress that today has sprawled into Thailand's second-largest city, the northern hub of business and tourism. Cooler and considerably less humid than Bangkok, Chiang Mai's pace of life is slower and the effects of Westernisation have yet to dominate the traditional charm. It is known as the centre of handicrafts — wood, silver, pottery, lacquer-ware and woven silks and cottons, with areas of the city devoted to particular crafts. The quality of workmanship has sadly suffered with the tourist demand, but the choice is excellent and it's easy to make careful selection.

Within the city and nearby surroundings are opportunities to visit old and beautiful temples, see elephants at work, explore caves and waterfalls, see hilltribe villages and catch glimpses of the northern styles of festival celebration and entertainment.

Opposite, *northern vistas: overlooking Mae Hong Sorn in the far north.*

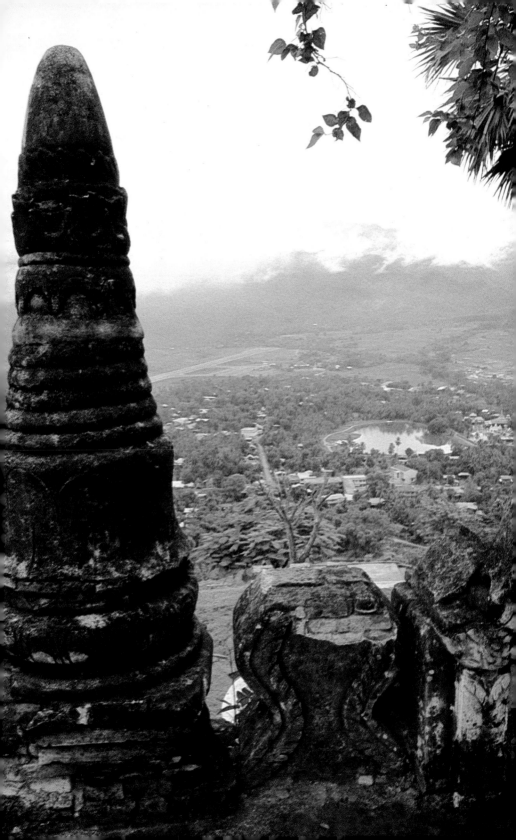

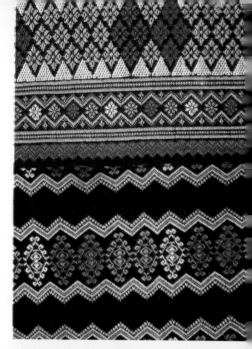

Just north of the city is **Doi Suthep**, with its revered old temple offering excellent views of the hills and valleys around. The temple is reached by a flight of almost 300 steps, flanked by *nagas*, the mythological seven-headed serpents, and the temple sanctuaries are beautifully maintained through the gifts of pilgrims who come to worship a relic of the Buddha. Nearby is the **Bhubing Palace**, open on weekends and public holidays when the Royal Family is not in residence. The gardens offer brilliant displays of both tropical and temperate flowers. On the way to Doi Suthep, one can visit the botanical gardens, the zoo, **Huay Kaew** waterfall and the **University** with its tribal museum. Half on hour's drive from Soi Suthep is the **Meo Camp** at **Doi Pui**, which the Tourism Authority has been reconstructing as an authentic village, hoping to lessen the effects of the constant visits by tourists.

A more artificial display of hilltribes is at the **Old Chiang Mai Cultural Centre**, where a gathering of families from several tribes live in reconstructed village settings. Here, every evening, there's a **Khan Tok** dinner party, with a banquet of northern style foods and an elaborate cultural show of hilltribe music and dances.

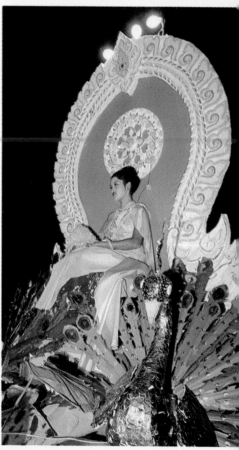

The "unspoilt" hilltribe stations are in the misty valleys of the hills and visits should only be arranged with the help of a reputable tour agent.

For elephant entertainment, there's a lumber camp around 60 kilometres to the north of the city. One watches elephants happily bathing, then hauling logs and giving rides to tourists. Here you can arrange an overnight elephant safari, with very rustic accommodation at a hilltribe village.

The Mae Sa Valley Resort, near the elephant camp, offers more sophisticated accommodation in bamboo huts and cottages, for at least 600 Baht (US$30) a night, plus meals, but the setting is delightful.

Longer trips out of Chiang Mai, to the west, can cover the **Doi Inthanon**

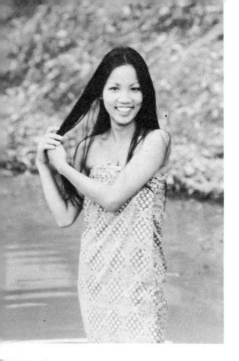

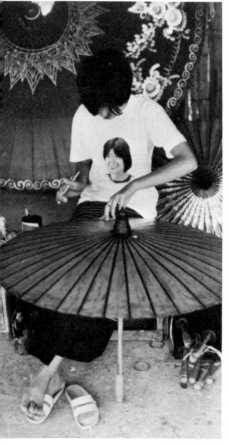

National Park and the ruggedly beautiful areas on the way to **Mae Hong Son**, framed in the north and west by the Shan states of Burma.

Far in the northern mountains is **Chiang Rai**, and the border town of **Chiang Saen** where one looks across the **Mekong River** to Laos. Just a few kilometres more, and you reach the **Golden Triangle**, the three-way border of Thailand, Laos and Burma, with the countries separated by the Mekong and its tributary, the Mae Sai. The Golden Triangle is also notorious for its traditional opium production.

Chiang Mai is easily reached by air, rail or road from Bangkok, and *Thai Airways* also serves the remoter towns of Chiang Rai and Mae Hong Son, with flights out of Chiang Mai. An organised programme for Chiang Mai and Chiang Rai can easily be arranged in Bangkok, through any major tour operator, solving the problems of transportation and hotel bookings. Some have regular departures, cheaper than making individual arrangements. For peak seasons, particularly November through February, one needs to make bookings well in advance as flight capacities and hotel rooms are limited. Chiang Mai hotels are good — ranging from simple guest houses to the first class properties of the **Rincome, Chiang Inn** and **Poy Luang** — but those outside the northern capital are limited in facilities of an international standard.

Dining outside the hotels in Chiang Mai is fun — the range of foods is limited but the settings are unusual. There's even an English pub, serving pies and puddings.

For those who want to explore up-country Thailand, particularly the scenic and cultural charms of the north, an excellent "around Thailand" programme has been developed. The trip takes seven days, with overnights at Khao Yai

Beauty: hill tribe embroidery: Chiang Mai bather: and right, *umbrella painting.*

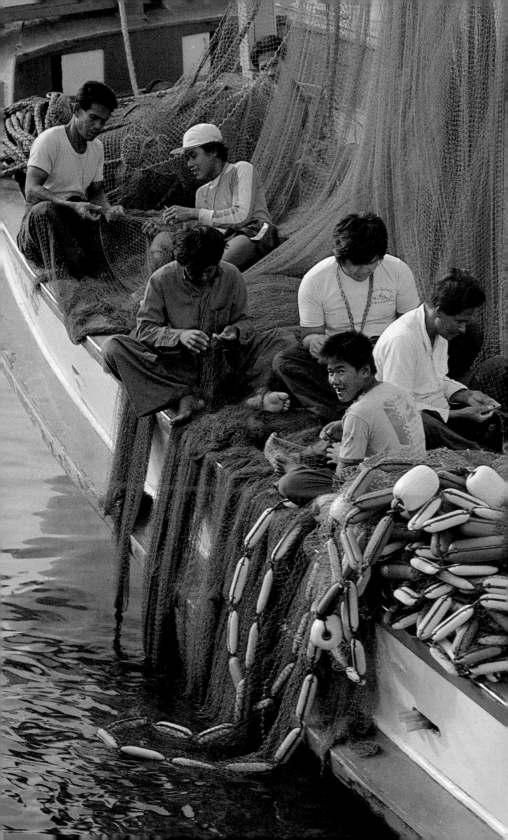

(visiting Korat and Phimai), Phitsanulok, the Bhumibol Dam (with visits to Sukhothai and Sri Satchanalai), Chiang Mai and Chiang Rai. Transportation is cleverly planned by rail, road, air and river (down the **Mae Kok River** from **Tha Thon** to Chiang Rai). Departures from Bangkok are every Wednesday, and you need to make bookings well in advance. Price is 11,000 Baht (US$550) per person (minimum 2) and all meals are included. Operated by Diethelm Travel, but you can book through any agent.

The Eastern Gulf

The growth of **Pattaya Beach** from a fishing village to a full-scale resort in less than 10 years is one of the greatest success stories of tourism in Asia. The long beach is fronted by almost a dozen top class hotels and there are more on a cliff-top nearby. There are also bungalow complexes ideal for families with children. Nightlife ranges from noisy to naughty — in fact, whatever you want it to be — and restaurants match Bangkok's for variety and flair, with an emphasis, of course, on fresh seafood.

Every imaginable water sport is available — sailing, fishing, wind surfing, skiing, scootering, or just swimming, and there's also the delight of para-sailing if you dare. Dive shops provide Scuba gear, and qualified instructors, and it's easy to arrange cruises by junk or fishing boat to off-shore coral islands. Some hotels have tennis and squash courts, and there are golf courses nearby. Inland tour pursuits include an elephant show and orchid farms. You can ride horses or motorcycles (check the insurance!), or simply soak up the sun at the beach or around the hotel swimming pool.

Pattaya is less than a two-hour drive from Bangkok and coach operators offer many daily departures, for around 120 Baht (US$6) each way. Even the top hotels are still relatively cheap — less than 1,100 Baht (US$50) for twin accommodation, but rates go up around 200 Baht during high seasons. Food is inclined to be more expensive than in Bangkok.

For those seeking quieter escapes to sea and sunshine, there are a number of other resorts along the same coast. Before Pattaya is **Bang Saen**, hectic with day-trippers at weekends and almost deserted during the week. The Tourism Authority operates the hotel, around 400 Baht (US$20) a twin room. The area's attractions include the monkey cliff on **Sammuk Hill**, a fishing village, a handicraft centre, oyster farms along the shore, and the nearby **Bang Phra** golf course, also operated by the TAT.

Bang Saray is down the coast from Pattaya, offering a good beach, limited facilities and bungalow accommodation. This is one of the best places for hiring fishing equipment and boats, and shell collectors can buy beautiful specimens from the fishermen.

An hour beyond Pattaya is **Rayong** with a private beach development called **Wang Kaew**. The small hotel and bungalows are often fully booked at weekends, but the beach is lovely and the restaurant offers simple, but tasty, Thai meals.

The other main attraction of the Eastern Gulf is the gem centre of **Chantaburi** — noted for sapphires. You can even hire your own plot and dig for gems yourself, but don't expect success.

The Southern Peninsula

Hua Hin is a traditional Thai resort that only recently has adequately catered to people who don't have their own beach cottages. The beach is wide, and long, and there's plenty of sea-space until late afternoon when the Thai people come out of the shade to swim. It is better to book accommodation in advance — especially in the hot summer season when children are on holiday (April and May). There's the **Railway Hotel** — ask for the "old

Opposite, a fishing boat at Hua Hin in the south.

51

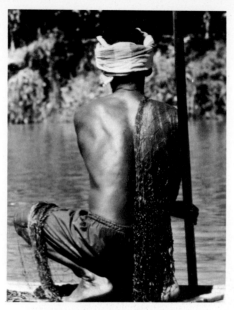

relaxed, with beaches that are devoted to the pursuit of sunshine rather than water-sport activity. There are two main beach-side hotels — the **Phuket Island Resort**, on its own private beach, and the **Patong**, on Patong Beach which also has a number of bungalow-style accommodations. Price for the hotels is around 550 Baht (US$27.50) a twin, higher during peak seasons. There is another good hotel in town, the Pearl, at around 500 Baht a twin, and regular hotel buses run to and from one of the beaches.

One can take tours around the island, climbing hills (**Laem Promthep** is lovely at sunrise or sunset) and visiting pearl farms and a tin dredge, but by far the most rewarding excursion is to **Phangnga Bay**, by coach and launch. The Bay is scattered with weird, towering limestone "islands," with cliffs that rise straight up from the clear, calm waters. Cruising by small boat is most appealing at dawn — one can watch dolphins playing on their way out to feed, and the area has an incredibly tranquil beauty. One "island," **Panyee**, has a Muslim fishing village on stilts, and you're welcome to visit. Another, **Pinggan**, was the location of the filming of the James Bond adventure "The Man with the Golden Gun." You'll recognise the hideway of the villain, Scaramanga.

wing" as the big, terraced rooms are charming and the "new" bungalows are sad by comparison — booked through Hualumpong Station; and the new **Sai Lom Hotel** that's expensive by Hua Hin standards at 750 Baht (US$36.50) a twin. Book at the **Rose Gardens Resort** office in **Siam Square**. Nightlife in Hua Hin is virtually nil and western food is, in general, not well prepared. Make sure you have breakfast in the Railway Hotel dining room during your visit; it's a worthwhile experience. There is a very extensive market and an excellent 18-hole golf course.

You can travel to Hua Hin by road or rail — trains leave Hualumpong around noon, 4.00 p.m. and 5.00 p.m. daily, arriving around four hours later. Most of the trains back leave Hua Hin extremely early in the morning, like 3.00 a.m. or 5.00 a.m.

Phuket, the southern island province, is most conveniently reached by air — TAC has at least one 737 jet flight daily. Road travel from Bangkok takes a tiring 14 hours and by the time one gets to the incredible coastal views of the **Andaman Sea** one has little appreciation of scenery. Phuket's economy is not, as yet, based on tourism and the seaside scene is calm and

Haad Yai is the brisk commercial centre of the south, full of markets and Malaysian tourists. There are many hotels, ranging from dingy old to garish modern, and most have good restaurants and facilities. Haad Yai's visitor attractions are mainly centred around shopping and Thai-style nightlife, but there is a very impressive reclining Buddha (at **Wat Haad Yai**), and one can watch bullfights (no matadors involved, just the bulls fighting each other). It is as much fun watching the gambling fever of the audience as the animals in their hefty battles.

Poses: left, a fisherman from the south and right, sculpture at Kanchanburi in the west.

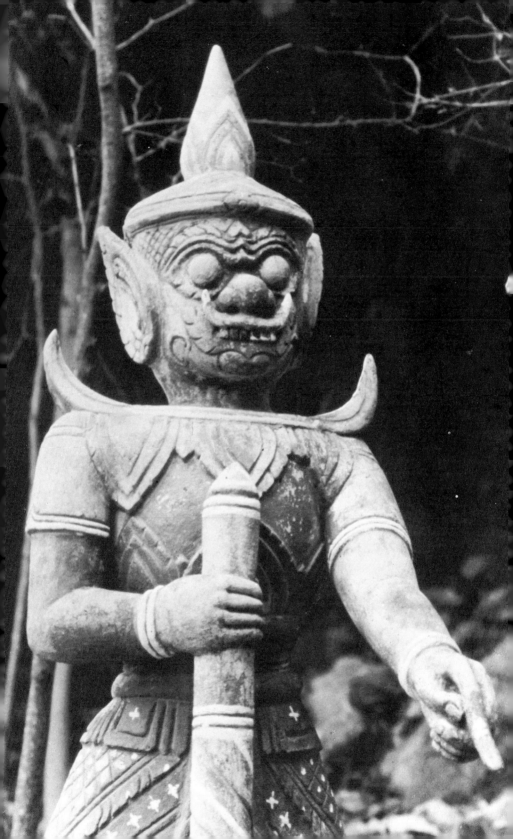

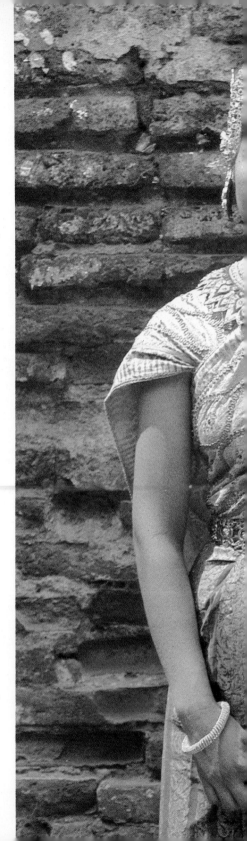

Haad Yai is also a good base for visiting the pretty resort of **Songkhla**, 30 kilometres away. **Samila Beach** has one good hotel, the Samila. Rooms are clean and comfortable and the terrace open-air dining room is a pleasant spot to relax. Along the beach is a fishing village, with the south's stylised, gaily decorated boats. The villages are Muslim and ladies will feel more comfortable wearing slacks than shorts or a skirt during a visit.

Songkhla also has a wide lagoon, which one can cross by ferry and climb a cliff (feels like many hundreds of stairs) to an old fortress at the top. The view of the lagoon and Samila Bay is impressive, especially when the fishing boats leave in the evening, with the crews letting off firecrackers to ask the spirits to provide a good catch.

Another southern Thai island is worthy of note — **Koh Samui**, Coconut Island, off the **Surat Thani** coast. Surat Thani can be reached from Bangkok by air, or by overnight train from the **Thonburi station**. One then takes a ferry across to the island. Accommodations are very simple and restaurants very modest, and the feeling is very escapist. There is little to do except explore the beaches, enjoy the sunshine and watch trained monkeys scampering up trees to harvest coconuts.

The Ancient Capitals

Ayuthaya, Siam's capital for four centuries before being overrun by the Burmese in 1767, is just 85 kilometres from Bangkok, along a good highway. Most people feel that a day trip out of Bangkok is sufficient, but an overnight stay (hotels are few, small and inexpensive, but clean) allows for not only more detailed exploration of the ruins but also the colourful experiences of a busy country town. There are two floating restaurants with waiters who speak enough English to guide you on the menu, and the opportunity to tour the major historical sites along the river surrounds by long-tailed boat. The

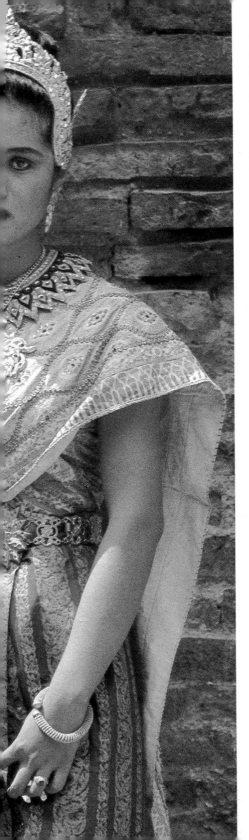

Tourism Authority's Bangkok office can advise on all details of getting there and getting around.

Sukhothai, Siam's first capital founded in 1238 is further north and less accessible. Most convenient way of touring is to fly from Bangkok to **Phitsanulok**, stay at the **Amarinakorn Hotel** and take day-time excursions from there. There is also a good new hotel, the **Phet**, around 300 Baht (US$15) a night in nearby **Kampaengphet**, one of the satellite cities of the Sukhothai era.

Sukhothai was abandoned, rather than destroyed by war, and some of the world's finest Buddhist art is still magnificently on display in the quiet surroundings of rural countryside. The old walled city is around 13 kilometres from "modern" Sukhothai town and is the main area of interest. Inside the walls is the **Ramkambaeng National Museum** with a fine collection of sculpture showing not only the Sukhothai refinements of Theravada Buddhism but the strong early influences of Brahmaism and the Khmer styles of art. Here too are the ruins of **Wat Mahathat**, the biggest and finest of the Sukhothai temples.

Outside the walls, at **Wat Sri Chum**, is one of Thailand's largest seated Buddhas, with each finger taller than a man. Other temple ruins worth a visit are **Wat Chetupon** and **Wat Saphan Hin**. Visitors are requested not to wander around the more isolated ruins without first reporting to police at the station opposite the **National Museum**.

Around 50 kilometres north of Sukhothai is **Sri Satchanalai**, with its old walled town reached by ferry across the **Yom River**. Here are some of the most beautiful Sukhothai era remains, including the kilns that produced the famous ceramics.

Old times: a Lopburi lady in traditional costume and over, *temple ruins in Central Thailand.*

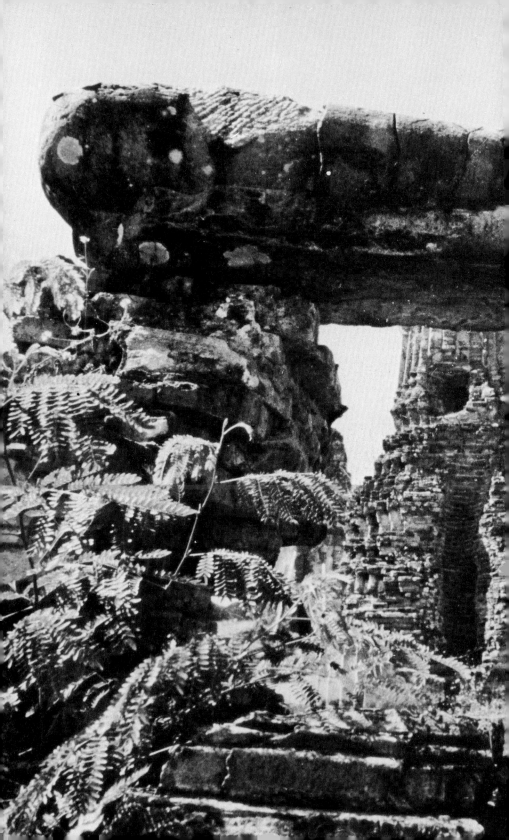

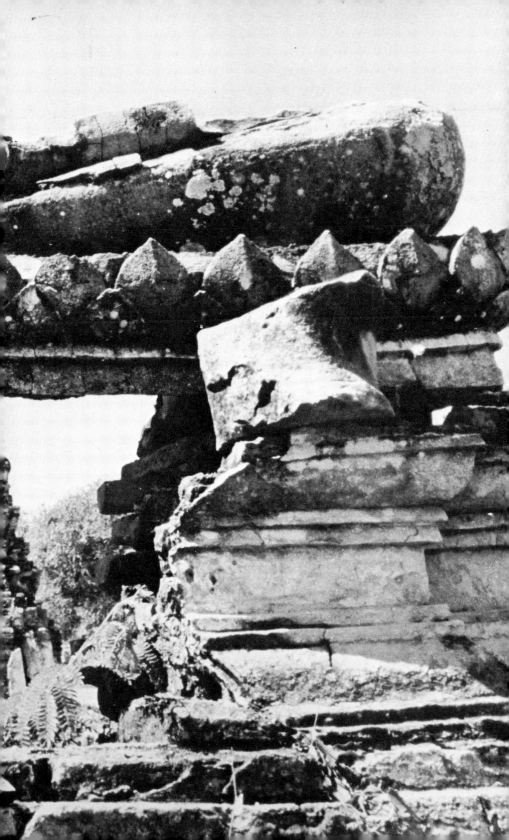

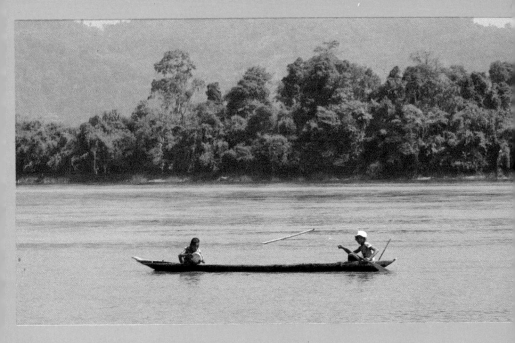

Passport to Adventure
Off the Beaten Track

For most visitors who take the time to explore a little beyond the standard travel patterns, Thailand can be called a country of adventure. Even a day spent just outside the cities can open up rare experiences of the countryside and its people while the traveller retains the basic comforts of hotel-style accommodation and conventional means of transportation. But beyond these mini-adventures are a number of opportunities to explore and experience the areas of Thailand that are little touched by the world outside. Venturing deep into the rugged jungles of the west and the misty, mysterious mountains of the north is, in general, not for the timid. For those with a strong spirit of adventure, fortitude and self-reliance along with an ability to accept the unexpected and adapt to often primitive living conditions, the rewards of new experiences and understanding can be enormous.

The Northern Mountains

As an introduction to the adventures of Thailand's far north, the **Mae Sa Valley**, just an hour's bumpy ride from **Chiang Mai**, provides a surprising degree of sophistication. A new accommodation project, opened early in 1980 in a valley setting at a cool 2,000 metres, offers a happy compromise between the remoteness of the mountains and the comforts of a city hotel. In fact, there is more a feeling of adventure rather than the pursuit of it, and even the more timid explorer will be able to relax.

The valley slope has been landscaped in a series of terraced gardens, with a collection of thatched-roof houses and simple bamboo cottages. Hotel-style comforts are provided in softly quilted beds, and bathrooms with hot water and modern fittings. The decor is a curious blend of Asian and European, which can only be described as Thai-Tyrolean. All vegetables served at the restaurant are grown on the hotel grounds, and the menu selection offers both Thai and western dishes. Accommodation is not cheap by up-country Thailand standards — a double room runs to around 600 Baht (US$30) and set meals are 250 Baht (US$12.50) per person each day. An overnight package out of Chiang Mai to the resort is offered for 1,700 Baht (US$85) per person, including a visit to an elephant camp, an hour's ride by elephant up to the resort, a visit to a hilltribe village and all meals. One can hike up into the hills around, or take arranged tours with a guide along. Bookings can be made at the **White Inn** in Bangkok, Soi 4, Sukhumvit Road, or in Chiang Mai, at the **North-West Tours** office in the **Suriwongse Hotel**.

At the elephant camp, a short hike down from the Mae Sa Valley Resort, it is possible to arrange safaris into the hills aboard the original Land-Rover, the elephant. The novelty of the journey soon wears off — elephants are surprisingly uncomfortable to ride for more than an hour or so at a time. Costs are around 2,500 Baht (US$125) per person for an overnight trip, with the night spent at a Meo hilltribe village. One needs a sleeping bag or at least a blanket. Contact in Chiang Mai is **Erawan Tours**.

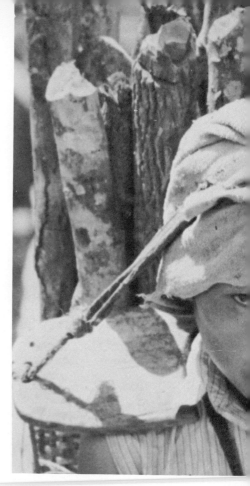

There are many hilltribe settlements in the northern areas, ranging from those of the least-sophisticated **Akha** to the villages of the **Meo** that have been pretty well commercialised by the frequent visits of foreign tour groups. In Chiang Mai one can arrange transportation and a guide to travel far into the hills, to villages that retain their basic cultures and traditions as yet little eroded by attempts to assimilate them into the mainstream of Thai life. Costs range from as little as 400 Baht (US$20) a day per person, but it should be noted that a guide familiar with the areas, and peoples, is essential. It is recommended that arrangements be made with a reputable tour agency (both **North-West Tours**, previously mentioned, and **Discovery Tours**, in the **Chiang Inn Hotel**, have already established good reputations for this style of programme).

Trekking programmes demand a good degree of fitness, confidence, and again, careful planning with a reliable agent. They can, however, offer some of the north's greatest scenic experiences, and the rare opportunity to visit an assortment of isolated and unique mountain tribes. A six-day itinerary out of Chiang Mai, with the actual trekking beginning in the area of **Fang**, can take one through areas of bamboo and teak forest, jungles and green valleys, and into settlements of the **Shan, Lisu, Akha, Meo** and **Yao**. The last day would involve a journey by jeep into **Chiang Rai**, for travel by air or bus back to Chiang Mai. Costs would be in the region of 6,000

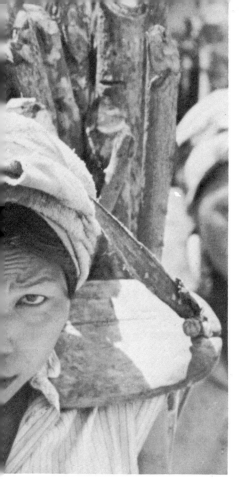

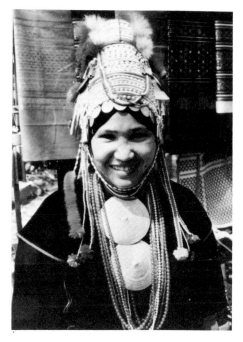

Baht (US$300) per person, with all accommodation and meals provided in the local villages. Conditions, at best, are primitive, and such a trip should only be undertaken by those with a proven ability to hike long distances, a curious mind, and a strong stomach to cope with alien foods.

Less arduous is a hike on foot or by pony up **Doi Inthanon**, Thailand's highest mountain which reaches almost 2,500 metres. The peak is in the **Doi Inthanon National Park**, around 70 kilometres from Chiang Mai. One needs to obtain approval from the park authorities in Chiang Mai, and in a three-day trip, one can see working elephants, and Karen and Meo villages. There are set camp-sites along the way, with simple accommodation and facilities.

One of the most popular overnight tours out of Chiang Mai is to **Chiang Rai**, riding the rapids of the **Mae Kok River** from Tha Thon, on the Burmese border. An exciting variation is to do the river section by bamboo raft, spending two nights on board one's own river house. Each raft is built especially for each trip arranged so costs are rather high. One of the largest Bangkok-based tour operators, Diethelm Travel (at the corner of Soi Ton Son on Ploenchit Road) does arrange special programmes including the Mae Kok trip by raft, but plenty of advance time is needed. An eight-day programme by train out of Bangkok, including all meals and nights in Chiang Mai, Chiang Rai and on the raft, is around 7,500 Baht (US$375) per person, based on a minimum of six participants.

Kanchanaburi

The province of **Kanchanaburi** is one of Thailand's most wildly beautiful areas, located some 130 kilometres northwest of Bangkok, bordering on Burma. Once

Endurance: Ekah hill tribe woman from Chiang Rai, and tribeswoman near the Burmese border. Over, the stars of the elephant round-up.

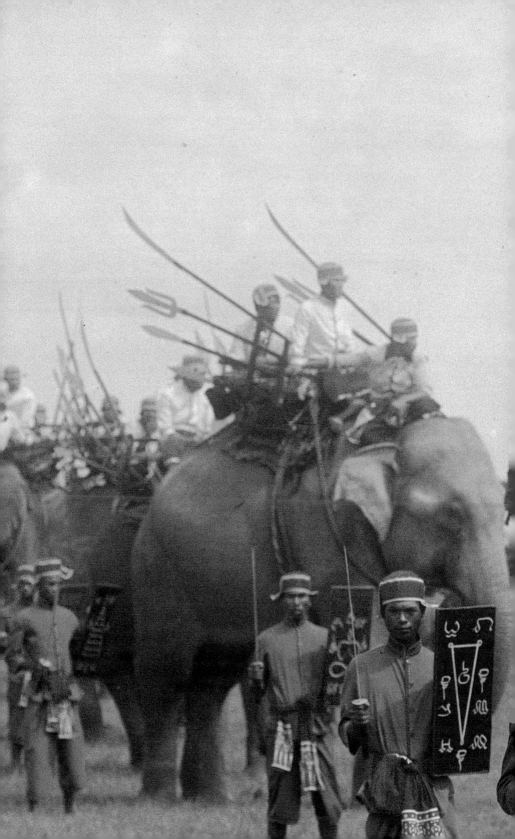

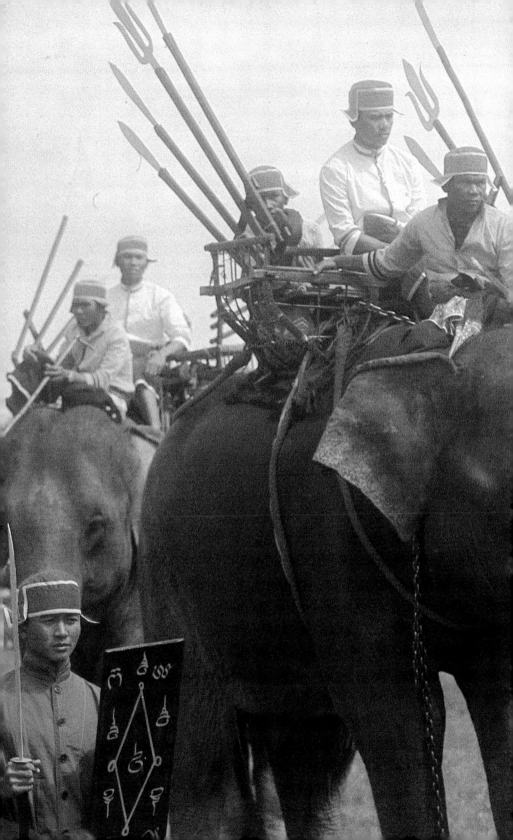

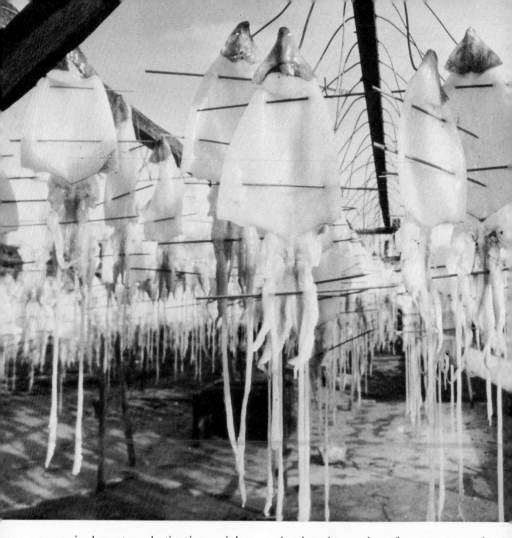

recognised as a tour destination mainly for its famous **Bridge over the River Kwai** and "Death Railway," its great growth in popularity over recent years is one of the success stories of Thai tourism. There is now a good riverside lodge, and numerous developments offering accommodation in bamboo cottages on on rafts anchored at the river bank. An imaginative collection of tour activities includes trips along the old railway and the river and into the jungle, and many of these excursions are trips into a wilderness world which is fast disappearing.

An enterprising Frenchman, Jaques Bes, responsible for the establishment of the first river-raft accommodation, has developed a number of even more exotic programmes, that offer even the most jaded explorer entirely new realms to discover. Most ambitous is a six-day expedition up into the mountainous area of the **Three Pagodas Pass**, the point where the railway built through Kanchanaburi by allied prisoners of war during World War II was to link Thailand with Burma. The trip involves travel by jeep and boat, with variations depending on the time of year and the height of the river, and hikes through the jungle to **Lao, Mon** and **Karen** villages for the overnight stays. Participants also explore limestone caves and remains of the tracks and waggons from the days of the railway's construction, now being

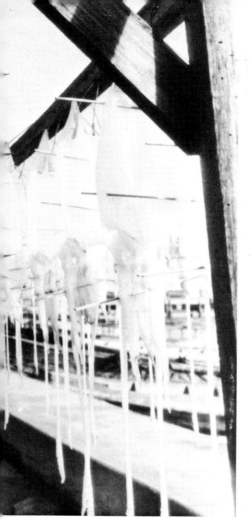

elephant and jungle experience without the thrills of the calls of the wild at night. Any overnight stay in the jungle is at a simple hut or local village. Definitely not for the nervous, or those who are picky eaters.

The mood of living on a bamboo raft quietly anchored at the river bank is considerably enlivened by the idea of actually cruising down the river. Allowing plenty of time for the raft construction, it is possible to arrange a two or three day "float," but costs are high for just a couple of people. Each raft costs around 6,000 Baht (US$300) to build, sleeping up to ten people, and one needs a boat to accompany it, at 1,000 Baht (US$50) per day. Journeys can begin or end at the Floatel rafts, with a cook and driver on board to take care of all the boat-keeping details. Meal costs are 185 Baht (US$9.25) a day, per person. The **Floatel office** in Bangkok is at the **Narai Hotel** on Silom Road.

Phuket

This southern island province is more noted for the tranquility of its beaches rather than any adventurous activity but mention should be made of the five or six day Scuba diving trips that can be arranged. The islands in the Andaman Sea, off the coast of **Ranong**, offer some of the most spectacular diving experiences anywhere but suspense is provided by the prevalence of pirates in the area. The islands are isolated and people are wary of strangers so engine trouble can leave one with a long row home. Apart from taking these hazards into account, the trip should also only be considered by well-experienced divers. Local agents in Phuket will be able to assist with arranging a boat and a crew and assembling all equipment and food.

covered by the relentless jungle. Prices are quoted for an eight-day programme, including travel to and from Bangkok and the first and last nights at the Floatel river-rafts. For two people, cost is 8,250 Baht (US$412.50) each; for four people, 5,200 Baht (US$260) each. Accommodation and meals are the "best available" at the local villages (delightful French cuisine at the rafts!), and people joining the trip are recommended to have a lightweight pack, sleeping bag, sturdy shoes, a first-aid kit and plenty of pluck.

Jungle trips by elephant are also arranged by Jaques Bes, at 1,200 Baht (US$60) each day per elephant, which carries two people. It can be a day's excursion for those who want the

Delights: opposite, squid drying at Hua Hin and over, the endless spectacle of dramatic coastline.

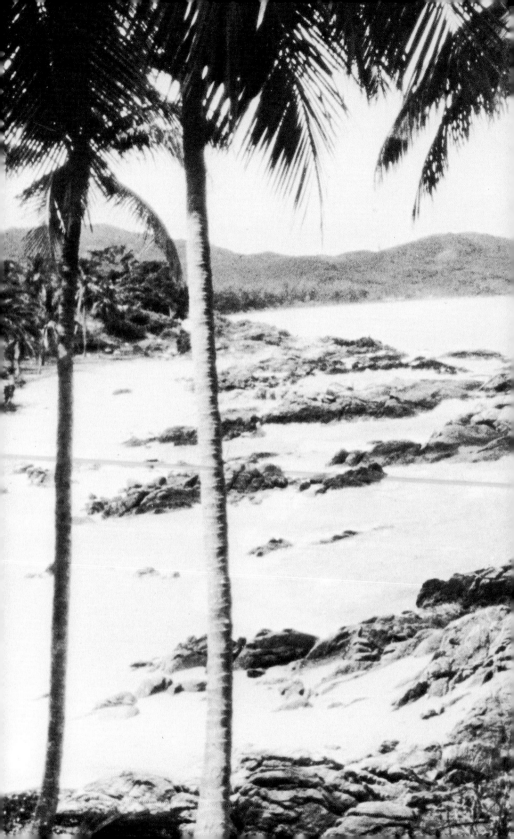

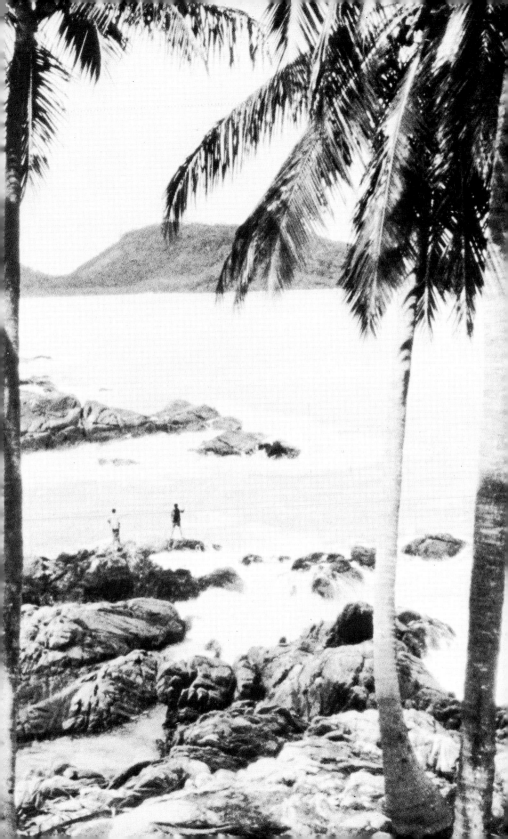

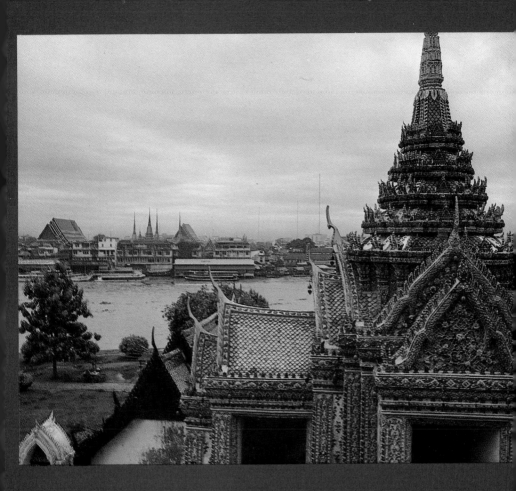

Travellers Tips

Passports/Visas

All visitors to Thailand must have a valid passport, but visas for most nationalities do not have to be obtained in advance for a stay of up to five days. For the "transit without visa" pass, passengers should have an onward ticket out of Thailand. There have been announcements that this 15-day pass will be extended to 30 days in the "near future" but this is not likely to be until 1982. At present, no extensions are permitted and a passenger must not overstay the 15 days. Exceptions can be made in cases of illness but one needs an official doctor's certificate, and the process of extending the visa is very complicated. For people who want to stay longer than 15 days, tourist visas can be obtained from Thai embassies and consulates abroad. These are good for up to two months with a possible one month extension.

The validity of a tourist visa is three months, which means the passenger must enter Thailand within three months of obtaining the visa. An exit visa is not required; airport departure tax is 50 Baht (US$2.50) per person. The Bangkok immigration office is on **Soi Suan Plu**, off Sathorn Tai Road, telephone 286-7003.

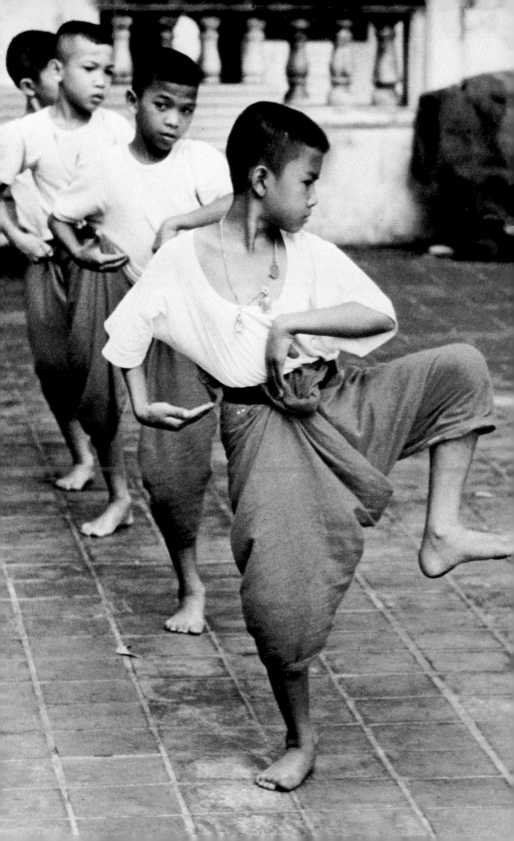

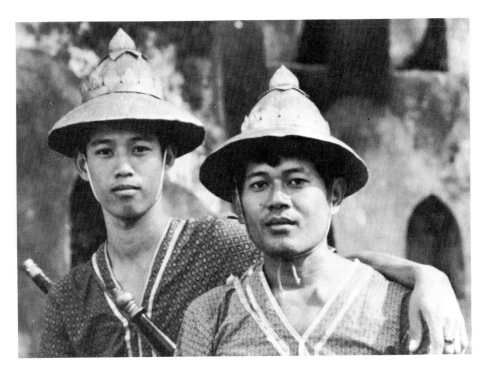

Health Regulations

It is no longer necessary to have certificates of smallpox and cholera innoculations to enter Thailand, unless one is arriving from an infected area. A general opinion is that one should have the innoculations anyway as with any cholera "scare" in the region, the need for certification is likely to be re-introduced.

Customs

Goods permitted to be brought in duty-free include 200 cigarettes, one litre of wine or spirits. The usual restrictions on weapons, drugs etc. apply.

Currency

A visitor can bring in any amount of money in travellers cheques but cash over US$2,000 should be declared on arrival. Foreign cash taken out must not be greater than the amount declared on arrival. No one can bring in, or take out, Thai currency of more than 500 Baht (US$25).

Thai Baht is in notes of 500 Baht (purple), 100 Baht (red), 20 Baht (green), and 10 Baht (brown). Coins are 5 Baht (round, silver, with a copper-coloured rim), one Baht (silver, round) and 50 stang and 25 stang, small brown coins. There are 100 stang to 1 Baht. Approximate exchange rates are:

US$1 = 20 Baht
A$1 = 22 Baht
DM$1 = 11 Baht
S$1 = 10 Baht

Most international credit cards are widely accepted in Bangkok and to a lesser degree in the major tourist centres of Pattaya and Chiang Mai. Change money at hotels (rates are usually quite low), licenced money changers and banks — branches of the Bangkok Bank generally give the best rates.

Unending drama: left, *boys learning Thai dancing* and above, *Lopburi Festival.*

71

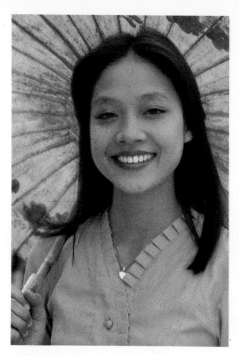

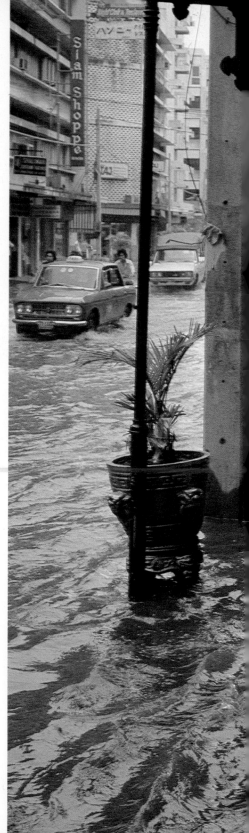

Weather

Most of Thailand has three distinct
seasons — the hot season spanning
March through May; the rainy season
June through October; and the "winter,"
November until February. The hot
season brings temperatures between
30°C and 40°C (not too many days
reaching the extreme peak), and during
the monsoon period the temperatures are
lower but the humidity is generally
higher. This season is the most erratic —
some days are clear and sunny while
others have torrential thunderstorms that
produce a surprising amount of water to
wade through on city streets. The cool
season is the most pleasant for exploring,
although temperatures in the north can
drop to 8°C and one definitely needs a
jacket.

Thailand's sunshine is very strong —
midday is not recommended for
sunbathing as one is sure to burn very
quickly. The climate down the southern
peninsula is less extreme, with the
weather generally sunny and humid all
year round. Rains are unpredictable,
likely to occur at any season.

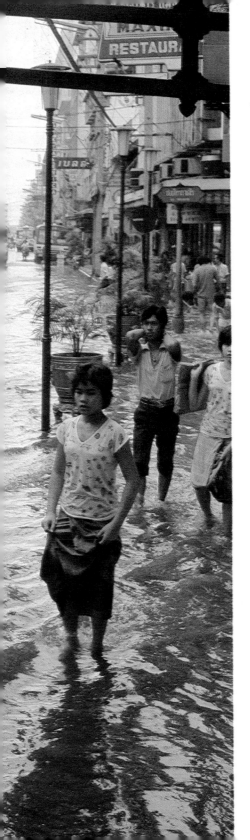

Clothing

Leave your nylon shirts and underwear at home; cool cottons are the most comfortable for Thailand. While to be "casual" is quite acceptable, Thais appreciate neatness and it is considered impolite to wear shorts and skimpy tops on city streets. And ladies should omit the "little black dress" from a Thailand wardrobe — black is the colour of mourning. Wear a hat while travelling under the sun, and always, comfortable shoes.

Transfers and Transportation

Thai International runs the transfer services from Bangkok's **Don Muang Airport** into town. A private limousine is 200 Baht; seat-in-the-coach 50 Baht, to any hotel.

Around Bangkok, available transport varies immensely in style and price. Local buses, non-airconditioned, are an experience to be avoided, especially at rush hours (early morning, late afternoon), but are delightfully cheap at one Baht for any journey. Air-conditioned buses are five Baht, and better value. Routes are all marked in Thai, but explanatory maps are available at book stores.

Local taxis are cheap but can be hair-raising. All have meters but these are never used (an over-sight of the law that introduced them), and a price must be settled before you get in. Minimum fare is 10 Baht, and that's for a very short journey; average would be 20 Baht; and from Silom Road to the old city area of the Grand Palace no more than 50 Baht. Fares are higher during rush hours. Be sure the driver understands exactly where you want to go (English language is a problem) — better to have your destination written in Thai.

Heavy weather: far left, sunshaded lady of Chiang Mai and left, coping with Bangkok's floods once again.

Hotel taxis are more expensive, but air-conditioned, and most drivers will speak a little English.

The three-wheeled *samlors*, called tuk-tuks, are not recommended for extensive travel around the city. Although cheaper than taxis (about 40 percent less), they're hazardous in city traffic.

Hire cars are available from **Avis** and **Hertz**, and a number of small local companies. Self-drive is not recommended, as driving in Bangkok traffic takes a lot of nerve and getting used to. **Avis** (at the **Rama Tower Hotel**, Silom Road, telephone 234-1010, ext 257) charges from 1,200 Baht (US$60) a day, including chauffeur, gas and full insurance; **Hertz** 750 Baht (US$37.50) a day, with chauffeur but excluding gas and two Baht charge per kilometre. It's approximately 250 Baht (US$12.50) more a day to keep the car overnight outside Bangkok. The Hertz office is on **Ploenchit Road**, telephone 252-4917. Avis has a number of "drive-way" holiday programmes available, to Pattaya Beach and Chiang Mai, and also has a Chiang Mai office.

Thailand's highways are good — especially the **Asian Highway** network — but as over 80 percent of the traffic is commercial — heavy trucks that defy any speed limit, and "orange-crush" buses that race to be ahead of schedule — road travel by local transport can only be described as "rather dangerous," especially at night. Tour coaches, with better safety standards (and drivers not paid incentives to get there ahead of time) do operate over main routes, but are recommended for day-time travel only.

The road to Pattaya Beach is now a dual highway, a great improvement since 1979, and the trip from Bangkok takes just two hours. Thai International operates coaches directly from Bangkok Airport to the resort, departing Don Muang daily at 11.00 a.m. and 9.00 p.m.; returning to the airport at 6.00 a.m. and 4.00 p.m. Cost is 130 Baht (US$6.50) per person, one way.

Many tour operators have regular

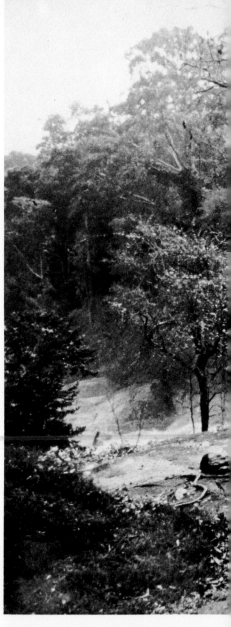

coach services from Bangkok hotels to Pattaya — as an example, **World Travel Service**, one of the best, has departures from Bangkok at around 8.00 a.m. 12.00 and 4.00 p.m. daily, for 120 Baht (US$6) each, way, or 220 Baht (US$11) round trip.

Air services around Thailand by the domestic carrier, **Thai Airways**, are plentiful, many by Boeing 737 jet, but

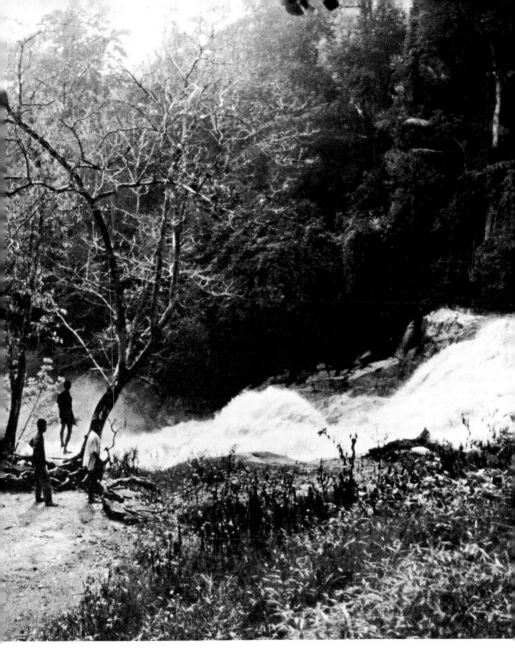

capacity is insufficient at peak holiday seasons (particularly November through January), so bookings should be made well in advance for the most popular routings of Chiang Mai and Phuket. One-way fare to Chiang Mai is 930 Baht (US$46.50); to Phuket 1,120 Baht (US$56); Haad Yai 1,270 Baht (US$63.50) and Udorn, in the northeast, 650 Baht (US$32.50). Fare increases are to be expected with the rises in fuel costs. Thai Airways office is at **6 Larn Luang Road**, telephone 281-1633.

Thailand's train services are highly recommended as a very pleasant compromise between the tedium and hazards of long journeys by road and the

Above, *waterfall: near Kanchanaburi, Western Thailand.*

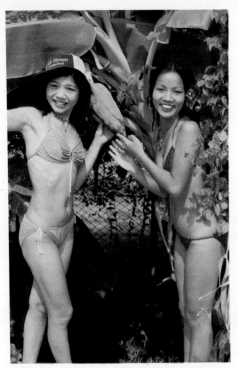

the tourist centres communication can be a problem. It is advisable to have your hotel address written out in Thai, and ask the hotel reception staff to write out in Thai any particular location you need to reach by bus or taxi.

Hotels

Bangkok has some of the region's finest hotels — over 10,000 rooms meeting international standards. Many have particular attributes, such as **The Oriental's** superb river-side location, the **Siam Inter-Continental's** spacious garden setting; and **The Ambassador's** extensive collection of restaurants, and all have many "luxuries" as standard service — swimming pools, 24-hour room service and a high staff-to-guest ratio. Apart from its top-line hotels, the city also has a vast range of cheaper accommodations, some of them with a charming "guest-house" atmosphere like the **White Inn** (Soi Nana 4, Sukhumvit Road).

Outside the capital, with the exception of Pattaya, the hotels are less lavish in their facilities, but all do promise a warm welcome and a high degree of personal attention.

The following hotels are all members of the **Thai Hotels Federation**, and offer the top accommodation available in each area indicated. Rates are approximate, as fluctuations occur between high and low seasons, and do not include the standard 10 percent service charge or 16.5 percent government tax. Rates are for a twin-bed room.

expense of air travel. Services on board are excellent, but food ranges between good and inedible (it can only be the luck of the day because it's hard to find a logical reason for the extreme variations). Avoid the risk by taking along packaged foods and fruit. The daily express service between Bangkok and Chiang Mai leaves Hualumpong Station at 6.00 p.m. and arrives Chiang Mai at 7.00 a.m. Costs are about 450 Baht (US$22.50) per person, one way, for first class (sharing an air-conditioned two-berth compartment), 250 Baht (US$12.50) for second class with berth, non-airconditioned. Bangkok — Haad Yai is around 530 Baht (US$26.50), one way, first class; 280 Baht (US$14) second class.

Language

Thai is the national language, with its own written form (based on Sanskrit) and regional variations in dialect. In hotels, the major restaurants, shops and offices, English is widely understood, but outside

Bangkok:

	Baht
Oriental	1,700
Montien	1,400
Siam Inter-Continental	1,400
Ambassador	1,400
President	1,300

Splashing out, above, at the Rincome Hotel, Chiang Mai and opposite, at a Bangkok hotel.

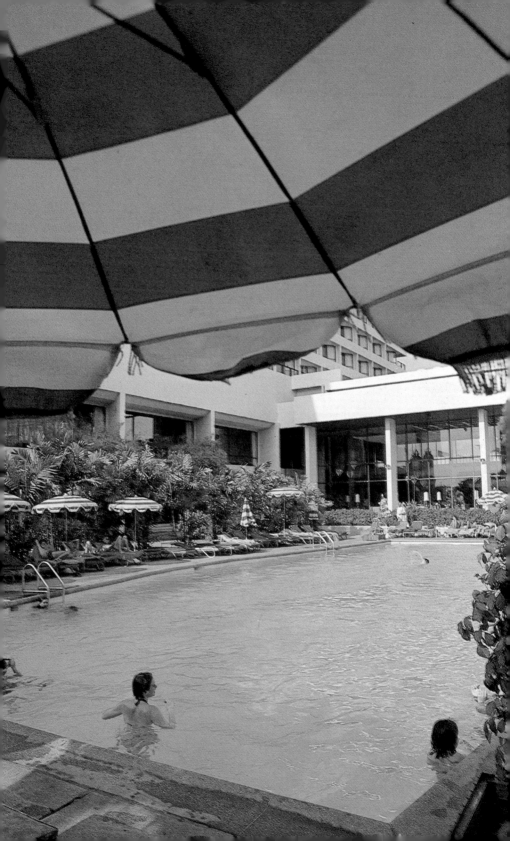

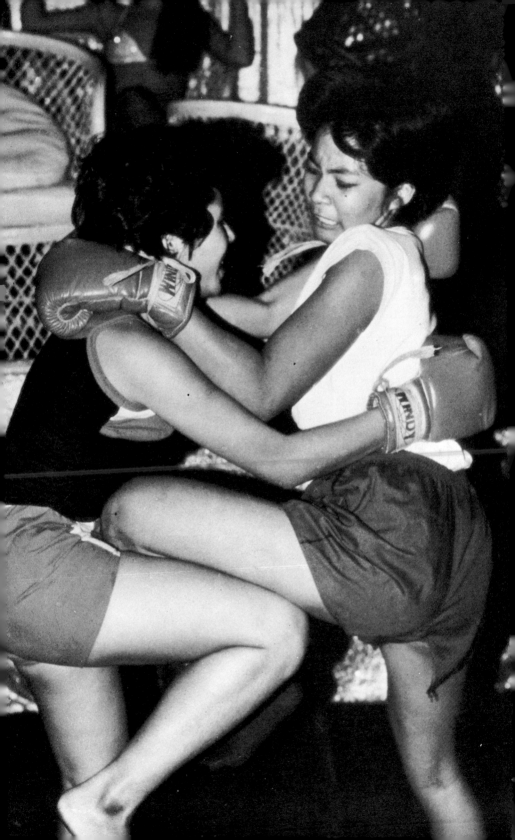

Dusit Thani	1,300
Erawan	1,300
Sheraton	1,200
Indra Regent	1,200
Rama Tower	1,200
New Imperial	1,100
Narai	950
Mandarin	1,100
Asia	1,100
First	950
Impala	600
Chavalit	950
Windsor	900

Pattaya:

Royal Cliff Beach	900
Pattaya Palace	900
Regent Pattaya	900
Asia Pattaya	800
Tropicana	780
Holiday Inn	800
Siam Bayshore	900
Wongse Amatya	800
Orchid Lodge	800
Ocean View	700
Royal Garden	800

Chiang Mai:

Rincome	900
Chiang Inn	800
Poy Luang	600
Suriwongse	700

Phuket:

Phuket Island Resort (beach-side location)	550
Pearl (in town)	500

Electricity

Thailand operates on 220 volt, 50 cycle AC power, but most hotels, at least in Bangkok, Pattaya and Chiang Mai, will be able to provide adaptors.

Water

Visitors should *not* drink tap water — the water is apparently good at its sources but pipes travel under the canals and there is concern about seepage. Hotels

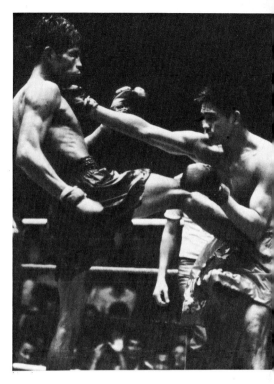

and restaurants provide bottled water for drinking and at the open-air markets and small restaurants, one is usually offered pale iced tea.

Business Hours

Government offices — most are open Monday through Friday 8.30 a.m. to 4.30 p.m., with a 12 noon to 1.00 p.m. lunch break.

Banks — Monday through Friday, 8.30 a.m. to 3.30 pm.

Post Offices — the Bangkok G.P.O. is on New Road (Charoen Krung) between Suriwongse and Siphya Roads, open from 8.00 a.m. to 8.00 p.m. Monday through Friday; until 1.00 p.m. on weekends and holidays. There is a 24-hour service for long-distance telephone calls and telegrams. All hotels have post office facilities.

Retail stores — there is no fixed rule but

So vicious: Thai boxing above: the bigtime game in a stadium and right, infighting at a Patpong bar.

the big department stores, such as
Central, open around 10.00 a.m. daily
and close around 7.00 p.m. Smaller
stores often open earlier and close later;
markets in general close up by 7.00 p.m.,
except those that feature the open-air
dining rooms.

Newspapers

There are three daily newspapers in
English, the **Bangkok Post** (with the
highest circulation and good coverage of
world news), **Bangkok World** (an
afternoon tabloid) and the **Nation
Review**. Many overseas newspapers and
magazines are available at hotel book-
stores.

Shopping

The Tourism Authority publishes a guide
to recommended retail stores in Bangkok
which is available at the reception desks
of most hotels. Main shopping areas are
around Silom and Suriwongse Roads,
Charoen Krung Road; Siam Square and
the Siam Centre opposite, Rajdamri
Road, along the upper end of Sukhumvit
Road and, of course, in the multitude of
markets. There are few fixed-price stores
and each price tag is only an indication of
what the seller hopes to get. As a general
rule, deduct 40 percent and work up from
there. One of the best buys in Thailand is
jewellery — precious and semi-precious
stones set in white or yellow gold. Shop

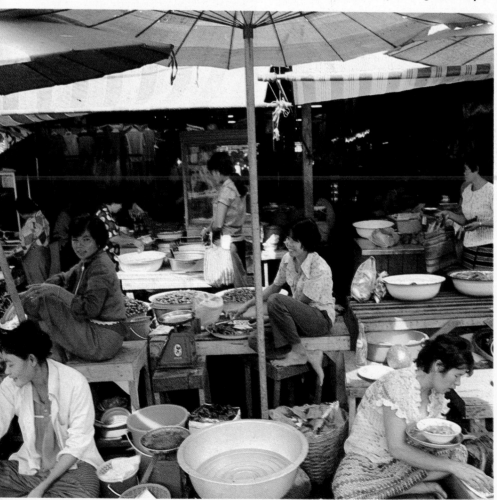

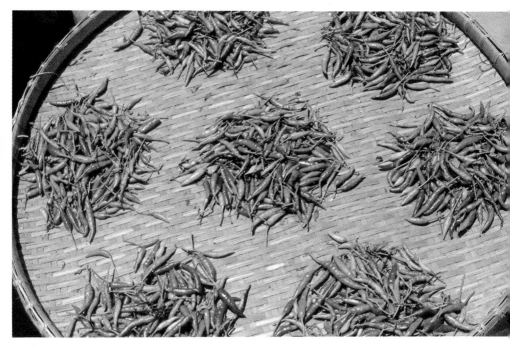

only at the recommended stores and insist on a guarantee. If you're spending big money on jewellery and you don't know gemstones, head for a shop with a firmly-established reputation, such as **Alex and Company** on Oriental Avenue. The owner is a gemologist, prices are high, but value is assured. This store will also do appraisals for you on jewellery you've purchased elsewhere.

Silk is everywhere in a glorious abundance of colours and patterns. The best selection, with a guarantee of the genuine product, is Jim Thompson's (the **Thai Silk Company**) near the Rama IV end of Suriwongse Road. Prices here are fixed, around 220 Baht (US$11) a yard for dress-weight silk, and there's also a good collection of ready made clothing, cushions, purses, ties, scarves and home accessories.

Handicrafts, in wood, bronze, neilloware, lacquer and basketry are popular buys, as are the distinctive creations in cloth, embroidery and silver by the various hilltribes. **Chiang Mai** is a major sales centre for hilltribe work, but in Bangkok one of the best overall collections is at the **Hill Tribe**

Foundation, just around the corner from **Siam Centre** on Phyathai Road.

Thai celadon pottery, copies of the art developed at the old capital of Sukhothai, is very beautiful but heavy to carry home. Best selection is at **Celadon House**, on Silom Road.

Over recent years, Thailand has developed the skill of leatherwork, and the quality matches that of many of the overseas, well-established leather manufacturers.

Be careful about buying antiques and religious objects. The Thai government has clamped down strongly on the export of religious art — both antique and modern. The export of Buddha images, even those made in Burma, is *totally forbidden* and for antiques an export permit is required, and not always granted. Most reputable dealers will help in the obtaining of permits, but the process is slow and one must allow at least a week.

Weekend market, Bangkok: opposite, *shellfish preparation and* above, *the little wrinkled chillies are the real heavy guys.* Over, *at Rayong town fair in Central Thailand.*

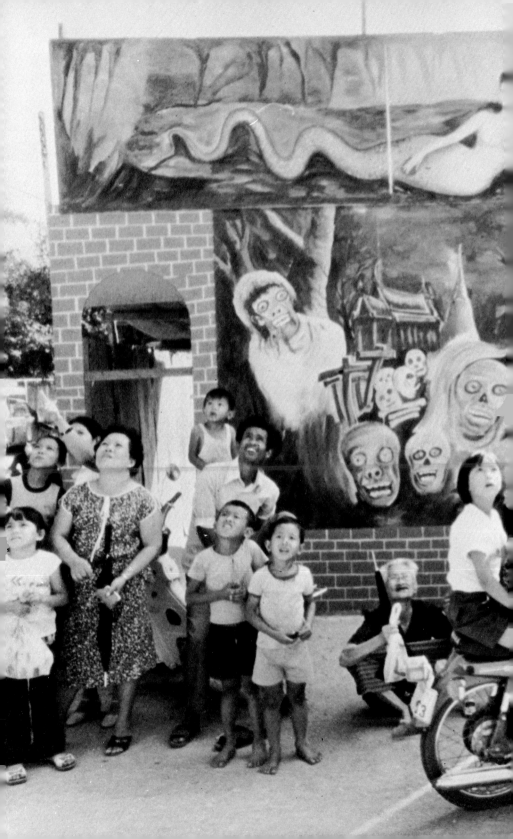

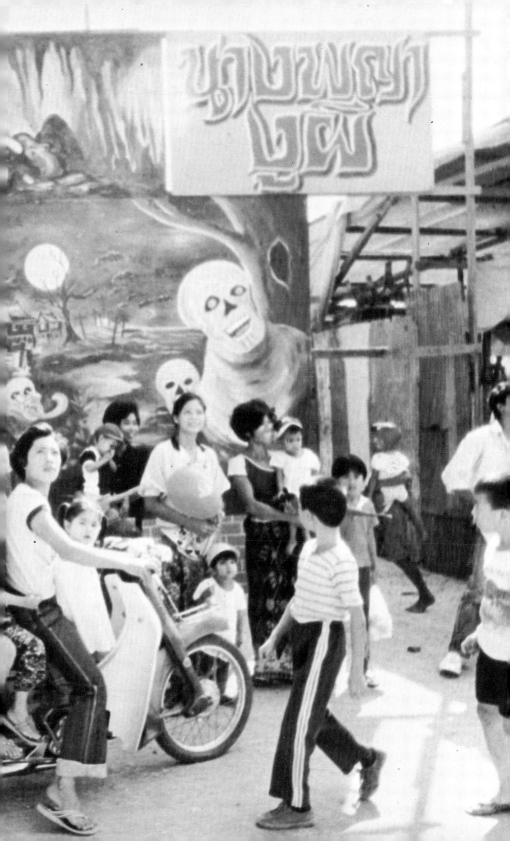

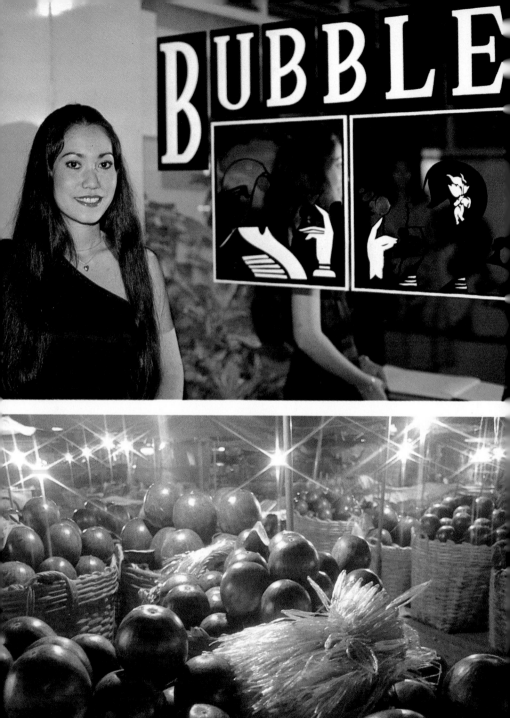
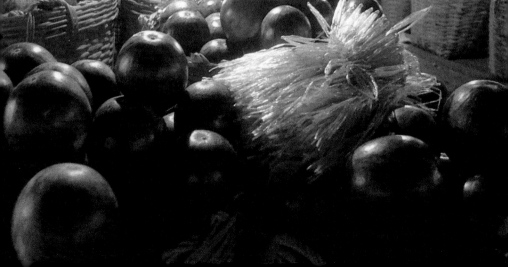

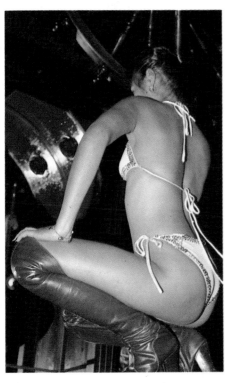

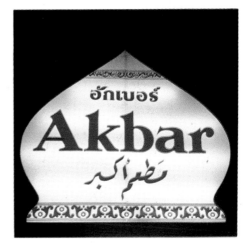

อักเบอร์

Akbar

مطعم اكبر

Nightlife

Bangkok's evening entertainment ranges from raunchy to sophisticated, covering all the naughty areas in between. The blocks around **Patpong Road**, between Silom and Suriwongse, are a neat little commercial district by day and a maze of bars with a-go-go, painted ladies, disco blare and bright lights by night. Great for a look at the seamier side of life, but with a happier atmosphere than found in similar areas elsewhere. Mixed couples will not feel out of place. For the truly seedy Bangkok nightlife scene, take a look around **Soi Cowboy**, off Soi 23 Sukhumvit Road, and the **Grace Hotel** coffee shop after midnight. For tamer pursuits, stay around the top hotels which all have bars and nightclubs but the scene is international rather than distinctly Thai.

One form of entertainment that cannot be ignored is that of the massage parlours. Literally hundreds offer the traditional massage or whatever one is prepared to pay for.

Outside Bangkok, the nightlife simmers down, except in **Pattaya** where the offerings rival the capital's array of hedonistic pursuits.

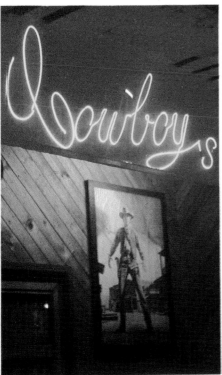

Appetites: flashing neon; succulent water melons; every want is catered for in Bangkok's night town.

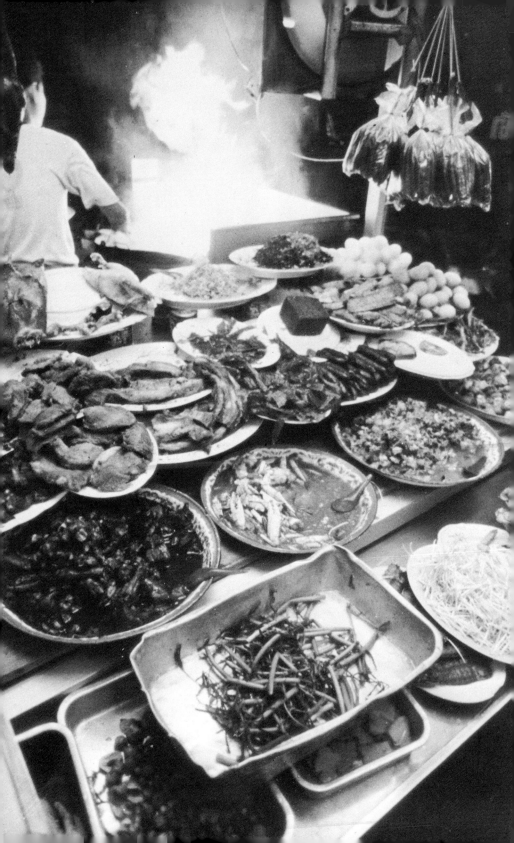

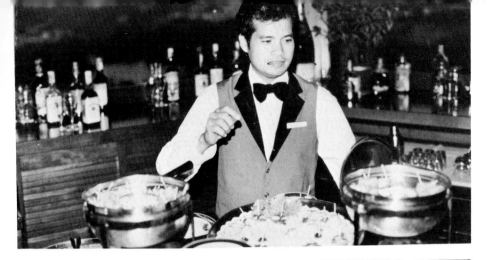

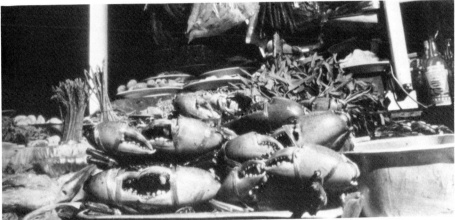

Dining Out

In Bangkok there's food to everyone's taste, in a collection of restaurants that specialise in every kind of Oriental and Western cuisine. Literally no culinary style is ignored and costs by international standards are relatively inexpensive, particularly in the restaurants not attached to hotels. In other tourist centres, western food is more restricted to the hotel dining rooms and coffee shops.

Thai food is best experienced by a novice at one of the restaurants catering to tourists. Many, like Bangkok's **Chit Pochana** on Soi 20 Sukhumvit, will tone down the chillis on request. Items to try at *Tom Yam*, a spicy soup with a distinctive flavour of lemon grass, made with shrimp, chicken or fish; *Gang Pet*, a hot curry of meat or fish with coconut milk; any of the noodle dishes, with *Barmi*, the yellow noodles, *Mee Krob*, the crispy noodles, or *Khoit Teo*, the wide rice noodles; *Kai Yat Sai*, an omelette stuffed with pork; and *Preo Wan*, the sweet and sour dish with chicken, pork or seafood.

Bangkok has a number of theatre-restaurants that offer performances of classical and folk dances and a set meal of typical Thai foods. Popular among these are **Baan Thai** at **7 Sukhumvit Soi 32** and **Piman** at **46 Sukhumvit Soi 49**. Cost is around 250 Baht (US$12.50) per person.

More appetisers: opposite, *flash-frying at a food shop;* above left, *preparing flashy food at the Dusit Thani Hotel, Bangkok;* right, *food to snare the passers-by in a food shop.*

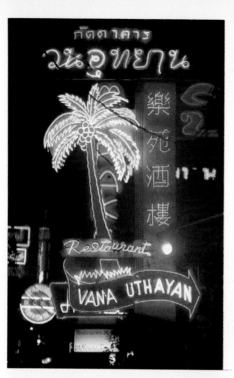

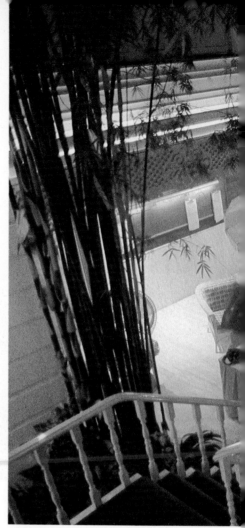

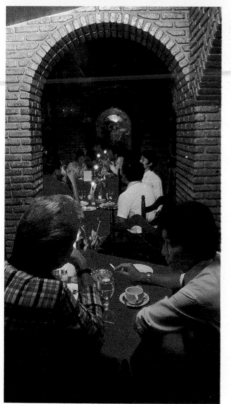

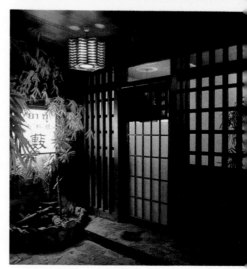

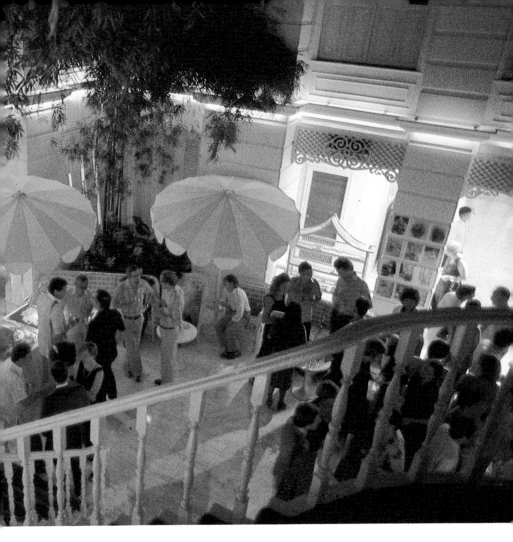

Tipping

Hotels and most restaurants add a 10 percent service charge to the bill so additional tipping is optional. It should be noted that a one Baht tip is considered rude and unless you feel that more is deserved, it's better not to tip at all.

Television

All television programmes are dubbed in Thai, but English soundtracks for the few American and British series programmes are available on FM radio. News also is in Thai, but both Channel 7 and Channel 3 do have short satellite coverage every evening with English soundtrack.

Cinema

A few years back the Thai Government raised import taxes on foreign films to an extraordinary degree, making it economically unfeasible for distributors to bring in the latest releases, except for those which are sure to have wide local audience appeal, such as "Superman." Old films already in the country from before the ban are re-run, which is great if you really want to see "West Side Story" again. Western films are shown with

Nights in style: far left top, *neon tempter;* bottom left, *Roberto's Italian Restaurant;* near left, *outside one of the many Japanese restaurants; and* above, *the Authors' Lounge at the Oriental Hotel.*

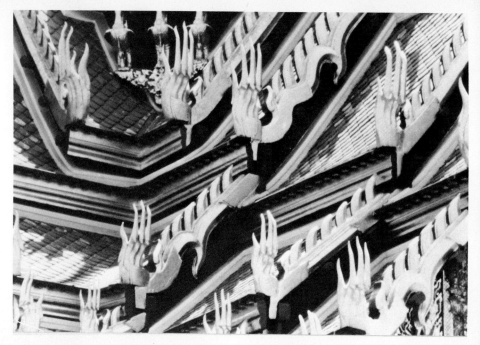

English soundtracks (Thai subtitles) in over a dozen Bangkok theatres that are air-conditioned and extremely comfortable. Highest ticket price is 40 Baht.

What the average Thai movie lacks in cinematic skill it makes up for in length and range of emotions covered. All seem to attempt to cater (in 2-1/2 hours or more) to every taste, with romance, brawls, music, slap-stick and incredibly gory violence, held together loosely by a confusing central theme. With the prohibitive tax on foreign films, some producers are making brave, and good, attempts at developing the art to a more sophisticated level, but lack of local popularity is rather defeating. There's also a good array of Chinese "sword-fighting" films, many with English sub-titles. Thai films have no English sub-titles.

One joy of the Thailand cinema is the enormous posters and displays produced as advertisements. These are Thailand's finest "pop art," in glorious technicolour, taking up whole sides of buildings and especially-erected billboards all over the city.

Church Services

Catholic — Assumption Cathedral, Oriental Avenue, or Holy Redeemer, Soi Ruam Rudee; **Episcopalian** — Christ Church, Convent Road; **Baptist** — Calvary Church, Soi 2, Sukhumvit Road; **Mormon** — Church of Christ, Soi 21, Sukhumvit Road; **Presbyterian** — International Church, Soi 19, Sukhumvit Road; **Seventh Day Adventist** — Soi Charoen Suk, Soi 63 Sukhumvit Road. The *Bangkok Post* lists times of services in English in the weekend editions.

Doctors/Hospitals

Medical care in Thailand is of a generally high calibre, and qualified treatment can be obtained at most hospitals. However, for those who would prefer the services of a European doctor, the following clinics in Bangkok are recommended: **P.S.E. Clinic**, 3/4 Nares Road (off Suriwongse) telephone 235-3981; **British Dispensary,**

Symmetry: above, sculpted roofs and opposite, fluid dancers. Over, the old rhythms continue unbroken outside Bangkok.

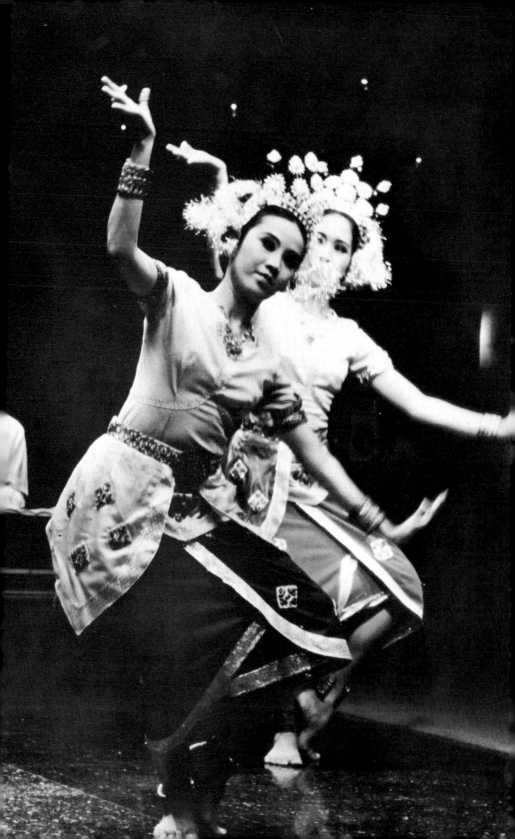

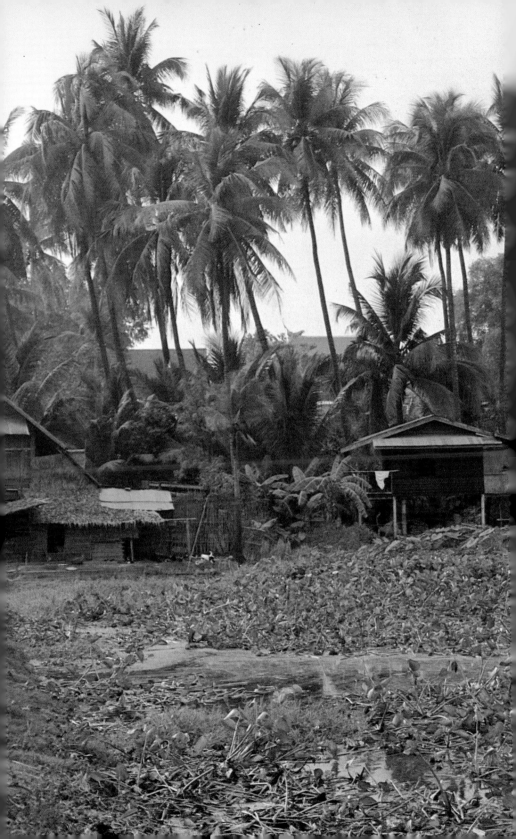

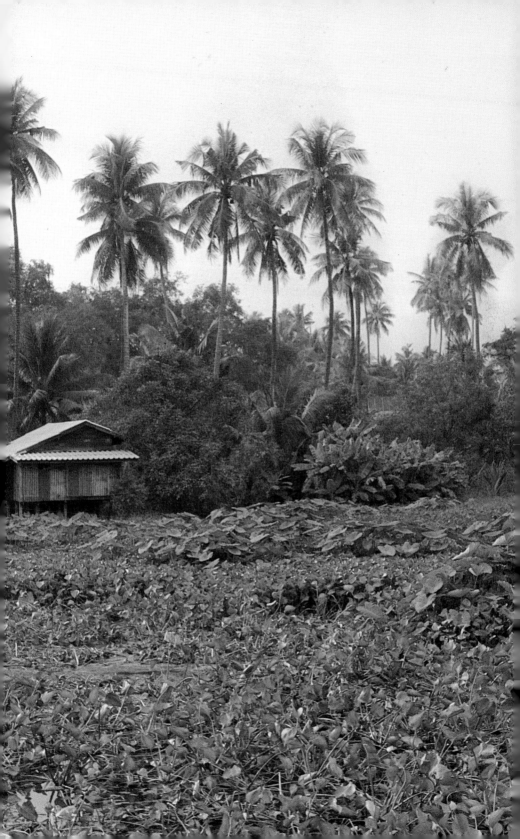

corner of Oriental Avenue, New Road, telephone 234-0174, or 108 Sukhumvit Road, near Soi 5, telephone 252-8056; **New French Dispensary**, (a husband and wife team of doctors), 691 Siphya Road, telephone 234-2790.

Recommended hospitals are: **Bangkok Nursing Home**, Convent Road (the most expensive); **Bangkok Christian** (corner of Silom and Patpong Roads); **Petchburi General**, 1126 New Petchburi Road, near the Wireless Road intersection.

Personal Security

Petty crime has risen greatly in Thailand over recent years, particularly in the cities that play host to the ever-increasing numbers of tourists. Things to watch out for are pickpockets (carry money in a pocket accessible only to you); handbag snatchers, even on busy city streets; and the pilfering from handbags on crowded buses. It is wise not to wear a lot of expensive-looking jewellery, and keep all travel documents and money in a hotel deposit box or safe. In the case of armed threat, do *not* resist the robbery, and report immediately as you can to the police. Your hotel will advise on the procedures to take. Such incidents can be avoided by using discretion when walking around the quieter parts of town, and taking taxis around at night rather than walking home to your hotel. A word about drugs — Thailand has now imposed among the world's severest penalties for buying or carrying narcotics, which are still both plentiful and cheap. Do *not* be tempted by the availability — most sources are known to the police and you can very easily get caught. Your embassy, or a lawyer, can do very little to help. Be cautious of touts who offer you girls, goods or guide services. You're invariably over-charged, if you're lucky enough to actually get anything for your money. Men should

Crumbling magnificence: temples slowly failing the test of time.

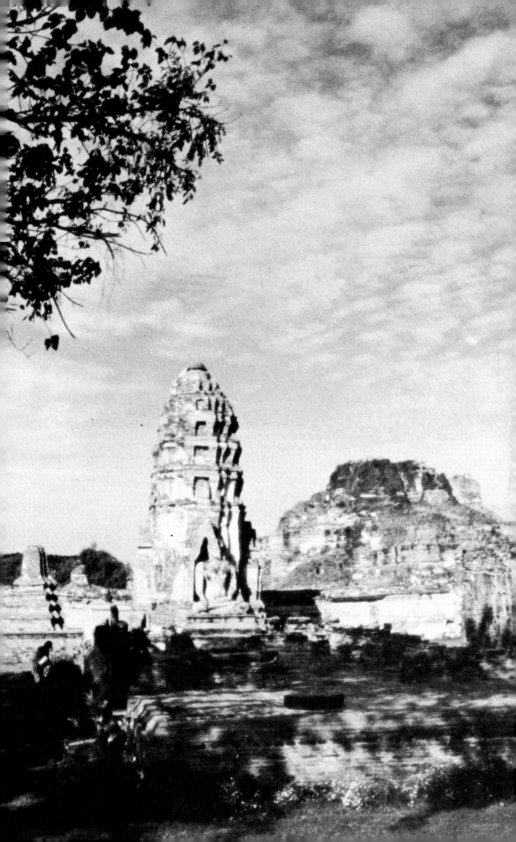

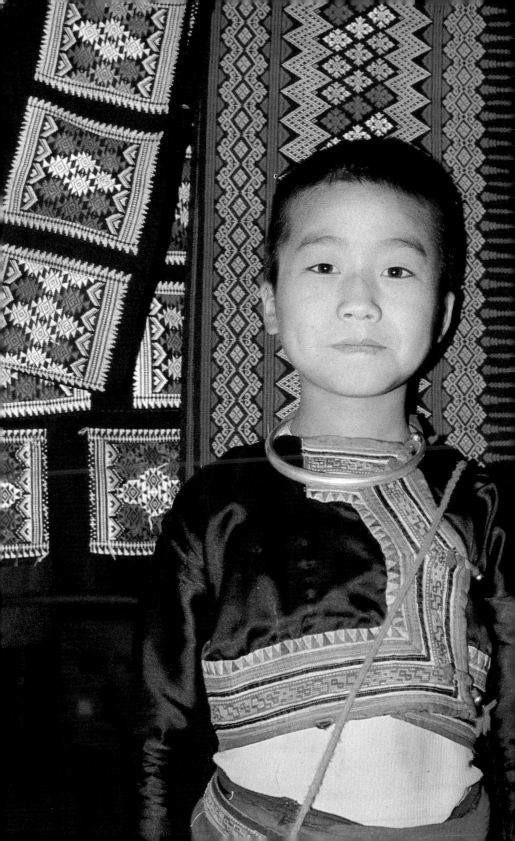

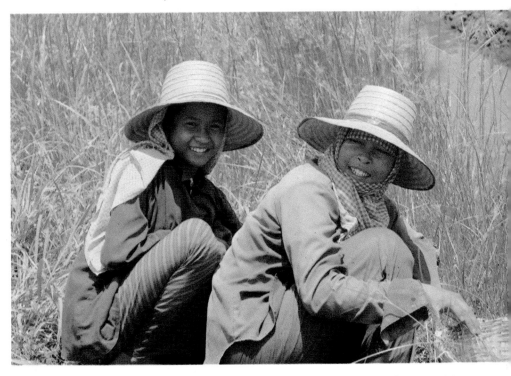

also beware of tall, attractive friendly ladies who come on a little strong — chances are that the beautiful she is a *he*!

Embassies and Consulates

Argentina
62 Silom Road
Tel: 234-6911

Australia
37 Sathorn Tai
Tel: 286-0411

Austria
Soi Athakarnprasit, Sathorn
Tel: 286-3011

Bangladesh
47 Rama IV
Tel: 279-3018

Belgium
44 Soi Pipad, Silom
Tel: 233-0840

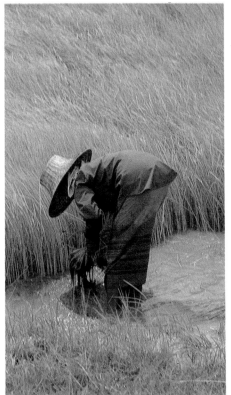

Rural life: opposite, *Meo hill tribe boy at Chiang Mai night bazaar;* above, *girls working in the fields of Central Thailand* and left, *gathering in the rice.* Over, *country boys north of Bangkok.*

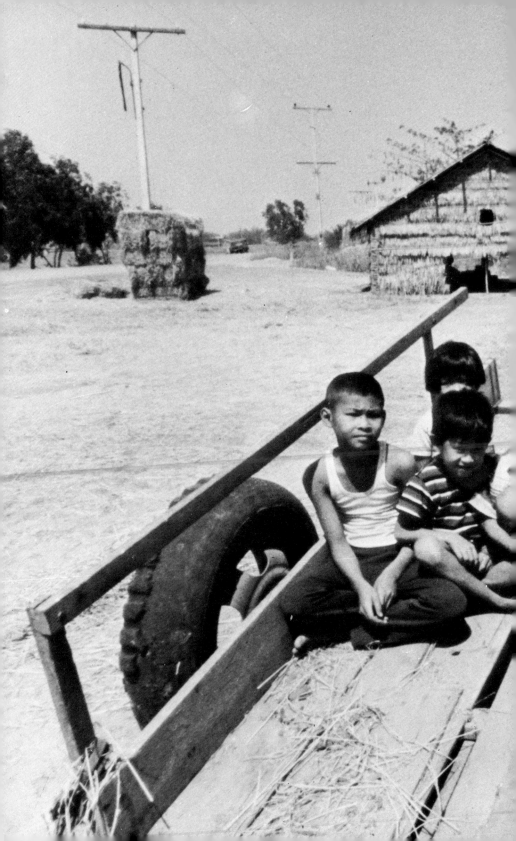

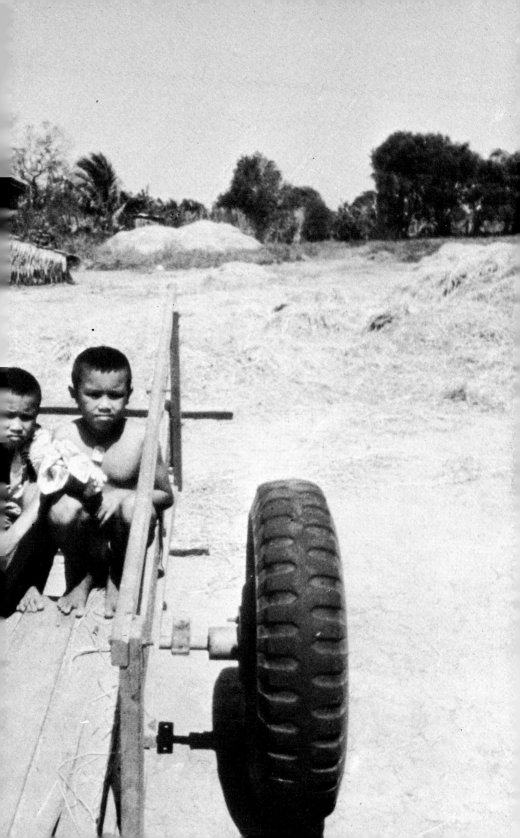

Brazil
518/2 Ploenchit
Tel: 252-9780

Burma
132 Sathorn Nua
Tel: 233-2237

Canada
Boonmitr Bldg, Silom
Tel: 234-1561

Denmark
10 Athakarnprasit, Sathorn
Tel: 286-3930

Czechosovakia
197/1 Silom Building
Tel: 234-1922

German Fed. Rep.
9 Sathorn Tai
Tel: 286-4223

Great Britain
Wireless/Ploenchit Roads
Tel: 252-7161

Finland
138 Silom
Tel: 234-1617

France
35 Customs House Lane, New Road
Tel: 234-0950

Greece
412/8-9 Siam Square
Tel: 252-1686˙

India
46, Soi 23 Sukhumvit
Tel: 392-4161

Indonesia
600-2 Petchburi Road
Tel: 251-6719

Israel
31 Soi Lang Suan, Ploenchit
Tel: 252-3131

Italy
92 Sathorn Nua
Tel: 234-9718

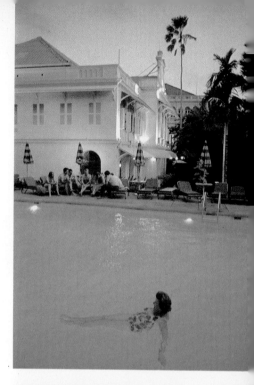

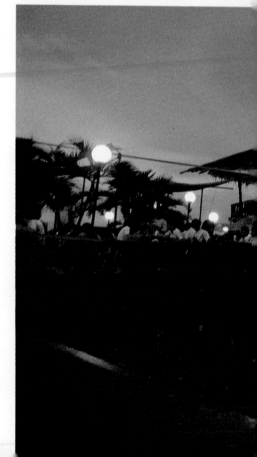

Sundowners: above far and near left, *at the Oriental Hotel;* bottom, *Rin Nam restaurant, a converted barge ideal for sipping mekong whisky after a day's work.*

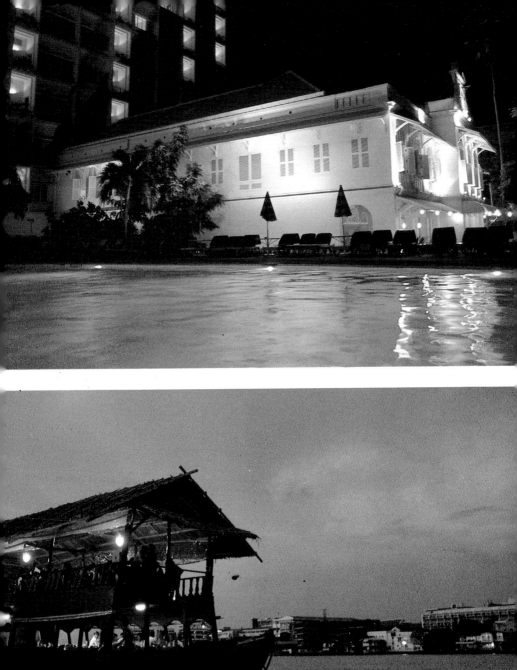
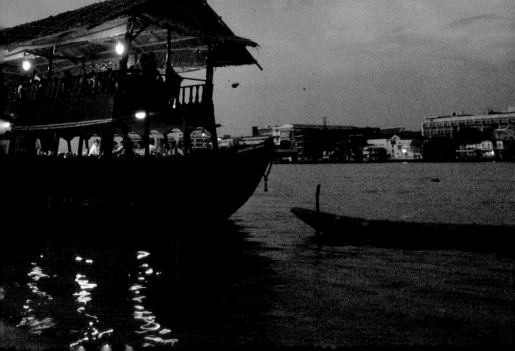

Japan
1674 New Petchburi
Tel: 252-6151

Korea
28/1 Surasak, Silom
Tel: 234-0723

Malaysia
35 Sathorn Tai
Tel: 286-1390

Nepal
189 Soi Puengsuk, Sukhumvit
Tel: 391-7240

Netherlands
106 Wireless
Tel: 252-6103

New Zealand
93 Wireless
Tel: 251-8165

Norway
690 Sukhumvit
Tel: 392-1046

Pakistan
31, Soi 3 Sukhumvit
Tel: 252-7036

Philippines
760 Sukhumvit
Tel: 391-0008

Poland
61 Soi 23 Sukhumvit
Tel: 391-2356

Portugal
26 Bush Lane, New Road
Tel: 234-0372

Saudi Arabia
138 Silom
Tel: 233-7941

Singapore
129 Sathorn Tai
Tel: 286-2111

Spain
104 Wireless
Tel: 252-6112

Sri Lanka
Nailert Bldg, Sukhumvit
Tel: 251-8554

Sweden
138 Silom
Tel: 234-3891

Switzerland
35 Wireless
Tel: 252-8992

Turkey
352 Paholyothin
Tel: 279-0999

United Arab Republic
49 Soi Ruam Rudee
Tel: 252-6139

U.S.A.
95 Wireless
Tel: 252-5040

U.S.S.R.
108 Sathorn Nua
Tel: 234-2012

Yugoslavia
28 Soi 61 Sukhumvit
Tel: 391-9090

Tourism Authority of Thailand

The main office of the TAT in Bangkok is on Raidamnoen Nok Avenue, and the information section is open every day from 8.30 a.m. to 4.30 p.m. Staff here are very helpful and can provide masses of detail on each area of Thailand and the convenient ways of getting there. Here also one can make bookings for the TAT-operated resorts — Khao Yai, Bang Saen Beach and the Bang Phra Golf Course. Telephone number is 282-1143. There is also a TAT information counter at the airport.
Other TAT domestic offices:

Chiang Mai
135 Praisani Road.
Tel: 235-334.

Kanchanaburi
Sueng Chuto Road.
Tel: 511-200.

Korat (Nakhon Ratchasima)
53/1-4 Mukkhamontri Road.
Tel: 243-427, 243-751.

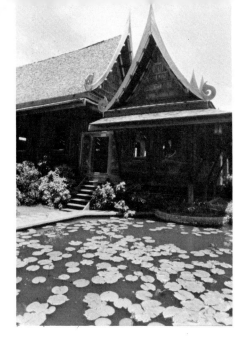

Pattaya
Chai Hat Road (along the main beach).
Tel: 418-750.

Phuket
73-75 Phuket Road.
Tel: 212-213.

Haad Yai
9 Prachathipat Road.
Tel: 243-747.

The Tourism Authority also has overseas offices in Los Angeles, New York, London, Frankfurt, Paris, Sydney, Tokyo and Singapore.

Tips on Behaviour

The Thai people are very tolerant of foreigners who, through a lack of knowledge of traditional customs, make what they consider social blunders. However, there are a number of do's and don'ts that, if observed, will make a Thailand holiday a little smoother. First, concerning the Buddhist religion and temples. *Do* dress with respect, especially for a visit to the **Grand Palace** and the revered **Wat Phra Keo**. Until recently, men had to wear a jacket and tie and women wearing slacks and open-toed shoes were not permitted to enter. It's now a little more relaxed, but Thais will appreciate your dressing up a little to match the occasion. Shoes *must* be removed before entering the gallery containing the main Buddha image of any temple and, most importantly, you should never touch the head of a Buddha image. If you want a photograph taken with a Buddha, please don't stand too close, and give the respect that the Thais believe it deserves.

A woman should *never* touch or pass anything directly to a monk, and should not enter the monk's quarters of a temple.

The head is considered the most important part of the body, and you should *never* touch a Thai on the head. This taboo is relaxed with small children.

The feet are the lowest part of the body and it is considered rude to point with one's foot, or sit cross-legged with a foot pointed at another person. For this reason, you will rarely see a Thai sitting cross-legged. Thai etiquette forbids the display of public affection; even holding hands is frowned upon in polite Thai society.

The Thai form of greeting is the *wai*, the charming gesture of folding the hands together in front of the face. There is rigid social custom associated with the height of the hands, depending on social rank, age and occupation — for example, a Thai will never be the first with a *wai* to a younger person; so it's better to avoid it or simply make a slight gesture when there's a need to return a *wai* greeting.

Thais address each other by first names with the preface of "Khun" which stands for Mr, Mrs or Miss or Ms. As Thai surnames are often unpronounceable for foreign tongues, you'll feel happier doing the same.

Tradition above, old Thai house at the Ancient City and over, *idle appreciation of bridge construction from the Oriental Hotel's riverside terrace at cocktail time.*

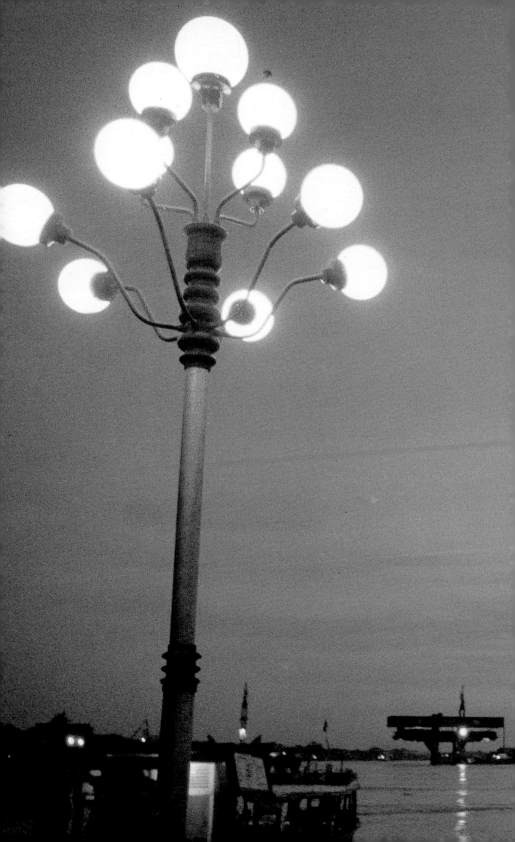

Index

Markets